MTP International Review of Science

Biochemistry
Series One

Consultant Editors
**H. L. Kornberg, F.R.S. and
D. C. Phillips, F.R.S.**

Publisher's Note

The MTP International Review of Science is an important new venture in scientific publishing, which is presented by Butterworths in association with MTP Medical and Technical Publishing Co. Ltd. and University Park Press, Baltimore. The basic concept of the Review is to provide regular authoritative reviews of entire disciplines. Chemistry was taken first as the problems of literature survey are probably more acute in this subject than in any other. Physiology and Biochemistry followed naturally. As a matter of policy, the authorship of the MTP Review of Science is international and distinguished, the subject coverage is extensive, systematic and critical, and most important of all, it is intended that new issues of the Review will be published at regular intervals.

In the MTP Review of Chemistry (Series One), Inorganic, Physical and Organic Chemistry are comprehensively reviewed in 33 text volumes and 3 index volumes. Physiology (Series One) consists of 8 volumes and Biochemistry (Series One) 12 volumes, each volume individually indexed. Details follow. In general, the Chemistry (Series One) reviews cover the period 1967 to 1971, and Physiology and Biochemistry (Series One) reviews up to 1972. It is planned to start in 1974 the MTP International Review of Science (Series Two), consisting of a similar set of volumes covering developments in a two year period.

The MTP International Review of Science has been conceived within a carefully organised editorial framework. The overall plan was drawn up, and the volume editors appointed, by seven consultant editors. In turn, each volume editor planned the coverage of his field and appointed authors to write on subjects which were within the area of their own research experience. No geographical restriction was imposed. Hence the 500 or so contributions to the MTP Review of Science come from many countries of the world and provide an authoritative account of progress.

Butterworth & Co. (Publishers) Ltd.

MTP International Review of Science

Biochemistry

Series One

Volume 10
Defence and Recognition

Edited by **R. R. Porter, F.R.S.**
University of Oxford

Butterworths · London
University Park Press · Baltimore

THE BUTTERWORTH GROUP

ENGLAND
Butterworth & Co (Publishers) Ltd
London: 88 Kingsway, WC2B 6AB

AUSTRALIA
Butterworths Pty Ltd
Sydney: 586 Pacific Highway 2067
Melbourne: 343 Little Collins Street, 3000
Brisbane: 240 Queen Street, 4000

NEW ZEALAND
Butterworths of New Zealand Ltd
Wellington: 26–28 Waring Taylor Street, 1

SOUTH AFRICA
Butterworth & Co (South Africa) (Pty) Ltd
Durban: 152–154 Gale Street

ISBN 0 408 70504 3

UNIVERSITY PARK PRESS

U.S.A. and CANADA
University Park Press
Chamber of Commerce Building
Baltimore, Maryland, 21202

Library of Congress Cataloging in Publication Data
Porter, Rodney Robert, 1917–
    Defence and recognition.

    (Biochemistry, series one, v. 10)
    1. Immunology. I. Title. II. Series.
    [DNLM: 1. Immunity. QW504 D313 1974]
    QP1.B48 vol. 10 [QR181] 574.1'92'08s[574.2'9]
    ISBN 0-8391-1049-9   73-16059

First Published 1973 and © 1973
MTP MEDICAL AND TECHNICAL PUBLISHING CO LTD
St Leonard's House
St Leonardgate
Lancaster, Lancs
and
BUTTERWORTH & CO (PUBLISHERS) LTD

Typeset and printed in Great Britain by
REDWOOD BURN LIMITED
Trowbridge and Esher
and bound by R. J. Acford Ltd, Chichester, Sussex

Consultant Editor's Note

The MTP International Review of Science is designed to provide a comprehensive, critical and continuing survey of progress in research. Nowhere is such a survey needed as urgently as in those areas of knowledge that deal with the molecular aspects of biology. Both the volume of new information, and the pace at which it accrues, threaten to overwhelm the reader: it is becoming increasingly difficult for a practitioner of one branch of biochemistry to understand even the language used by specialists in another.

The present series of 12 volumes is intended to counteract this situation. It has been the aim of each Editor and the contributors to each volume to provide authoritative and up-to-date reviews and also carefully to place these reviews into the context of existing knowledge, so that their significance of the developments relative to the overall advances in biochemical understanding can be understood by advanced students and non-specialist biochemists. It is particularly hoped that this series will benefit those colleagues to whom the whole range of scientific journals is not readily available. To keep abreast of future developments further volumes will be published as and when this is felt to be appropriate.

In order to give some kind of coherence to this series, we have viewed the description of biological processes in molecular terms as a progression from the properties of macromolecular cell components, through the functional interrelations of those components, to the manner in which cells, tissues and organisms respond biochemically to external changes. Although it is clear that important topics may have been ignored in a collection of articles chosen in this manner, we hope that the authority and distinction of the contributions will compensate for the shortcomings of thematic selection. We certainly welcome criticisms, and solicit suggestions for future reviews, from interested readers.

It is our pleasure to thank all who have collaborated to make this venture possible—the volume editors, the chapter authors, and the publishers.

Leicester   H. L. Kornberg

Oxford   D. C. Phillips

Preface

The defence of an animal against invading organisms and the recognition between cells both of the same and of different individuals are associated phenomena in which knowledge and interest are growing very quickly. It is only in recent years that the opportunities of a biochemical approach to these topics has become apparent. Now, however, this has become an area of very rapid development and immunology the principle science concerned with these problems has become a topic of study for most students of biochemistry. This book has been written primarily for biochemists who wish to familiarise themselves with present knowledge and with the many problems awaiting investigation.

The major difficulty, as always in studying new fields, lies in memorising the unfamiliar terminology and there is no doubt that for most biochemists the nomenclature of the complement system and of histocompatibility antigens to mention only two of the topics in this book, does offer difficulty. However, an effort has been made by the authors to define the words used, to follow the most generally accepted usage and to be consistent. It is hoped that this will minimise the effort needed for biochemists to read this introduction to immunology.

It is a subject which ranges from histology to genetics and yet is so interlocked that study of isolated aspects, which may appear to be of particular interest to biochemists and are sometimes separated as immunochemistry, loses much of the interest. An attempt has been made, therefore, to cover as many aspects as seemed feasible but there are regrettable omissions. However, it is hoped that sufficient has been included to give an adequately balanced view of what must at present be one of the most quickly developing fields of biology.

Oxford   R. R. Porter

Contents

1
Interferon

D. C. BURKE
University of Warwick

1.1 INTRODUCTION

Interferon is the name given to a group of antiviral proteins, which are made in eucaryotic cells after treatment with a wide variety of agents, and which inhibit the multiplication of many animal viruses. Interferon, or more correctly, interferons, for the name describes a whole group of substances, was discovered by Isaacs and Lindenmann[1] during a study of viral interference. In this phenomenon, which has been known and studied for many years (see Henle[2] for a review), treatment of cells with one animal virus ('the interfering virus') protected the cells against the subsequent action of another virus ('the challenge virus'). Since the growth of challenge virus could be inhibited even though it was unrelated to the interfering virus, the effect was not mediated by antibody nor was it due to destruction of the cellular receptors for the challenge virus. Moreover, the interfering virus did not even have to multiply, for virus which had been inactivated by heat or ultraviolet irradiation was still an efficient interfering agent. Little more was known about the mechanism involved, until Isaacs and Lindenmann[1] showed that cells treated with an interfering virus released a soluble factor into the medium, which when added to new cells would protect them against the effect of the challenge virus. The factor was named 'interferon' by Isaacs, who remarked that since the physicists had a whole range of fundamental particles, the neutron, proton, etc., he did not see why the biologist should not have his fundamental particle!

Isaacs and his colleagues went on to characterise their interferon preparations and to attempt to purify them. Other laboratories in Europe and the United States started work and a very large number of papers have resulted. These have been summarised in books[3-5] and reviews[6-7] which should be consulted for more detail.

Research has concentrated on two main areas—an explanation of the formation and action of interferon in molecular terms, and the use of interferon as a possible clinical antiviral. As will be described below, the formation of interferon involves the derepression of a cellular gene, and much still remains to be learnt about this process. Study of the mode of action of interferon requires the use of purified interferon, since many early studies investigated not the effects of interferon, but the effects of the impurities present in the interferon preparation! Despite intensive effort, interferon has still not been obtained pure, but it has been obtained sufficiently pure to use in investigation of its mode of action, and recently used to obtain a clear-cut answer. Research on the clinical use of interferon has followed two lines—the preparation of sufficient partially purified interferon to obtain an effect in animals and man, and the administration of agents which act as inducers of interferon. Both approaches have been used in clinical trials but neither is yet ready for general use.

1.2 BIOLOGICAL PROPERTIES OF INTERFERON

1.2.1 Criteria for accepting a viral inhibitor as an interferon

The name interferon was originally given by Isaacs and Lindenmann[1] to a substance obtained when pieces of chick chorio-allantoic membranes were treated with heat-inactivated influenza virus. Other workers used other cells and other agents, both viral and non-viral, inducers, to obtain preparations which inhibited virus multiplication. But were these interferon? And were other viral inhibitors, such as those found in body fluids, interferons? It was obviously necessary to establish criteria for accepting a viral inhibitor as an interferon. The difficulty was that it became apparent that interferon was not a single substance but a group of substances which shared a number of properties but were not necessarily identical. It has therefore been necessary to establish a set of criteria to identify an interferon—most of which are met by most preparations of interferon. These criteria are:

1.2.1.1 *The virus inhibitor must be a protein*

All partially purified interferons have been shown to be protein. This is most readily demonstrated by treatment of the crude preparations with a proteolytic enzyme, such as trypsin. This criterion distinguishes interferons from the Facteur Inhibiteur, described by Nagano and co-workers[8], which is mainly carbohydrate.

Because they are proteins, interferons would be expected to be antigenic. Probably because of the small amounts of interferon present in the crude preparations it has proved very difficult to prepare antisera (Section 1.6.2.2). The molecular weights generally fall in the range 20 000–100 000, but some with molecular weights of up to 160 000 have been reported (see Section 1.6.2).

1.2.1.2 *Its antiviral effect must not result from non-specific toxic effects on cells*

Many agents, e.g. ammonium sulphate, will inhibit virus multiplication by killing the cells in which the virus grows. However, interferons produce no gross toxic effect although many crude preparations will show some effect if refined tests for disturbed cell function are used.

1.2.1.3 *It must be active against a wide range of unrelated viruses*

Interferon is active not only against the virus which induced its formation but also against a wide variety of animal viruses. This shows that interferon acts against some process common to the multiplication of all viruses, but since interferon is non-toxic, this process must not be of importance to the host-cell. It is clearly important to find out exactly how interferon inhibits the growth of viruses. However, for reasons which cannot as yet be explained, different viruses, different strains of the same virus, and even variants of the same strain of virus are inhibited to different extents in interferon-treated cells. The particular method used to assess the sensitivity of viruses to interferon certainly has an important influence, but even more important is the choice of the particular cells in which the comparison is made. A careful comparison[9] has been made of the capacity of homologous interferon preparations to inhibit plaque formations by vaccinia, Semliki forest (SFV) Sindbis and vesicular stomatitis viruses (VSV) in cultures of mouse embryo, hamster kidney, rabbit kidney, human embryo lung and bat embryo cells. Vaccinia virus was the most sensitive of the four viruses when tested in hamster and mouse cells, but it was the least sensitive in human, bat and rabbit cells. SFV was the least sensitive of the four viruses in hamster and mouse cells, and was relatively sensitive in bat and rabbit cells. VSV was never the most sensitive nor the most resistant. The protective effects of interferon is not limited to virus infections: some non-viral agents are also inhibited by interferon, e.g. members of the trachoma-inclusion conjunctivitis (TRIC) group of agents[10-12], the eucaryote protozoan *Toxoplasma gondii*, and some rickettsiae and bacteria[14]. Nothing is known about the mechanism of this effect.

1.2.1.4 It must inhibit virus replication by a process involving RNA and protein synthesis

Interferon is only effective if it is incubated with cells for several hours at 37°C. The interferon may then be removed without any loss of the protective effect. No protective effect is obtained if the cells are incubated at 0°C, or if the challenge virus is added together with the interferon. This shows the necessity for some metabolic process to occur and distinguishes interferon from the virus inhibitors found in serum which are only active while in contact with the cells. The use of metabolic inhibitors, such as actinomycin[15], *p*-fluorophenylalanine[16] and puromycin[17] showed that this metabolic process required both RNA and protein synthesis, and its nature is discussed in more detail below (Section 1.7.1).

1.2.1.5 Most interferons are only formed in response to a specific stimulus

This stimulus may be virus or a wide variety of other compounds (see Section 1.3) and the mechanism of formation is discussed in Section 1.5. There are, however, a few reports of spontaneous interferon formation[18].

1.2.1.6 Most interferons are much more active in cells of the homologous species than in other cells

Tyrrell[19] reported that calf interferon was inactive in chick allantoic cells, and chick interferon was inactive in calf kidney cells. Various other interferons have since been found inactive in cells from heterologous cells[20, 21], and it has often been said that interferons are only active in cells of the homologous species of animal, i.e. they are species specific. However, this is an over simplification. Bucknall[22], using human cells and monkey cells from three different species of monkeys, found that human and monkey interferons were almost equally active in both human and monkey cells. There was thus complete cross-reaction at the level of a taxonomic family. Moehring and Stinebring[23], as a result of experiments with interferons from five avian species, suggested that there was 'order specificity' and not 'species specificity'. However, there are several reports[24, 25] of the activity of human interferon in rabbit kidney cells, although this is not true of all preparations of human interferon[9, 26, 27]. Interferons are not antigenic in allogenic systems[28], and there is some evidence that interferons which show heterospecific activity share common antigens[25]. Thus the phrase 'species specific', which has been used by many workers, is misleading. However, it remains a fact that many preparations of interferon do have maximum activity in cells of the homologous species, and less or no activity in cells of others. The explanation of this phenomenon is discussed in detail later (Section 1.7.1).

1.2.1.7 Most interferons are stable at pH 2

Many interferons have been reported to be stable at pH 2, but this is not a sufficient basis for calling a viral inhibitor an interferon, since there are other viral inhibitors which are stable at pH 2[29], and the interferons formed in immunologically-competent cells (see Section 1.3.4) are unstable at pH 2[30].

1.2.2 The assay of interferon

1.2.2.1 The inhibition of virus growth in interferon-treated cells

Interferons are characterised by their ability to inhibit virus growth. However, the extent of this inhibition is governed by many factors. One of these is the time and temperature of incubation with the cells (see Section 1.2.1.4), another whether the cells are homologous to the interferon or not (see Section 1.2.1.6). Frequently the antiviral effect differs in different cells from a single species, for example, differences in the sensitivity to interferon of various sub-lines of HeLa and L cells have been reported[31-33]. Since the ability of a cell to respond to interferon involves a particular gene or genes (see Section 1.7.1), it is not surprising that cells respond differently. It may be that a cell line lacking this gene(s) will be isolated. This variation in response may be due to the inactivation or suppression of the interferon gene(s), or possibly due to its loss.

When cells are treated with interferon and then infected with a challenge virus, less virus is formed than in controls and damage to cells may be delayed or prevented. The lower yields of virus in interferon-treated cells result from the combined effect of a reduction in the number of cells producing virus and in the amount of virus produced in the remaining cells[34-36]. It is this reduction in yield that is the basis of the assay for interferon.

1.2.2.2 Methods for assaying interferon

Apart from the particular way used to assess virus growth, nearly all interferon assays are carried out in the same general way. The interferon preparation concerned is diluted in the appropriate cell culture medium, and each dilution is tested in one or more replicate cultures. These are incubated, usually overnight, so that the interferon produces its antiviral effect in the cells, the fluids are removed and the cells washed before addition of the challenge virus. The washing is important in order to remove other virus inhibitors which may be present in crude interferon preparations. Control cultures treated with diluent alone are included in the assay. In some methods, all are challenged (virus control cultures), while in other methods, some are left uninfected (cell control cultures). When the infected cultures have been incubated for a suitable period of time, the extent of virus growth in control and interferon-treated cultures is measured in some way. A relationship is then established between the extent of virus growth and some function of the interferon dose, usually graphically.

Three principal methods of assessing virus growth have been used in interferon assays. These are plaque-reduction, cytopathic effect (c.p.e.)-inhibition and yield-reduction. In the first two methods the extent of virus growth is scored directly either as the number of plaques, or the extent of c.p.e. In the yield-reduction method, the virus yield has to be titrated in fresh cells, and another step is involved. C.p.e.-inhibition can be measured directly by visual scoring, or more conveniently, by the uptake of the vital-dye, neutral red. When the virus yield obtained in the first two methods is plotted against the logarithm of the interferon dilution, a series of parallel S-shaped lines are obtained which are linear over the range corresponding to 25–75% virus growth. It is convenient in such assays to take the dilution of an interferon preparation at which virus growth is 50% of that in the infected control cultures as the titre. In contrast, in yield reduction assays, the log reduction in virus yield may be linearly related to the log dilution of interferon over a wide range[38], and the dilution at which virus yields are $0.5 \log_{10}$ less than in controls has usually been taken as the titre. The sigmoidal dose response curve of the plaque-reduction assay can be transformed into a straight line relationship by use of probit graph paper[39].

A large number of variants of these three methods, plus others, have been used by different workers and an assessment of their pros and cons is outside the scope of this article. The reader is referred to excellent reviews by Finter[40, 41].

1.2.2.3 Interferon standards

It is most important to include a standard preparation of interferon in each assay in order to assess the reproducibility of the assay. Clearly, reproducible assays are desirable, but reproducibility should not be confused with precision, which is also desirable. It is also most important to relate the interferon titres obtained by one group of workers to those obtained by others, and this is best done by assaying a reference research standard in both laboratories and reporting all results in terms of these units. The qualities necessary for suitable standards have been discussed[42], and research reference standards for chick, mouse, rabbit and human interferons are now available (see Appendix of Ref. 5).

1.3 SUBSTANCES WHICH STIMULATE THE FORMATION OF INTERFERON

Until 1963, the viruses were the only substances known to stimulate the formation of interferon. However, since then many more substances have been discovered.

1.3.1 Viruses

Members of practically every major virus group have now been shown to induce interferons in some system (see Ref. 43 for a list). These include the myxoviruses, togaviruses (arboviruses), enteroviruses, reoviruses, RNA tumour viruses, adenoviruses, herpes viruses and pox viruses. These viruses will induce interferons in man, mice, rabbits, chicks, rats, monkeys, hamsters, guinea-pigs, horses, cattle, sheep, tortoises, fishes or bats, or in cells derived from these animals. Certain generalisations can be made from the accumulated data.

1.3.1.1 Some viruses are better inducers than others

The myxoviruses and togaviruses (arboviruses) are good inducers of interferon. Both groups are RNA viruses with a ribonucleoprotein core surrounded by a lipoprotein envelope. They will infect many different animals and cells, and usually do not shut off the cellular synthetic processes required for interferon formation. Those viruses, such as the more virulent strains of polio virus, which inhibit cellular RNA and protein synthesis are poor inducers for this reason. However, it is much less clear why the DNA viruses, such as the herpes and pox viruses, are such poor inducers. The adenoviruses are good inducers in chick cells[44, 45].

1.3.1.2 Some inactivated viruses are good interferon inducers

Interferon was discovered using heat-inactivated influenza virus as an inducer. The virus did not multiply at all in the interferon-producing cells, showing that virus multiplication was not necessary for induction. Ultraviolet (u.v.) inactivated influenza[46], parainfluenza[47], reo[48], vaccinia[49] and adenoviruses[50] are also good inducers. The explanation of this phenomenon is considered below (Section 1.5.2.1).

1.3.1.3 Whole animals are good producers of interferon

All the early work on interferon and much of that concerned with the mechanism of interferon formation has been done using cell cultures. However, Baron and Buckler[51] found that intravenous innoculations of Newcastle Disease Virus (NDV) into mice produced very high titres of interferon within 4–8 h. The virus interacts with the interferon-forming tissues of the reticuloendothelial system without preliminary virus replication, and since this virus is inactivated by serum substances, relatively little infectious virus contaminates the interferon preparation. This system has provided a convenient source of high-titre mouse interferon.

1.3.1.4 Fungal viruses

These will be considered separately because of their importance in subsequent work. At a time when many fungal culture filtrates were being tested for the presence of new antibiotics, two, termed statolon and helenine, were found to have activity against several unrelated viruses[52,53], and in 1964 statolon was shown to be an interferon inducer[54]. Helenine was also found to induce interferon[55], and fractionation of the extracts showed that the activity was due to a fungal virus which contained double-stranded RNA[56-58].

1.3.2 Nucleic acids

Isaacs suggested in 1961[59] that interferon formation was a response to foreign nucleic acids, but the experiments[60,61] were difficult to repeat and the idea was abandoned[62]. However, in 1967, Hillemann and his co-workers made the important observation that double-stranded ribonucleic acids (ds-RNA) from various sources were potent inducers of interferon *in vivo* and *in vitro*[57,63-66]. The observation was first made with ds-RNA extracted from helenine, and similar results were obtained using reovirus RNA and the double-stranded replicative form from *E. coli* infected with the coliphage, MS2. They also found that *synthetic* ds-RNAs were active as interferon inducers, and that poly rI:rC (polyriboinosinic acid annealed to polyribocytidylic acid) was the most active of those tested. This discovery of a synthetic interferon inducer provided the stimulus for a search for a correlation between structure and biological activity which is discussed later (Section 1.5.3.1). The activity of poly rI:rC is greatly enhanced by the addition of DEAE-dextran, and some cells will only produce interferon when it is present[67]. This material probably functions both to inhibit nuclease breakdown of ds-RNA[68] and to increase uptake by the cells[69].

1.3.3 Endotoxin

Intravenous injection of rabbits or mice, or treatment of certain types of cell cultures with endotoxin leads to the formation of interferon[70-73]. However, this process is much less sensitive to the effects of inhibitors of protein and

RNA synthesis than the response to viruses[74, 75] and it has been suggested that two fundamentally different mechanisms may be involved in these responses, endotoxins causing 'release' of preformed interferon and viruses leading to *de novo* synthesis (see Section 1.5.1). Viruses can induce interferon in many different types of cell in tissue culture, but endotoxins are only effective in cultures of reticuloendothelial cells, such as peritoneal macrophages[18, 76], spleen cells[72] and leucocytes[73]. The results suggest that many of the effects of endotoxin may result from the reaction of immunocompetent cells carrying a specific receptor for endotoxin.

1.3.4 Mitogens, cell transformation and interferon induction

Phytohaemagglutinin (PHA) induces interferon formation in cultures of human white blood cells[77]. The PHA had to be kept in contact with the cells if interferon production was to continue[78, 79], and the response was related to the extent to which lymphocyte growth was stimulated, while if the cultures failed to transform, no interferon was produced[79]. The correlation between interferon formation and transformation was also observed when white cells from immune donors were treated with specific antigens[79], interferon production and transformation both taking place at the same interval after treatment. Lymphocytes from non-immune donors did not respond. It has also been demonstrated that specific antilymphocyte globulins[80, 81] and its divalent F (ab')$_2$ fragments[81] are able to induce interferon synthesis. The interferon produced appears to differ in charge and molecular weight from virus induced interferon made in the same cells[82]. This mechanism may be an important way of producing interferon *in vivo*.

1.3.5 Synthetic polymers

Regelson[83] showed that a number of synthetic polycarboxylates had antiviral activity in mice, and several groups have shown that these compounds induce interferon[83-85]. One of the compounds (pyran copolymer) has been studied in some detail. Primary cells and cell lines did not form interferon in response to pyran copolymer, but peritoneal macrophages formed small amounts if pyran copolymer was complexed with arginine[84]. A comparison of the activity of a series of different polymers indicated that the mol. wt. had to be greater than 3000 and that a high density of free anionic groups was required[84]. Other, as yet unidentified configurational requirements are necessary.

1.3.6 Other substances

A number of carbohydrates, many of which contain anionic groups, are interferon inducers *in vivo* or in cultures of mouse macrophages[75]. The antibiotics cycloheximide and kanamycin will also induce interferon *in vivo*[86, 87].

The doses of cycloheximide which induce interferon are invariably lethal. Interferons have been found in the serum of chickens and mice after intravenous injections of large numbers of certain Gram-negative bacteria, and also after injection of two trachoma-inclusion conjunctivitis (TRIC) agents, several protozoa and rickettsiae[75]. Nothing is known about the mechanism, but this list certainly widens the range of interferon inducers!

1.4 FACTORS INFLUENCING INTERFERON FORMATION

A very large number of factors affect interferon formation[88], some of which will be summarised in this section.

1.4.1 Influence of cell and animal strain

Primary tissue culture cells, cell strains and cell lines vary markedly in their capacity to produce interferon and no useful generalisations can yet be made. However, Vero cells, a line derived from the kidney of an African green monkey, are genetically incapable of producing interferon, although they are sensitive to it[24]. Cell-fusion studies, which are just beginning and which are discussed elsewhere (Section 1.5.2.2) should cast light on the genetic basis of the interferon response.

Working with strains of inbred mice, De Maeyer and De Maeyer-Guignard[89] showed that C57 B1 mice made 5–10 times more interferon than Balb/C or C3H/He mice, and by using appropriate genetic crosses, that interferon production was governed by a single partly dominant autosomal factor.

1.4.2 Influence of age

Carver and Marcus[90] found that chick cell cultures aged for 7 days *in vitro* produced up to 32 times more interferon than cultures 1–2 days old, and a similar effect was reported by Kato and Eggers[91], who isolated a factor, which when incubated with 1-day-old cultures increased the yield of interferon. They considered that this factor was not interferon, but since latent virus infections could give rise to interferon, which itself can increase the yield of virus-induced interferon by the 'priming' effect (Section 1.4.5.2), this data needs to be treated with caution.

The situation is not clear either *in vivo*. Isaacs and Baron[92] suggested that young embryos were less capable of forming interferon than older embryos of mature animals, but since infective virus was used to induce interferon formation, and since embryos of different ages certainly differ in their capacity to support virus multiplication, no firm conclusion can be drawn. More recently, Gandhi and Stewart[93] found no differences in the amount of interferon formed in response to u.v.-irradiated influenza virus from chick embryo tissue of different ages.

1.4.3 The influence of temperature

The production of interferon is a metabolic process that would be expected to occur within an optimum temperature range, which is usually *ca.* 35–40 °C. Similar results have been obtained in tissue culture systems and animals[88].

1.4.4 Influence of hormones

Since they regulate metabolic processes, hormones would be expected to influence interferon production, particularly in those organs where their effects are most evident. The corticosteroids have been studied extensively and, in general, reduce the amount of interferon formed *in vitro* and *in vivo*[88]. ACTH and pituitary growth hormone have been found to have no effect. Since the mode of action of hormones is so little understood, their use throws little light on the mechanism of interferon formation.

1.4.5 The effect of other factors

1.4.5.1 'Blocker' and 'Enhancer'

'Blocker' is the name given to a factor[94] which inhibited the formation of interferon. It is probably identical with the 'enhancer' (of virus multiplication) described by Kato *et al.*[95]. Little is known about the nature or mode of action of these factors.

1.4.5.2 The effect of interferon on interferon formation

Interferon treatment can have two effects on subsequent interferon formation. Pre-treatment with small doses increases the amount of interferon formed subsequently, while large doses decreases the amount[96, 97]. The stimulation of the subsequent interferon response is known as 'priming' and has been studied by several groups. Interferon is made earlier and faster in primed cells[97, 98], and it appears that priming by interferon either enables the cell to by-pass one of the sequential processes in induction or removes some restriction of the induction process[99].

1.4.5.3 The effect of viruses on interferon formation

It has been observed that some viruses grow better in cells that are already infected with another virus, and in some instances at least, this may be because the first virus inhibits interferon production[100, 101]. On the other hand, pre-treatment with viruses, particularly inactivated viruses, can stimulate the subsequent formation of interferon. It is not known whether this priming effect is similar to priming by interferon.

1.4.5.4 Carcinogens and antimetabolites

De Maeyer and De Maeyer-Guignard[102] observed that several carcinogenic polycyclic aromatic hydrocarbons reduced interferon formation while other structurally related, but non-carcinogenic, compounds had no effect. Several other carcinogenic compounds also inhibited production; nothing is known about this mechanism.

Many antimetabolites inhibit interferon formation[88], but since they have often been used to elucidate the mechanism of interferon formation, they will be discussed later (Section 1.5.2.3).

1.4.6 Formation of interferon in animals

1.4.6.1 Which cells are responsible for the formation of interferon?

Several approaches have been made to this problem. The organs have been removed from a rabbit or rat and slices of kidney, spleen, lung, etc. tested for their ability to produce interferon. The results obtained depend upon conditions (the inducer used, the method of preparing the tissue etc.), but in general those organs containing large amounts of reticuloendothelial cells are the most productive.

The results obtained when an inducer is injected into the whole animal are more complex. They depend on the route of administration and the fate of the inoculum, but again the cells of the reticuloendothelial system are indicated. It is clear that no single organ is involved since neither adrenolectomy, thymectomy nor spleenectomy destroys the capacity to produce interferon.

More specific information was obtained by means of x-irradiation. Whole-body irradiation depresses the capacity to form interferon[103], which can be restored by transplanting bone marrow immediately after irradiation. Transplantation of Wistar rat marrow cells into irradiated C3H mice produced rat-mouse chimaeras which subsequently produced rat but not mouse interferon[104]. The authors concluded that interferon was mainly produced by cells derived from bone marrow.

1.4.6.2 The tolerance phenomenon

If mice or rabbits, which have been stimulated to form interferon by injection of a particular inducer, are given a further injection then no second yield of interferon is obtained. This phenomenon is called tolerance. Generally speaking, the greater the number of previous injections, the greater the depression of the response to an interferon inducer. The effect lasts 4–6 days. The tolerance phenomenon has been used to determine whether the same cells are involved in the production of interferon after treatment with different types of inducers (endotoxin, viruses, or poly rI:rC), by using one inducer for the first injection and another for the second. The results are complex and no simple interpretation is possible[88]. The mechanism of this effect is unknown but it has clear implications for the use of interferon inducers in antiviral chemotherapy.

1.5 THE MECHANISM OF INTERFERON

1.5.1 Two general mechanisms of interferon formation

There appear to be two general mechanisms of interferon formation, which are referred to as 'synthesis' and 'release'. The distinction between them is largely based on work with metabolic inhibitors.

1.5.2 Interferon production by viruses

Virus-induced interferon formation is inhibited by actinomycin[105, 106], a widely studied inhibitor of DNA-dependent RNA synthesis, and by two other inhibitors with a similar effect[107]. Since actinomycin is effective in inhibiting interferon formation induced by RNA viruses, whose own multiplication is unaffected by the inhibitor, it has been concluded that interferon synthesis is coded for by the cell genome rather than the virus inducer. This implies that virus-induced interferon formation involves the unmasking of a cellular gene with consequent production of an interferon messenger RNA and its subsequent translation. As expected if *de novo* synthesis is involved, interferon production is inhibited by low doses of several inhibitors of protein synthesis, notably puromycin, *p*-fluorophenylalanine[109] and cycloheximide[86]. This theory explains why interferons show characteristic species specificities (see Section 1.2.1.6), and the report that an apparently identical interferon is induced in chick cells by both an RNA and a DNA virus[110]. This mechanism is frequently referred to as a derepression mechanism, although it is highly unlikely that it is similar to the familiar Jacob–Monod scheme[111].

Similar results have been obtained when the effects of metabolic inhibitors on virus-induced interferon production in animals was measured—actinomycin[86, 112], puromycin[86, 113] and cycloheximide[86] all inhibited interferon formation, although results were complicated by the toxic effects of the antimetabolites.

Virus-induced interferon formation may therefore be divided into three stages: (a) Virus invasion, followed by dissolution of the virion and release of the interferon inducer; (b) Interaction of the inducer, either directly or indirectly, with the host cell genome, leading by a derepression mechanism to; (c) Synthesis of interferon messenger RNA, its translation and the release of interferon from the cell.

These stages will now be considered in turn.

1.5.2.1 Events preceding derepression

What component of the virus is responsible for triggering the sequence of processes that leads to the formation of interferon? The destruction of the inducing capacity of myxoviruses by excessive heat or u.v.-irradiation suggested that the inducer was either nucleic acid or protein, and the reduced yields of interferon obtained when incomplete influenza virus (which has a smaller amount of nucleic acid than usual) was used for infection[114], and, more importantly, the inducing ability of naturally occurring and synthetic ds-RNA, suggested that the inducer was the virus nucleic acid. Thus the virus nucleic acid was responsible for initiating two chains of events—those leading to virus multiplication and those leading to interferon formation.

The general approach has therefore been to discover what stages in virus multiplication are essential for interferon formation. Interpretation has proved to be much simpler in those systems where the virus does not multiply but only induces interferon, and most of the work has been done in tissue culture systems. Skehel and Burke[115] used a system in which chick cells were infected with the togavirus, Semliki Forest virus (SFV), at 37 °C and the cells were then incubated at 42 °C. Under these conditions, interferon, but not virus, was formed. Using virus that had been progressively inactivated with hydroxylamine, they showed that the capacity to produce interferon was inactivated at the same rate as the other virus functions, and they concluded that functional virus RNA was necessary for interferon formation. If so, what function did the virus RNA have to carry out? Further investigation[116] showed that incubation at 37 °C was essential for interferon formation, and that during this incubation, virus RNA synthesis occurred. Since this virus RNA synthesis included synthesis of a double-stranded replicative form, they suggested that the formation of double stranded RNA was the first step to the induction of interferon. Further attempts to elucidate the processes involved made use of temperature-sensitive mutants of the related virus Sindbis[117] or SFV[118], but no clear-cut interpretation was possible.

If formation of double-stranded virus RNA is essential for the formation of interferon, how do the non-infective preparations of the myxoviruses induce interferon? Since these preparations, which are obtained by treatment of the virus with heat, ultraviolet irradiation or β-propiolactone under controlled conditions[119], are completely non-infective, it has been suggested[120] that the inducer was the single-stranded virus RNA. However, there has been some dispute as to whether a *limited* amount of virus RNA synthesis occurred in interferon-producing cells[121, 122], which was finally resolved when it was found that the virus particle contained an RNA-directed RNA polymerase[123], and that virus preparations that were able to induce interferon formation still contained a small amount of RNA polymerase activity[119, 124]. Thus in this system too, interferon production depends on a limited amount of virus RNA synthesis, but whether it is the process of RNA synthesis or the partially double-stranded RNA product which is the inducer is not yet certain.

Little is known about the mechanism of induction by DNA viruses. Double-stranded polydeoxyribonucleotides are not interferon inducers (Section 1.5.3.1), so that interferon formation may depend on the formation of ds-RNA. However, the ds-RNA found by Colby and Duesberg[125] in chick cells infected with vaccinia virus does not appear to be involved in interferon formation[49].

1.5.2.2 The derepression event

If interferon is formed by derepression of the interferon gene, then the inducer molecule must interact specifically with the cell genome, either by entering the nucleus, or through some cytoplasmic intermediate. Nothing is known about this mechanism. There is, however, some evidence for an interferon gene. When tissue culture cells are irradiated with u.v.-light, the capacity to produce interferon is lost with single-hit kinetics, suggesting that a single gene is involved[126-129]. Attempts to identify the chromosome responsible for interferon production by cell-fusion experiments are just beginning[130-132].

1.5.2.3 Transcription and translation of the interferon gene

Information about the kinetics of transcription of a messenger RNA can be obtained by addition of actinomycin and measuring its effect at different times. Once transcription of the messenger RNA is complete, actinomycin will cease to have an inhibiting effect and if the product continues to be formed, then it may be concluded that the messenger RNA is stable. This type of experiment has shown that the synthesis of the interferon messenger RNA is complete within a few hours after infection and it is stable for up to 18 h[133]. Recently much more direct evidence for the existence of an interferon messenger RNA has been obtained by extraction of RNA from an interferon-producing cell and translation in other cells[134]. The release of interferon from cells does not require protein synthesis but does depend on proteins containing biologically active SH groups[135].

1.5.3 Interferon production by polynucleotides

1.5.3.1 Relationship between structure and function

Measurement of interferon inducing capacity of a large number of synthetic polynucleotides has enabled a number of conclusions to be drawn (See Ref. 133 for a detailed discussion). They are:

(a) *Double-strandedness*—The double-stranded polynucleotides are much more active than the corresponding single-stranded polynucleotides, which are probably active because of the small amounts of secondary structure that they contain. The double-stranded polynucleotides will, of course, be much more resistant to nuclease in the medium and on the cell surface. Triple-stranded polynucleotides are inactive[133].

(b) *Stable secondary structure*—All the biologically active polyribonucleotides have a thermal midpoint transition temperature (T_m) of at least 50 °C[136]. There is, however, no simple correlation between T_m and biological activity, since poly rI:rC is the most active inducer, yet it has a T_m of only 62.5 °C while poly rG:rC has a T_m of 136 °C, yet is much less active than poly rI:rC[133]. It is likely that this requirement reflects the necessity for the polynucleotide to stay in helical form at the temperature of incubation with the cell (37 °C)[137].

(c) *Ribonuclease resistance*—When the phosphate group of poly r AU was replaced by thiophosphate to give poly r (As Us), the product had the same T_m but was considerably more stable to the action of ribonuclease[138], and was also a more effective interferon inducer[139]. However, poly r AU is nine times more sensitive to the action of ribonuclease than is poly rA:rU, but it has a higher T_m and is a more active inducer[133]. Thus ribonuclease resistance alone is not enough.

(d) *Molecular weight*—Lampson *et al.*[140] found that poly rI:rC samples of mol. wt. 6×10^6 and 2.7×10^5 were active, but that biological activity was lost when the molecular weight was 1.5×10^5. Wacker *et al.*[141] measured the biological activity of poly rI complexed with oligonucleotides of poly rC, and of poly rC complexed with oligonucleotides of poly rI. They found that biological activity was greatly depressed when the chain length fell below 20–30 nucleotides and that the complex formed from oligonucleotides of poly rI and poly rC (mol. wt. $= 3 \times 10^4$) had little biological activity. There is therefore a lower limit for the molecular weight in order to retain biological activity, but there does not appear to be an upper limit. Tytell *et al.*[142] studying the effect of variation in size of the individual chains in the complex, came to the important conclusion that biological activity was much more dependent on the integrity of the poly I strand than poly C strand. Data obtained by Niblack and McCreory[143] did not support this conclusion, but it is likely that the polydispersity of their product affected their results. More recent work[144, 145] in which the effect of or breaks in one chain were investigated, also support this conclusion. These authors all found that poly rI:poly (1-vinylcytosine) was also active, again suggesting that the poly C strand plays a less important role. It suggests that the function of the poly C strand may be to form a double-stranded structure and so provide ribonuclease resistance, but that of the poly I strand is to initiate the formation of interferon.

(e) *2′-OH group*—The 2′-OH of ribose is essential: polydeoxyribonucleotides[133], poly rI:poly 2-O′ methyl C[146] and poly 2-O′ acetyl C and poly 2-O′ acetyl I[147] are all inactive. Mixed polymers in which one chain was poly rI and the other poly dC had little or no activity[148, 149].

(f) *Comment*—It is not yet possible to explain why certain double-stranded polynucleotides are so active, and it has been suggested that the intracellular receptor must be very specific. It is notable that the effect of substituents attached to the purine and pyrimidine rings is small while that of those attached to the ribose ring is large. The former are in the centre of the double-stranded chain, while the latter are on the outside and able to interact with other components. However, it should also be remembered that the inducer has to survive nuclease attack in solution and on the cell surface, interact correctly with the cell surface and then probably interact with a cytoplasmic receptor. The optimal structure may be different for each of these interactions, and the observed structure–function relationship the sum of them.

1.5.3.2 Interaction of polynucleotides with cells

Radioactive polynucleotides have been used extensively to study this interaction and to attempt to trace the inducer molecule inside the cell. Colby and

Chamberlin[150] showed that, in spite of their different antiviral activities, poly rI:rC, poly rA:rU and poly rI:dC were bound to chick embryo cells at similar rates, and that poly rI:rC and poly rI:dC were degraded intracellulary to acid-soluble material, at about the same rate. Bausek and Merigan[69] showed that poly rI:rC first bound to the cell surface, a step occurring equally well at 4°C as at 37°C, and that binding was greatly enhanced by the addition of DEAE-dextran (see Section 1.3.2). Binding was followed by a temperature-dependent step which was essential for subsequent interferon formation, during which only a small proportion of radioactivity entered the cell. Attempts to follow the fate of the intracellular poly rI:rC by autoradiography were unsuccessful and it was concluded that only a small fraction of the bound poly rI:rC entered the cell. The question is, does any? That is, does poly rI:rC have to enter the cell or does it induce from the cell surface? Although poly rI and poly rC are almost inactive on their own, when they are added to the cell sequentially interferon is produced[150]. The single-stranded polynucleotide probably persists at the cell surface until the second single-stranded polynucleotide is added and the two combine to form poly rI:rC. This certainly suggests that the ds-RNA may induce from the cell surface, but since virus ds-RNA is infective[151], it must be able to enter the cell. The question whether poly rI:rC *needs* to enter the cell to induce interferon formation is a major unsolved problem.

1.5.3.3 How do polynucleotides induce interferon formation?

The major question here has been whether polynucleotides induce interferon by a process similar to the viruses (Section 1.5.2) or like endotoxin, which stimulates the 'release' of preformed interferon (Section 1.5.4). This question has been investigated mainly by comparing the sensitivity of the processes to metabolic inhibitors. Several groups of workers found that the interferon induced by ds-RNA was less sensitive to actinomycin and cycloheximide than the virus induced process[48, 133], but the differences may have been due to the heterogeneity of the cell cultures which were used—some cells responding to one inducer and some to another. The different effects of antimetabolites were therefore due to the different sensitivity of these cells to their action—and a careful study, using mouse L cells and cultures of primary and secondary mouse cells, has shown that the processes induced by ds-RNA and virus are equally sensitive to the effect of antimetabolites in L cells[152], but that primary mouse kidney cultures contain cells which are only able to respond to ds-RNA and are more resistant to inhibitors of protein synthesis.

Remarkable results have been obtained using poly rI:rC as an inducer in primary rabbit kidney cells. Addition of antimetabolites immediately after exposure of the cells to the ds-RNA reduced the yield of interferon, but later addition caused a marked stimulation of the yield[153, 154]. This super-induction phenomenon has been explained by postulating that interferon formation was shut off by the action of a protein, whose formation was inhibited by the antimetabolites.

Very varied results have been obtained when the effects of antimetabolites on interferon induced in animals by poly rI:rC have been investigated (see

Ref. 133 for a summary). Ho and Ke[155] have attempted to explain some of the inconsistencies by suggesting that poly rI:rC stimulates interferon by a two-step reaction, involving first, the synthesis of 'pre-interferon' by a process involving protein synthesis and, secondly, its conversion to interferon by a process not involving protein synthesis. They used this hypothesis to explain (i) how cells treated with small amounts of poly rI:rC become resistant to virus infections, and (ii) how prior treatment with poly rI:rC accentuates the response to endotoxin, postulating that poly rI:rC induces formation not only of interferon but also of pre-interferon, which endotoxin can convert to interferon.

1.5.4 Interferon production by endotoxin

In contrast to the viruses and ds-RNA, endotoxin only induces interferon formation *in vivo* and in cells of reticuloendothelial origin in culture. Neither does the process show the sensitivity to actinomycin and cycloheximide that is characteristic of the other two classes of inducers. It has been suggested that endotoxin 'releases' preformed interferon (see Ref. 75 for summary).

The component of endotoxin essential for its interferon-inducing action was shown to be lipid by use of endotoxin prepared from a series of bacterial mutants[156, 157].

1.6 PURIFICATION AND PHYSICO-CHEMICAL PROPERTIES OF INTERFERONS

1.6.1 Introduction

Purification of interferon is important for a number of reasons: first, it is important to know what interferon is—for this obviously has a bearing on its mechanism of production; secondly, it has become clear that work on the mode of action of interferon is fraught with hazards unless purified interferons are used since many of the earlier results were found later to be due to contaminating substances[158]; third, any interferon that is to be inoculated into man must obviously be free of as much contaminating material as possible.

Purification of interferon has however proved to be very difficult, and no interferon has been obtained in the pure state. The difficulties arise from a number of causes: all samples have of course to be assayed for biological activity, and thus all purification work is laborious and time-consuming; the very high specific activity of interferon (see below) means that the crude material actually contains very little interferon by weight and, therefore, very large volumes of crude interferon have to be used, and finally it has become clear that interferon preparations are not necessarily homogeneous either in molecular weight or iso-electric point. Thus the molecular weight depends on the inducer used, the cells in which the interferon is made in tissue culture, the organ or tissue involved when interferon is formed *in vivo*, the time of sampling, and the degree of stimulation with the inducer.

If interferon is made in tissue culture under controlled conditions it is likely that it will be relatively homogeneous in molecular weight, but interferon made *in vivo* is much more difficult to control in this way. Less work has been done on the microheterogeneity in iso-electric point, but this will obviously seriously hamper fractionation of interferon on ion-exchange columns.

Early work showed that interferons had the normal properties of proteins— they were destroyed by proteolytic enzymes, precipitated by ammonium sulphate, adsorbed to and eluted from ion-exchange columns etc., and the general approach has been to fractionate crude interferon preparations by conventional methods. These have included precipitation, ion-exchange chromatography, gel-filtration and electrophoresis. It has been relatively simple to measure the effect of various specific reagents, or to establish molecular weights by filtration down a calibrated Sephadex column. It has been much more difficult to attempt to produce highly purified interferon, and because large amounts of high-titre interferon preparations are required, work has been almost completely restricted to virus-induced interferons. The results obtained with different interferons will now be briefly described.

1.6.2   Purification and properties of individual interferons

1.6.2.1   Chick interferon

Chick interferon was the first interferon to be partially-purified by a multi-stage process, and Fantes[158, 159] purified interferons from allantoic and tissue-culture fluids 20 000- and 3400-fold, respectively to obtain from both sources material with a specific activity of 1.6×10^6 units/mg protein. However, polyacrylamide gel electrophoresis at an acid pH showed that most of this protein was present as impurity[160, 161], and it was not possible to estimate how pure the best preparations were.

All the molecular weight values for chick interferon fall within the range 25 000–35 000, although there are a few reports of minor species of higher molecular weight[158]. Fantes[162] found, by electrofocusing, that chick interferon was heterogeneous in iso-electric point. There were probably five or more different components, with iso-electric points ranging from pH 6.4 to *ca.* 7.3. However, the interferons accounting for most of the activity were iso-electric in the pH 6.6–7.0 region, a value also obtained by direct determination with the unfractionated interferon, and one in agreement with most other published data. It is not known whether this heterogeneity is due to polymorphism of individual interferon components, or whether there is only one interferon with a variety of charged substituents such as sialic acids.

Experiments utilising specific reagents have shown that chick interferon has at least one essential disulphide group, amino group and methionine group, but that hydroxyl or sulphydryl groups are ʼot essential[163].

1.6.2.2   Mouse interferon

Early work (summarised in Ref. 158) achieved 6500-fold purification of mouse tissue culture interferon. More recent work has used serum-free medium to prepare mouse tissue culture interferon, and purification by two different groups[164, 165] yielded material with a specific activity of 6.4×10^6 and 3.1×10^6 units/mg protein. Further purification of this latter material raised the specific activity to 5.3×10^7 units/mg protein, but electrofocusing of radio-active preparations showed that a considerable proportion of the radio-activity was carried by inert protein[166], and that when preparations obtained from non-stimulated cells were purified by a similar scheme, the product contained biologically-inactive, mainly intracellular proteins that were indistinguishable by electrofocusing from the interferon preparations. It was suggested that normal cells continuously produce interferon-like proteins, and that virus stimulation only activates and releases these proteins.

Most virus-induced mouse interferons have molecular weights in the range 23 000–38 000. Carter[167] has shown that mouse interferon may exist either as a monomer, mol. wt. 19 000 or a dimer both of which are active. However, heavier interferons (mol. wt. up to 62 000) have been reported in mouse serum. Many mouse interferons induced by non-viral substances have relatively high molecular weights. Mouse interferons, like chick interferons, show considerable heterogeneity in iso-electric point[168]. The values range from pH 6 to 10 although most of the material is iso-electric from pH 6.75 to 7.7. Unlike chick interferon, mouse interferon is destroyed by 8 M urea. However, like chick interferon, mouse interferon has essential disulphide bonds[169].

As expected, interferon is antigenic, although purified and concentrated preparations have to be used to raise antibody, probably because of the small amount of interferon present. Antibody has been used to show that mouse interferons, induced by virus or endotoxin, do not show significant antigenic dissimilarities[170].

1.6.2.3 Human interferon

The purification of human interferon is obviously of importance for clinical trials, but it has proved much more difficult to purify than chick or mouse interferons. However, by a combination of steps, interferon prepared in human leucocytes has been purified *ca.* 75-fold to give a product with a specific activity of up to 10^6 units/mg protein[171].

Human interferons show a considerable range of molecular weights. Most of the values range between 18 000 and 33 000, and Carter[167] has also shown that human interferon may exist either as a monomer or a dimer. Several larger interferons have been described: the value of 160 000 for the molecular weight of the interferon obtained by treatment of human amnion cells with Sendai virus is among the highest so far reported[158].

Human interferons also show a range of iso-electric points, with the majority of the material iso-electric between pH 6 and 5.5[158].

1.6.2.4 Rabbit interferon

Some recent work by Wagner's group[172] used interferon prepared by treat-ment of primary rabbit cells with Newcastle Disease Virus in a serum-free medium in which two of the amino acids were tritium labelled. The initial material had a specific activity of 2×10^4 units/mg protein, and using methods that had been used for the purification of chick interferon, a product with a specific activity of 48×10^6 units/mg protein was obtained, which, on polyacrylamide gel electrophoresis, gave a single peak that contained all the biological activity and most of the radioactivity. However, purified material from uninfected cells gave a radioactive peak in the same position, suggesting either that the inducer activated a pre-existing interferon-like protein, or that the product was still impure.

The molecular weights of rabbit interferon extend over a range from 28 000 to >100 000, the value depending on both the cells and the inducer. Many of the preparations contained interferons of more than one molecular weight[158]. Rabbit interferon have iso-electric points ranging from pH 5.07 to 6.68[173]. Treatment with neuramidase increased the proportion of the less acidic components at the expense of the more acidic ones, suggesting that the microheterogeneity was due to varying numbers of sialic acid residues.

Rabbit interferons contain an essential methionine residue and probably also carbohydrate. Disulphide bonds may be essential for activity[158].

1.6.2.5 Other interferons

Monkey, rat and calf interferons have all been partially purified, although not as extensively as those discussed above. No new principles have emerged from these studies.

1.6.3 Comment

The purification of interferon has proved to be very difficult and comparatively little progress has been made recently. No interferon has been obtained pure, and the two most recent studies, on mouse[168] and rabbit[172] interferons, indicate that interferon may be formed by modification of a pre-existing protein. If this is so, it has consequences for the mechanism of interferon formation, which has been shown to be susceptible to inhibitors of protein synthesis, and which is usually thought of as involving *de novo* protein synthesis (Section 1.5.2). On the other hand, it may be that even the best preparations are still relatively impure, and that interferon of very high specific activity is formed by *de novo* synthesis.

1.7 THE MECHANISM OF INTERFERON ACTION

When cells are treated with an appropriate interferon, they become resistant to virus infection. This resistance extends to both DNA and RNA viruses, yet there is no toxic effect on the cells. Interferon must therefore affect some process which is common to all viruses, yet is absent from the host cell. The evidence increasingly suggests that this process is virus protein synthesis.

Interferon acts, not by inactivating the virus, but by rendering the cell resistant to virus infection. Two questions can then be asked: how does interferon render the cell virus-resistant? and, what events in the virus growth cycle are affected in the resistant cell? In attempting to answer these questions, it is essential that purified interferon be used since much conflicting and false information has resulted from the use of crude interferon preparations which contain substances which have multiple effects on cell metabolism[174].

1.7.1 The interaction of interferon with cells

It appears that only small amounts of interferon need bind to the surface of a cell for resistance to develop. When interferon was assayed after a series of serial transfers, it was found that only *ca.* 7% of the original interferon was removed after four transfers[175]. The higher figures reported by other authors may be due to non-specific adsorption[176, 177]. The rate of loss of heterologous interferon appears to be less than that of homologous interferon[178, 180], and this is one way in which the characteristic species specificity is shown.

This interaction can be separated into two stages. The initial reaction takes place in the cold, takes *ca.* 10–20 min, and results in the binding of interferon to a superficial site. The second stage requires incubation at 37 °C but can proceed even if interferon is no longer present in the medium[179]. However, it is not known whether interferon enters the cell.

It is this second stage that is blocked by actinomycin[15] and inhibitors of protein synthesis[174], although there is some difficulty about the interpretation of the results obtained with inhibitors of protein synthesis. Thus, host cell RNA and protein synthesis are required before interferon can be effective. These results have been interpreted in several ways. First, that it is not interferon itself that is the virus inhibitor but a newly-synthesised protein that is synthesised by the host cell as response to treatment with interferon which is the effective antiviral agent[174]. Synthesis of this antiviral protein would provide a method of amplifying the effect of interferon. Second, that the newly-synthesised protein was required to facilitate the transport of interferon into the cell[180]. If this were the case, interferon itself would be the active antiviral agent. Third, that interferon may be modified in some way before it is active. No choice can be made between these alternatives at present.

In general, cells need to be exposed to interferon for several hours before virus challenge in order to obtain the maximum antivirus effect. This effect is at least partly due to the time required for synthesis of cellular RNA and protein to occur, and slower growing viruses may be inhibited without pretreatment of the cells with interferon.

1.7.2 Duration of the anti-virus effect

Interferon appears to be more effective in resting cells than in metabolically active cells[174], presumably because interferon, like all other cellular proteins, is turned over within the cell. Experiments using metabolic inhibitors suggest that synthesis of cellular RNA and protein is required for maintenance, as well as for the development of resistance[181]. The explanation of this effect is not known.

Cells exposed to interferon seem to recover their susceptibility to viruses in a stepwise manner. L cells, which had been treated with interferon for 24 h, regained their full susceptibility to virus infection after about seven generations. Before this, cells appeared which could produce virus protein but not infectious virus, and later cells were found which formed relatively small amounts of virus[182].

1.7.3 Effect of interferon on virus multiplication

Interferon reduces both the number of virus-producing cells and the yield of virus from those cells that do produce virus. Further investigation of mechanism of interferon action has depended on biochemical investigations.

1.7.3.1 RNA viruses

Adsorption of viruses to interferon treated cells is unimpaired, and since virus growth initiated by infective RNA is inhibited as effectively as that by virus, the interferon sensitive stage must lie beyond the stages of adsorption, penetration and uncoating[174]. Interferon does not inhibit the release of new virus nor does it cause accumulation of the products of virus multiplication[174]. Its action must therefore lie early in the virus multiplication cycle.

Synthesis of both virus RNA and protein is inhibited in infected cells treated with interferon[183-185]. This result would be expected whether interferon inhibited either virus RNA or protein synthesis because of the nature of RNA virus multiplication. The RNA of the infecting virus acts as a messenger RNA for synthesis of virus proteins which include the virus RNA-directed-RNA polymerase. This polymerase then synthesises more virus RNA which can, in turn, act as messenger. Thus inhibitors of virus RNA synthesis lead to inhibition of virus protein synthesis and vice-versa, and it has been difficult to distinguish at which site interferon acts. Evidence indicating that the effect was on virus protein synthesis was obtained by Friedman[185], who studied the synthesis of virus protein under conditions where virus RNA synthesis was inhibited by incubation at 42 °C. By using large amounts of virus to infect the cells, the synthesis of virus proteins using the RNA of the infecting virus as messenger could be studied. This was inhibited in interferon-treated cells. However, other evidence indicates an effect on virus RNA synthesis. Some RNA viruses contain an RNA-directed-RNA-polymerase and in this case, the messenger RNA is complementary in base sequence to the virus RNA. Synthesis of this virus messenger RNA can then be studied in infected cells treated with cycloheximide to inhibit translation of the newly-formed messenger RNA. Interferon pre-treatment was found to inhibit such virus RNA synthesis[186], indicating an effect on virus RNA synthesis rather than on virus protein synthesis. However, the interferon doses were high and it is possible the effect may be a secondary one.

1.7.3.2 DNA viruses

The DNA virus that has been most studied in relation to interferon action is vaccinia. Uncoating of this virus is a complex process, proceeding in two stages. First, the outer membrane is removed by host enzymes. Then a DNA-directed-RNA-polymerase enzyme within the virus particle synthesises a virus RNA which is translated on host ribosomes. The protein thus formed then brings about the second stage of uncoating, with subsequent further RNA and protein synthesis. These events occur in the cytoplasm and, by appropriate choice of conditions, can be studied without interference due to host cell RNA synthesis. Further, infection produces a very rapid inhibition of host cell protein synthesis with disaggregation of host cell polyribosomes, so that there is little interference from host cell protein synthesis either.

Using this system, inhibition of the virus DNA-directed-RNA-polymerase has been reported[187], but the effects were obtained at quite high interferon concentrations. This suggested that interferon inhibited virus transcription, and a similar conclusion was reached as a result of a study with SV40 virus[188]. A subsequent study[189] using much lower doses of interferon, showed that there was no inhibition of virus RNA synthesis (thus confirming earlier work[190]) but substantial inhibition of virus protein synthesis. This was because viral messenger RNA failed to form virus polysomes, due either to a defect in the ribosome or in the messenger RNA. Thus there is conflicting evidence as to whether interferon inhibits virus transcription or virus translation, and it is possible that it acts at both levels,

Using the DNA tumour virus SV40, it was found that synthesis of SV40 protein was inhibited in infected cells when they were treated with interferon, but not when the cells had been transformed with SV40, or when the cells were infected with a hybrid virus of adenovirus and SV40[191]. This must mean that there is nothing in the sequence of nucleotides specifying a virus protein which prevents its translation in interferon-treated cells. Resistance or sensitivity must be determined by some other character of the viral RNA such as configuration, the ribosome binding site or the initiation mechanism.

1.7.3.3 Cell-free systems

A number of attempts have been made to study the function of virus messenger RNA in cell-free systems. Two methods have been used. In the first, the binding of radioactively-labelled RNA to ribosomes derived from interferon-treated and control cells has been compared, and the behaviour of any ribosome–messenger RNA complex so formed has been studied in a cell-free system. In the second, the ability of virus RNA to stimulate amino acid incorporation into polypeptides in cell-free systems has been measured.

Using the first type of approach, Marcus and Salb[192, 193] proposed that a new protein, the translational inhibitory protein (TIP), was synthesised in interferon-treated cells. They suggested that this attached to ribosomes, specifically impairing their ability to translate virus as opposed to cellular messenger RNA. In addition, the ribosomes had a reduced capacity to bind virus RNA. These two changes in the ribosome could be distinguished by treatment with trypsin, which restored their capacity to translate but not to bind virus RNA. The reduced binding capacity of ribosomes from interferon-treated cells was also reported by another group[194, 195].

Using the second type of approach, the same two groups reported that virus RNA failed to stimulate amino acid incorporation when the ribosomes were obtained from interferon-treated cells[192, 195].

These results, which appeared to give a clear-cut answer, have encountered a number of criticisms. Two other groups have been unable to repeat the experiments of Marcus and Salb, finding no difference between the rate of attachment of virus RNA to ribosomes from control or interferon-treated ribosomes, or any difference in behaviour of such RNA-ribosome complexes[196, 197].

Recently much more clear-cut results have been obtained as a result of the progress made in the characterisation of products from cell-free systems containing virus messenger RNA. Cell-free systems, obtained from either uninfected or virus infected mouse L cells, were able to translate both haemoglobin messenger RNA and a virus messenger RNA to give products similar to those found *in vivo*. Treatment of cells with sufficient highly-purified mouse interferon to inhibit virus growth by more than 99% had no effect on the translation of the virus messenger RNA. However, when interferon-treated, virus-infected cells were used, inhibition of virus messenger RNA translation was noted[198]. This result shows that an effect of interferon is only detectable in virus-infected cells. The mechanism is unknown but it clearly provides a ready explanation for the lack of toxicity of interferon to uninfected cells.

1.7.3.4 The effect of interferon on the cytotoxicity due to viruses

Infection with certain viruses leads to a rapid inhibition of cellular RNA and protein synthesis, and also cytotoxity, although these two effects do not appear to be causually related. Both effects can be inhibited by treatment of the cells with interferon, although much more interferon is needed to inhibit cytotoxicity than is required to inhibit virus multiplication. The reason for this difference is not known[199].

1.7.4 The effect of interferon on uninfected cells

Many studies have shown that interferon has no gross effect on uninfected cells. Small changes have been reported, but it is difficult to exclude the possibility that these were due to impurities in the interferon preparations[174]. There have also been reports that highly purified interferon slowed the growth rate of cells[200, 201] and their tumour and colony forming ability[202]. It is possible then that interferon does have some effect on host cells, but less than that on virus multiplication. A better test would be to measure the effect of interferon treatment on the synthesis of a *new* cellular protein.

1.7.5 Factors affecting the action of interferon

The most important factors are given below.

1.7.5.1 Factors antagonising the action of interferon

A number of interferon antagonists have been extracted from either infected or uninfected cells[174]. None of them have been well characterised.

1.7.5.2 Age of the cell culture

Cells increase in sensitivity to interferon with increased age in culture. Chick embryos too appear to become more sensitive to interferon as they age[174]. The basis of both effects is unknown.

1.7.6 The site of interferon action

Evidence discussed above indicates that, in the interferon-treated cells, the translation of virus polyribosomes is inhibited. Is this due to an effect on the ribosome or on the messenger RNA, or on some other component of the translational apparatus?

Careful comparison of ribosomes from interferon-treated and control cells has failed to reveal any difference[203, 204]. Nor were any differences observed when comparisons were made of the rate of sedimentation of the ribosomes or their sub-units in sucrose gradients, in the ratio of monosomes to polysomes, or in the density of the ribosomes[205]. It appears unlikely that the ribosome is involved in interferon action, and a more likely site is the initiation of virus protein synthesis. Inhibition of some necessary processing of the virus nucleic acid, impairment of the action of an initiation factor or of an initiator transfer RNA could all explain the action of interferon.

1.8 THE ACTION OF INTERFERON IN ANIMALS AND MAN

Soon after their discovery, interferons were found to be active against many different viruses and to have little or no toxicity. It was therefore natural to investigate their use in medicine, and many studies have been carried out with interferon and with interferon inducers, although only the former will be discussed here. In these studies, it is important to use partially purified interferon if possible, especially for work in man, and also to use *enough* interferon. The latter has been achieved only by bitter experience.

1.8.1 The action of interferon in animals

Interferon was first shown to be active in animals by its injection into the rabbit skin followed later by challenge with vaccinia virus at the same place[206, 207]. There have since been many studies in which interferon has been shown to be active against a challenge virus inoculated into the same place, including skin, muscle and subcutaneous tissue[208]. These have been useful for establishing dosage, time of protection etc. but they are of little relevance to clinical practise, except for virus infections of the eye where interferon will protect against infection with vaccinia or herpes simplex[209].

The next step was to see whether interferon would protect against systemic infection, and a large number of studies have shown protection in mice, rats, rabbits, chicks and monkeys against a wide variety of challenge viruses, including tumour viruses[209, 210]. Mice have been used most often: they are cheap and convenient, there are suitable model virus infections and a high-titre mouse interferon can readily be obtained from mouse serum. The effects of a number of variables has been investigated; different doses of interferon, different routes of administration, different amounts of challenge virus and challenge at different intervals after treatment with interferon[209].

It has been more difficult to obtain protection against respiratory virus infections. These virus infections are of course of enormous importance, but it is not possible to protect by injection of interferon intramuscularly or intravenously. Interferon has to be given by spray or aerosol, or as drops into the nose or trachea. This is a relatively inefficient method and the protective effects obtained are much less marked.

In none of these studies has there been any evidence of toxicity due to the interferon preparations, which were often very crude, or of antigenic reactions.

1.8.2   The action of interferon in man

Viruses, double-stranded polynucleotides and pyran copolymer will all induce interferon in man, but the titres obtained have been surprisingly small[211]. Similar results were obtained in monkeys, and it is possible that the system for interferon production is more highly developed in mice and rabbits than in primates and some other animals (e.g. the ferret). Human interferon can however be prepared readily in human leukocytes or in monkey kidney cells in culture (monkey interferon is active in human cells). Interferon from this latter source was used for the first demonstration of interferon activity in man, with a vaccinia challenge at the site of injection[212]. A highly-significant protection was obtained. Monkey and human interferon has been used to treat virus infections of the eye[211]; positive protection was obtained. Human interferon has been used in large-scale Russian trials during an outbreak of influenza due to an A2 virus[213]. Striking protection was obtained with unconcentrated crude human leukocyte interferon—a startling result in view of the failure of a trial in Britain against a series of respiratory viruses[214]. There is no evidence of any toxicity due to interferon, and trials against respiratory infections—the most immediate attractive goal for antiviral chemotherapy—are continuing, the production of large amounts of partially-purified interferon being the main problem.

1.9 THE SIGNIFICANCE OF INTERFERON

Interferon was discovered as a result of treating chick chorioallantoic membranes maintained *in vitro* with an inactivated virus—a highly artificial system. However, interferon is formed in animals and man as a response to a wide variety of inducers, which include the viruses but also a number of other agents such as rickettsiae, protozoa and bacteria (see Section 1.3.6). Since interferon is also active against many of these agents, as well as against the viruses, it raises the question whether interferon is just an antiviral agent or whether it has some wider function in the control of cellular processes. The second view is strengthened by finding that interferon is produced by antigenically-competent cells.

Certainly, interferon appears to play a part in the recovery from normal virus infections. Interferon is produced in animals and man, not only after injection of large doses of an inducer, but also in response to vaccination and natural infection with viruses[211]. Interferon is formed relatively quickly after virus infection, before antibody formation, and it has been suggested that it is the first host defence process to be mobilised. In contrast, immunological mechanisms may not be essential for recovery, but they limit the spread of virus through body fluids during primary infection, and prevent reinfection[215]. Stevens and Merigan[216], as a result of a study of factors associated with the course of herpes zoster in human patients, concluded that at least two factors controlled the course of the infections: local interferon production (possibly mediated by sensitised lymphocytes) and humoral antibody. Interferon certainly plays a role in the maintenance of persistent infections *in vitro*, in which a delicate balance is maintained between virus and cell multiplication and it may play a role in such infections *in vivo*. But whether it plays any other role in the control of cellular processes is unknown.

Note added in proof

A recent clinical trial[217], using two batches of partially purified human interferon, showed that the onset of influenza virus infection could be delayed and infection with common cold virus prevented by spraying interferon into the upper respiratory tract before infection. This is the first successful propylactic trial in man with a respiratory virus infection: future trials will determine whether interferon can be used therapeutically.

References

1. Isaacs, A. and Lindenmann, J. (1957). *Proc. Roy. Soc. (London) Ser. B.*, **147**, 258
2. Henle, W. (1950). *J. Immunol.*, **64**, 203
3. *Interferons* (1966) (N. B. Finter, editor) (Amsterdam: North-Holland Publishing Company)
4. Vilcek, J. (1969). *Interferon* (Wien, New York: Springer-Verlag)
5. *Interferons and Interferon Inducers* (1973) (N. B. Finter, editor) (Amsterdam: North-Holland Publishing Company)
6. Colby, C., Jr. (1971). *Progress in Nucleic Acid Research and Molecular Biology*, Vol. II, 1 (J. N. Davidson and W. E. Cohn, editors) (New York and London: Academic Press)

7. De Clercq, E. and Merigan, T. C. (1970). *Ann. Rev. Med.*, **21**, 17
8. Nagano, T., Kojima, Y., Arakawa, J. and Kanashiro, R. S. (1966). *Jap. J. Exp. Med.*, **36**, 481
9. Stewart, W. E. II, Scott, W. D. and Sulkin, S. E. (1969). *J. Virol.*, **4**, 147
10. Sueltenfuss, E. A. and Polland, M. (1963). *Science*, **139**, 595
11. Hanna, L., Merigan, T. C. and Jawetz, E. (1966). *Proc. Soc. Exp. Biol. Med.*, **122**, 417
12. Reinicke, V., Mordhorst, C. H. and Schonne, E. (1967). *Acta Pathol. Microbiol. Scand.*, **69**, 478
13. Remington, J. S. and Merigan, T. C. (1969). *Proc. Soc. Exp. Biol. Med.*, **131**, 1184
14. Merigan, T. C. (1973). *Interferons and Interferon Inducers*, **251** (N. B. Finter, editor) (Amsterdam: North-Holland Publishing Company)
15. Taylor, J. (1964). *Biochem. Biophys. Res. Commun.*, **14**, 447
16. Friedman, R. M. and Sonnabend, J. A. (1964). *Nature (London)*, **203**, 366
17. Lockart, R. Z., Jr. (1964). *Biochem. Biophys. Res. Commun.*, **15**, 513
18. Smith, T. J. and Wagner, R. R. (1967). *J. Exp. Med.* **125**, 559
19. Tyrrell, D. A. J. (1959). *Nature (London)*, **184**, 452
20. Merigan, T. C. (1964). *Science*, **145**, 811
21. Baron, S., Barban, S. and Buckler, C. E. (1964). *Science*, **145**, 814
22. Bucknall, R. A. (1967). *Nature (London)*, **216**, 1022
23. Moehring, J. M. and Stinebring, W. R. (1970). *Nature (London)*, **226**, 360
24. Desmyter, J., Rawls, W. E. and Melnick, J. L. (1968). *Proc. Nat. Acad. Sci. USA*, **59**, 69
25. Levy-Koenig, R. E., Golgher, R. R. and Paucker, K. (1970). *J. Immunol.*, **104**, 791
26. Michaels, R. H., Weinberger, M. M. and Ho, M. (1965). *New. Engl. J. Med.*, **272**, 1148
27. Merigan, T. C., Gregory, D. F. and Petralli, J. K. (1966). *Virology*, **29**, 515
28. Levy-Koenig, R. E., Mundy, M. J. and Paucker, K. (1970). *J. Immunol.*, **104**, 785
29. Paucker, K. (1965). *J. Immunol.*, **94**, 371
30. Wheelock, E. F. (1965). *Science*, **149**, 310
31. Cantell, K. and Paucker, K. (1963). *Virology*, **19**, 81
32. Lockart, R. Z., Jr. (1965). *J. Bacteriol.*, **89**, 117
33. Wagner, R. R. (1965). *Amer. J. Med.*, **38**, 726
34. Ho, M. (1962). *Virology*, **17**, 262
35. Lockart, R. Z. Jr. and Sreevalsan, T. (1963). *Symposium on Fundamental Cancer Research at the University of Texas. M. D. Anderson and Tumour Institute, Houston, Texas*, 447 (Baltimore: Williams and Wilkin)
36. Fleischmann, W. R., Jr., and Simon, E. H. (1969). *Bact. Proc.*, 169
37. Finter, N. B. (1969). *J. Gen. Virol*, **5**, 419
38. Billiau, A. and Buckler, C. E. (1970). *Symp. Series Immunobiol. Standard*, Vol. 14, 37 (F. T. Perkins and R. H. Regamey, editors) (Basel: Karger)
39. Gifford, G. E., Toy, S. T. and Lindenmann, J. (1963). *Virology*, **19**, 294
40. Finter, N. B. (1966). *Interferons*, 87 (N. B. Finter, editor) (Amsterdam: North-Holland Publishing Company)
41. Finter, N. B. (1973). *Interferons and Interferon Inducers*, 135 (N. B. Finter, editor) (Amsterdam: North-Holland Publishing Company)
42. *Symp. Series Immunobiol. Standard*, Vol. 14 (F. T. Perkins and R. H. Regamey, editors) (Basel: Karger)
43. Ho, M. (1973). *Interferons and Interferon Inducers*, 29 (N. B. Finter, editor) (Amsterdam: North-Holland Publishing Company)
44. Béládi, I. and Pusztai, R. (1967) *Z. Naturforsch.*, **22b**, 165
45. Ho, M. and Kohler, K. (1967). *Arch. Gesamte Virusforsch.*, **22**, 69
46. Burke, D. C. and Isaacs, A. (1958). *Brit. J. Exp. Pathol.*, **39**, 452
47. Ho, M. and Breinig, M. K. (1965). *Virology*, **25**, 331
48. Long, W. F. and Burke, D. C. (1971). *J. Gen. Virol.*, **12**, 1
49. Bakay, M. and Burke, D. C. (1972). *J. Gen. Virol.*, **16**, 399
50. Pusztai, R., Béládi, I., Bakay, M. and Mucsi, I. (1969). *J. Gen. Virol.*, **4**, 169
51. Baron, S. and Buckler, C. E. (1963). *Science*, **141**, 1061
52. Powell, H. M., Culbertson, C. G., McGuire, J. M., Hoehn, M. M. and Baker, L. A. (1952). *Antibiot. Chemotherapy*, **2**, 432
53. Shope, R. E. (1953). *J. Exp. Med.*, **97**, 601

54. Kleinschmidt, W. J., Cline, J. C. and Murphy, E. B. (1964). *Proc. Nat. Acad. Sci. USA*, **52**, 741
55. Rytel, M. W., Shope, R. E. and Kilbourne, E. D. (1966). *J. Exp. Med.*, **123**, 577
56. Kleinschmidt, W. J. and Ellis, L. F. (1968). *Interferon*, 39 (G. E. W. Wolstenholme and M. O'Connor, editors) (London: J. and A. Churchill)
57. Lampson, G. P., Tytell, A. A., Field, A. K., Nemes, M. M. and Hilleman, M. R. (1967). *Proc. Nat. Acad. Sci. USA*, **58**, 782
58. Banks, G. T., Buck, K. W., Chain, E. B., Darbyshire, J. E., Himmelweit, F., Ratti, G., Sharpe, T. J. and Planterose, D. N. (1970). *Nature (London)*, **227**, 505
59. Isaacs, A. (1963). *Advances in Virus Research*, Vol. 10, 1 (K. M. Smith and M. A. Lauffer, editors) (New York: Academic Press)
60. Isaacs, A., Cox, R. A. and Rotem, Z. (1963). *Lancet, ii*, 113
61. Rotem, Z., Cox, R. A. and Isaacs, A. (1963). *Nature (London)*, **197**, 564
62. Isaacs, A. (1965). *Aust. J. Exp. Biol. Med. Sci.*, **43**, 405
63. Tytell, A. A., Lampson, G. P., Field, A. K. and Hilleman, M. R. (1967). *Proc. Nat. Acad. Sci. USA*, **58**, 1719
64. Field, A. K., Tytell, A. A., Lampson, G. P. and Hilleman, M. R. (1967). *Proc. Nat. Acad. Sci. USA*, **58**, 1004
65. Field, A. K., Lampson, G. P., Tytell, A. A., Nemes, M. M. and Hilleman, M. R. (1967). *Proc. Nat. Acad. Sci. USA*, **58**, 2102
66. Field, A. K., Tytell, A. A., Lampson, G. P. and Hilleman, M. R. (1968). *Proc. Nat. Acad. Sci. USA*, **61**, 340
67. Dianzani, F., Cantagalli, P., Gagnoni, S. and Rita, G. (1968). *Proc. Soc. Exp. Biol. Med.*, **128**, 708
68. Dianzani, F., Gagnoni, S. and Cantagalli, P. (1970). *Ann. N.Y. Acad. Sci.*, **173**, 727
69. Bausek, G. H. and Merigan, T. C. (1969). *Virology*, **39**, 491
70. Ho, M. (1964). *Science*, **146**, 1472
71. Stinebring, W. R. and Youngner, J. S. (1964). *Nature (London)*, **204**, 712
72. Kobayashi, S., Yasui, O. and Masuzumi, M. (1969). *Proc. Soc. Exp. Biol. Med.*, **131**, 487
73. Kono, Y. (1967). *Arch. Gesamte Virusforschung.*, **21**, 277s
74. Finkelstein, M. S., Bausek, G. H. and Merigan, T. C. (1968). *Science*, **161**, 465
75. Merigan, T. C. (1972). *Interferons and Interferon Inducers*, 45 (N. B. Finter, editor) (Amsterdam: North-Holland Publishing Company)
76. Borecký, L. (1968). *Medical and Applied Virology*, 181 (M. Sanders and E. H. Lennette, editors) (St Louis: Warren H. Green Inc.)
77. Wheelock, E. F. (1965). *Science*, **149**, 310
78. Friedman, R. M. and Cooper, H. L. (1967). *Proc. Soc. Exp. Biol. Med.*, **125**, 901
79. Green, J. A., Cooperband, S. R. and Kilbrick, S. (1969). *Science*, **164**, 1415
80. Falcoff, E., Falcoff, R., Catinot, L., Vomecourt, A. and Sanceau, J. (1972). *Europ. J. Clin. Biol. Res.*, **17**, 20
81. Falcoff, R., Oriol, R. and Iscaki, S. (1972). *Europ. J. Immunol.*, **2**, 476
82. Falcoff, R. (1972). *J. Gen. Virol.*, **16**, 251
83. Regelson, W. (1967). *Advan. Exp. Med. Biol.*, **1**, 315
84. Merigan, T. C. and Finkelstein, M. S. (1968). *Virology*, **35**, 363
85. De Somer, P., De Clercq, E., Billiau, A., Schonne, E. and Claesen, M. (1968). *J. Virol.*, **2**, 886
86. Youngner, J. S., Stinebring, W. R. and Taube, S. E. (1965). *Virology*, **27**, 541
87. Lukáš, B. and Hrušková, J. (1968). *Acta Virol.*, **12**, 263
88. Ho, M. (1973). *Interferons and Interferon Inducers*, 73 (N. B. Finter, editor) (Amsterdam: North-Holland Publishing Company)
89. De Maeyer, E. and De Maeyer-Guignard, J. (1970). *Ann. N.Y. Acad. Sci.*, **173**, 228
90. Carver, D. H. and Marcus, P. I. (1967). *Virology*, **32**, 247
91. Kato, N. and Eggers, H. J. (1969). *Virology*, **37**, 545
92. Isaacs, A. and Baron, S. (1960). *Lancet, ii*, 946
93. Gandhi, S. S. and Stewart, R. B. (1968). *Canad. J. Microbiol.*, **14**, 1305
94. Isaacs, A., Rotem, Z. and Fantes, K. H. (1966). *Virology*, **29**, 248
95. Kato, N., Eggers, H. J., Ohta, F. and Kobayashi, T. (1969). *J. Gen. Virol.* **5**, 195
96. Lockart, R. Z., Jr. (1963). *J. Bacteriol.*, **85**, 556
97. Friedman, R. M. (1966). *J. Immunol.*, **96**, 872

98. Stewart, W. E. II, Gosser, L. B. and Lockart, R. Z., Jr. (1971). *J. Virol.*, **7**, 792
99. Stewart, W. E. II, Gosser, L. B. and Lockart, R. Z., Jr. (1972). *J. Gen. Virol.* **15**, 85
100. Hermodsson, S. (1963). *Virology*, **20**, 333
101. Cantell, K. (1966) in *Medical and Applied Virology*, 31 (M. Sanders and E. H. Lennette, editors) (Missouri: Green)
102. De Maeyer, E. and De Maeyer-Guignard, J. (1968). *Interferon*, 218 (G. E. W. Wolstenholme and M. O'Connor, editors) (London: J. and A. Churchill)
103. Jullien, P. and De Maeyer, E. (1966). *Int. J. Radiat. Biol.*, **11**, 567
104. De Maeyer, E., Jullien, P. and De Maeyer-Guignard, J. (1967). *Int. J. Radiat. Biol.*, **13**, 417
105. Heller, E. (1963). *Virology*, **21**, 652
106. Wagner, R. R. (1963). *Annu. Rev. Microbiol.*, **17**, 285
107. Walters, S., Burke, D. C. and Skehel, J. J. (1967). *J. Gen. Virol.*, **1**, 349
108. Wagner, R. R. and Huang, A. S. (1965). *Proc. Nat. Acad. Sci. USA*, **54**, 1112
109. Buchan, A. and Burke, D. C. (1966). *Biochem. J.*, **98**, 530
110. Lampson, G. P., Tytell, A. A., Nemes, M. M. and Hilleman, M. R. (1963). *Proc. Soc. Exp. Biol. Med.*, **112**, 468
111. Jacob, F. and Monod, J. (1961). *J. Molec. Biol.*, **3**, 318
112. Ho, M. and Kono, Y. (1965). *Proc. Nat. Acad. Sci. USA*, **53**, 220
113. Ke, Y. H., Singer, S. H., Postic, B. and Ho, M. (1966). *Proc. Soc. Exp. Biol. Med.*, **121**, 181
114. Burke, D. C. and Isaacs, A. (1958). *Brit. J. Exp. Pathol.*, **39**, 78
115. Skehel, J. J. and Burke, D. C. (1968). *J. Gen. Virol.*, **3**, 35
116. Skehel, J. J. and Burke, D. C. (1968). *J. Gen. Virol.*, **3**, 191
117. Lockart, R. Z. Jr., Bayliss, N. L., Toy, S. T. and Yin, F. H. (1968). *J. Virol.*, **2**, 962
118. Lomniczi, B. and Burke, D. C. (1970). *J. Gen. Virol.*, **8**, 55
119. Sheaff, E. T., Meager, A. and Burke, D. C. (1972). *J. Gen. Virol.*, **17**, 163
120. Gandhi, S. S. and Burke, D. C. (1970). *J. Gen. Virol.*, **6**, 95
121. Huppert, J., Hillova, J. and Gresland, L. (1969). *Nature (London)*, **223**, 1015
122. Gandhi, S. S., Burke, D. C. and Scholtissck, C. (1970). *J. Gen. Virol.*, **9**, 97
123. Huang, A. S., Baltimore, D. and Bratt, M. A. (1971). *J. Virol.*, **7**, 389
124. Clavell, L. A. and Bratt, M. A. (1971). *J. Virol.*, **8**, 500
125. Colby, C. and Duesberg, P. H. (1969). *Nature (London)*, **222**, 940
126. De Maeyer-Guignard, J. and De Maeyer, E. (1965). *Nature (London)*, **205**, 985
127. Burke, D. C. and Morrison, J. M. (1966). *Virology*, **28**, 108
128. Cogniaux-Le Clerq, J. A., Levy, A. H. and Wagner, R. R. (1966). *Virology*, **28**, 497
129. Coppey, J. and Muel, B. (1970). *Int. J. Radiat. Biol.*, **17**, 431
130. Guggenheim, M. A., Friedman, R. M. and Rabson, A. S. (1969). *Proc. Soc. Exp. Biol. Med.*, **130**, 1242
131. Carver, D. H., Seto, D. S. Y. and Midgeon, B. R. (1968). *Science*, **160**, 558
132. Cassingena, R., Chany, C., Vignal, M., Suarez, H., Estrada, S. and Lazar, P. (1971). *Proc. Nat. Acad. Sci. USA*, **68**, 580
133. Burke, D. C. (1973). *Interferon and Interferon Inducers*, 107 (N. B. Finter, editor) (Amsterdam: North-Holland Publishing Company)
134. De Maeyer-Guignard, J., De Maeyer, E. and Montagnier, L. (1972). *Proc. Nat. Acad. Sci. USA*, **69**, 1203
135. Tan, Y. H., Jeng, D. K. and Ho, M. (1972). *Virology*, **48**, 41
136. De Clercq, E., Eckstein, F. and Merigan, T. C. (1969). *Science*, **165**, 1137
137. Pitha, P. M. and Carter, W. A. (1971). *Nature New Biol.*, **234**, 105
138. Matzura, H. and Eckstein, F. (1968). *Europ. J. Biochem.* **3**, 448
139. De Clercq, E., Eckstein, F., Sternbach, H. and Merigan, T. C. (1970). *Virology*, **42**, 421
140. Lampson, G. P., Field, A. K., Tytell, A. A., Nemes, M. M. and Hilleman, M. R. (1970). *Proc. Soc. Exp. Biol. Med.*, **135**, 911
141. Wacker, A., Singh, A., Svěc, J. and Lodeman, E. (1969). *Naturwissenschaften*, **56**, 638
142. Tytell, A. A., Lampson, G. P., Field, A. K., Nemes, M. M. and Hilleman, M. R. (1970). *Proc. Soc. Exp. Bio. Med.*, **135**, 917
143. Niblack, J. F. and McCreary, M. B. (1971). *Nature New Biol.*, **233**, 52
144. Pitha, J. and Pitha, P. M. (1971). *Science*, **172**, 1146
145. Carter, W. A., Pitha, P. M., Marshall, L. W., Tazawa, I., Tazawa, S. and Ts'o P. O. P. (1972). *J. Molec. Biol.*, **70**, 567

146. De Clercq, E., Zmudzka, B. and Shugar, D. (1972). *FEBS Lett.*, **24**, 137
147. Steward, D. L., Herndon, W. C. Jr. and Schell, K. R. (1972). *Biochim. Biophys. Acta*, **262**, 227
148. Vilcek, J., Ng., M. H., Friedman-Kien, A. E. and Krawciw, T. (1968). *J. Virol.*, **2**, 648
149. Colby, C. and Chamberlin, M. J. (1969). *Proc. Nat. Acad. Sci. USA*. **63**, 160
150. De Clercq, E. and De Somer, P. (1972). *J. Virol.*, **9**, 721
151. Ralph, R. K. (1969). *Advances in Virus Research*, **15**, 61 (K. M. Smith, M. A. Lauffer and F. B. Bang, editors) (New York: Academic Press)
152. Stewart, W. E. II, Gosser, L. B. and Lockart, R. Z., Jr. (1971). *J. Gen. Virol.*, **13**, 35
153. Vilček, J., Rossman, T. G. and Varacalli, F. (1969). *Nature (London)*, **222**, 682
154. Tan, Y. H., Armstrong, J. A., Ke, Y. H. and Mo, H. (1970). *Proc. Nat. Acad. Sci. USA* **67**, 464
155. Ho, M. and Ke, Y. H. (1970). *Virology*, **40**, 693
156. Youngner, J. S. and Feingold, D. S. (1967). *J. Virol.*, **1**, 1164
157. Feingold, D. S., Youngner, J. S. and Chen, J. (1968). *Biochem. Biophys. Res. Commun.* **32**, 554
158. Fantes, K. H. (1973). *Interferons and Interferon Inducers*, 171 (N. B. Finter, editor) Amsterdam: North-Holland Publishing Company)
159. Fantes, K. H. (1967). *J. Gen. Virol.*, **1**, 257
160. Fantes, K. H. (1968). *Medical and Applied Virology*, 223 (M. Sanders and E. H. Lenette, editors) (Missouri: Green)
161. Fantes, K. H. and Furminger, I. G. S. (1967). *Nature (London)*, **216**, 71
162. Fantes, K. H. (1969). *Science*, **163**, 1198
163. Fantes, K. H. and O'Neill, C. F. (1964). *Nature (London)*, **203**, 1048
164. Fitzgeorge, R., Allner, K. and Bradish, C. J. (1970). Personal communication
165. Paucker, K., Berman, B. J., Golgher, R. R. and Stanček, D. (1970). *J. Virol.*, **5**, 145
166. Stanček, D., Golgher, R. R. and Paucker, K. (1970). *Symp. Series Immunobiol. Standard*, Vol. 14, 55 (F. T. Perkins and R. H. Regamey, editors) (Basel: Karger)
167. Carter, W. A. (1970). *Proc. Nat. Acad. Sci. USA.*, **67**, 620
168. Stanček, D., Gressnerová, M. and Paucker, K. (1970). *Virology*, **41**, 740
169. Merigan, T. C., Winget, C. A. and Dixcn, C. B. (1965). *J. Molec. Biol.*, **13**, 679
170. Boxaca, M. and Paucker, K. (1967). *J. Immunol.*, **98**, 1130
171. Fantes, K. H. (1970). *Ann. N.Y. Acad. Sci.* **173**, 118
172. Yamazaki, S. and Wagner, R. R. (1970). *J. Virol.*, **5**, 270
173. Schonne, E., Billiau, A. and De Somer, P. (1970). *Symp. Series Immunobiol. Standard*, Vol. 14, 61 (F. T. Perkins and R. H. Regamey, editors) (Basel: Karger)
174. Sonnabend, J. A. and Friedman, R. M. (1973) *Interferons and Interferon Inducers*, 201 (N. B. Finter, editor) (Amsterdam: North-Holland Publishing Company)
175. Buckler, C. E., Baron, S. and Levy, H. B. (1966). *Science*, **152**, 80
176. Merigan, T. C. (1964). *Science*, **145**, 811
177. Sheaff, E. T. and Stewart, R. B. (1969). *Canad. J. Microbiol.*, **15**, 941
178. Gifford, G. E. (1963). *J. Gen. Microbiol.*, **33**, 437
179. Friedman, R. M. (1967). *Science*, **156**, 1760
180. Sheaff, E. T. and Stewart, R. B. (1969). *Canad. J. Microbiol.* **15**, 941; **16**, 1087, 1303
181. Baron, S., Buckler, C. E., Dianzani, F. (1968). *Interferon*, 186 (G. E. W. Wolstenholme and M. O'Connor, editors) (London: J. and A. Churchill)
182. Paucker, K. and Cantell, K. (1963). *Virology*, **21**, 22
183. Taylor, J. (1965). *Virology*, **25**, 240
184. Gordon, I., Chenault, S. S., Stevenson, D. and Acton, J. D. (1966). *J. Bacteriol.*, **91**, 1230
185. Friedman, R. M. (1968). *J. Virol.*, **2**, 1081
186. Marcus, P. I., Engelhardt, D. L., Hunt, J. M. and Sekellick, M. J. (1972). *Science*, **174**, 593
187. Bialy, H. S. and Colby, C. (1972). *J. Virol.*, **9**, 286
188. Oxman, M. N. and Levin, M. J. (1971). *Proc. Nat. Acad. Sci. USA*. **68**, 299
189. Metz, D. H. and Esteban, M. (1972). *Nature (London)*, **238**, 385
190. Joklik, W. K. and Merigan, T. C. (1966). *Proc. Nat. Acad. Sci. USA*. **56**, 558
191. Oxman, M. N., Baron, S., Black, P. H., Takemoto, K. K., Habel, K. and Rowe, W. P. (1967). *Virology*, **32**, 122
192. Marcus, P. I. and Salb, J. M. (1966). *Virology*, **30**, 502

193. Marcus, P. I. and Salb, J. M. (1968). *The Interferons*, 111 (G. Rita, editor) (New York: Academic Press)
194. Carter, W. A. and Levy, H. B. (1967). *Arch. Biochem. Biophys.*, **120,** 563
195. Carter, W. A. and Levy, H. B. (1968). *Biochim. Biophys. Acta*, **155,** 437
196. Lockart, R. Z. Jr. (1967). Personal communication
197. Kerr, I. M., Sonnabend, J. A. and Martin, E. M. (1970). *J. Virol.*, **5,** 132
198. Friedman, R. M., Esteban, R. M., Metz, D. H., Tovell, D. R., Kerr, I. M. and Williamson, R. (1972). *FEBS Lett.*, **24,** 273
199. Haase, A. T., Baron, S., Levy, H. and Kasel, J. A. (1969). *J. Virol.*, **4,** 490
200. Paucker, K. and Golgher, R. (1970). *Colloque No. 6, Institut National de la Sante et de la Recherche Médicale*, 119 (Paris: Institut National de la Recherche medicale)
201. Gresser, I., Brouty-Boyé, D., Thomas, M. T. and Macieira-Coelho, A. (1970). *Proc. Nat. Acad. Sci. USA.*, **66,** 1052
202. Gresser, I., Thomas, M. T., Brouty-Boyé, D. and Macieira-Coelho, A. (1971). *Nature New Biol.*, **231,** 20
203. Kerr, I. M., Martin, E. M., Sonnabend, J. A. and Metz, D. H. (1970). *Colloque No. 6, Institut National de la Santé et de la Recherche Médicale*, **85** (Paris: Institut National de la Santé et de la Recherche Médicale)
204. Bodo, G. (1969). Personal communication
205. Kerr, I. M., Sonnabend, J. A. and Martin, E. M. (1970). *J. Virol.*, **5,** 132
206. Lindenmann, J., Burke, D. C. and Isaacs, A. (1957). *Brit. J. Exp. Pathol.*, **38,** 551
207. Isaacs, A. and Westwood, M. A. (1959). *Lancet, ii,* 324
208. Finter, N. B. (1966). *Interferons*, **232** (N. B. Finter, editor) (Amsterdam: North-Holland Publishing Company)
209. Finter, N. B. (1973). *Interferons and Interferon Inducers*, **295** (N. B. Finter, editor) (Amsterdam: North-Holland Publishing Company)
210. Oxman, M. H. (1973). *Interferons and Interferon Inducers*, 391 (N. B. Finter, editor) (Amsterdam: North-Holland Publishing Company)
211. Finter, N. B. (1973). *Interferons and Interferon Inducers*, **363** (N. B. Finter, editor) (Amsterdam: North Holland Publishing Company)
212. Scientific Committee on Interferon (1962). *Lancet, i,* 873
213. Soloviev, V. D. (1969). *Bull. World Health Organ.*, **41,** 683
214. Scientific Committee on Interferon (1965). *Lancet, i,* 505
215. Baron, S. (1973). *Interferons and Interferon Inducers*, **267** (N. B. Finter, editor) (Amsterdam: North-Holland Publishing Company)
216. Stevens, D. A. and Merigan, T. C. (1972). *J. Clin. Invest.* **51,** 1170
217. Merigan, T. C., Reed, S. E., Hall, T. S. and Tyrrell, D. A. J. (1973). *Lancet, i,* 563

2
Anatomy of the Lymphoid System

J. J. T. OWEN
University College, London

2.1 INTRODUCTION

In just over a decade there have been remarkable advances in knowledge of the 'functional' anatomy of the lymphoid system which have paralleled major advances in immunology as a whole. This chapter will primarily be concerned with some of these functional aspects of lymphoid anatomy and no attempt will be made to give an account of the detailed descriptive anatomy of lymphoid organs and vessels—such accounts are available in a number of other sources[1-3].

2.1.1 Lymphocytes and immune responses

Conclusive evidence for the role of lymphocytes in immune responses has only been available since the late 1950s. Indeed, until this time it was widely believed that lymphocytes were 'end' cells and so not capable of further division and differentiation. In 1959, Hungerford *et al.*[4], who mainly were interested in obtaining dividing blood cells for chromosome preparations, found that a plant extract, phytohaemagglutinin, could stimulate division in lymphocytes *in vitro*. Although this stimulation was found to be of a non-immunological nature, the discovery precipitated a huge volume of work on the activation of lymphocytes by 'mitogens', a number of which have now been described[5]. This work has been paralleled by the demonstration of 'specific' immunological activation of lymphocytes by antigens both *in vivo* and *in vitro* and by experiments showing that depletion or addition of lymphocytes may impair or impart immunological responsiveness, respectively, in a number of animal models (for an account of the definitive experiments see Gowans and McGregor[6]).

These experiments demonstrated the central role of lymphocytes in immune responses as 'immunologically-competent cells'[7]. The basis of this role can now be understood in terms of the main elements of the clonal selection theory[8]. Briefly, this theory postulates that the variety of immune responses which an animal makes to innumerable antigens depends upon the presence of an array of lymphocytes each of which is genetically restricted so as to respond by clonal expansion to only one, or, at most, a few antigens. The basis for this restriction is now thought to lie in the uniqueness of antigen-recognition receptors expressed on the surface of individual lymphocytes. However, the mechanisms by which diversity of receptors is generated during lymphocyte maturation and, to some extent, the nature of the receptors themselves are still matters for discussion (see Chapter 10).

2.1.2 Two types of immune response—two major lymphocyte classes

The notion that there are two broad categories of immune response dates back to early studies on acquired immunity to bacteria and to the vexed question as to whether circulating antibodies or phagocytic cells were of greater importance in providing defence. Today, the question is usually re-phrased in terms of whether circulating antibody or direct lymphocyte participation is the predominant element in a given immune response. If the former, the response is classified as an example of 'humoral immunity'; if the latter, it is classified as an example of 'cellular' or 'cell-mediated' immunity. It is usual to define 'humoral immunity' as those responses transferable by sera from immune to non-immune animals and this category includes immediate hypersensitivity or allergic responses as well as defensive reactions to bacteria and some viruses. 'Cell-mediated' immunity is defined as those responses transferable by cells but not sera and includes skin graft rejection and graft-versus-host reactions as well as 'delayed hypersensitivity' responses to a variety of invading pathogens (for more detailed discussion see Chapter 3).

Although to some extent these definitions are inadequate, even 'humoral immunity' must ultimately depend upon cells, the concept of two types of immune response has proved useful. Thus, evidence has been obtained in a number of species that neonatal thymectomy profoundly affects capacity for cell-mediated responses[9, 10]; on the other hand, removal of a lymphoid organ unique to birds, the bursa of Fabricius, predominantly interferes wth humoral antibody production[11]. It is now known that the thymus and bursa separately control the maturation of two distinct lymphocyte populations known as T and B lymphocytes respectively and that T lymphocytes, either by direct participation or by activation of ancillary cells, are essential for cell-mediated responses[12, 13], while B lymphocytes are precursors of the antibody secreting cell line[14, 15]. Although no organ comparable to the avian bursa of Fabricius has been identified in mammals, there is substantial evidence for two mammalian lymphocyte classes which are probably analogous to the avian populations (see Section 2.3.3.2).

The discovery of these separate lymphocyte classes has necessitated a re-interpretation of many immunological phenomena as will be clear from reading other chapters in this volume and from accounts elsewhere[16]. It has also been realised that interaction between the two lymphocyte systems is necessary for many immune responses, especially for those involving humoral antibody production (see Section 2.4.3).

2.1.3 Primary and secondary lymphoid organs

It is now possible and useful to subdivide the lymphoid system into 'primary' or 'central' organs, where lymphocytes are generated and matured (e.g. thymus and avian bursa of Fabricius) and 'secondary' or 'peripheral' organs to which lymphocytes are seeded and where immune reactions take place (e.g. lymph nodes, spleen, etc.). However, it must be stated that there is evidence, at least in some species, that immune responses may take place in 'primary' organs and certainly there is considerable support for the notion that lymphocyte maturation may continue in 'peripheral' sites (see 19). Nonetheless, there is much support for such a demarcation and the concept of 'primary' and 'secondary' lymphoid organs will be used here.

2.1.4 Lymphocytes: phylogenetic aspects

Until quite recently it was thought that immunological reactions were unique to vertebrates. However, certain invertebrates have now been found to mount primitive immune reactions characterised by specificity and an elevated response to a second antigenic challenge[17]. At the moment there is no evidence that these responses are mediated by lymphocytes or immunoglobulin molecules, but they are associated with an infiltration of macrophage-like cells and there is some tentative evidence for the production of soluble effector molecules which show at least partial specificity. It is clear that specific immune responsiveness evolved in invertebrates before the development of lymphocytes and immunoglobulin molecules which characterise vertebrate responses. The mechanisms involved in these invertebrate responses are of obvious importance to an understanding of the phylogenesis of immunity and constitute an interesting area for future investigation.

Among vertebrates, even the most primitive living forms, hagfish and lamprey, show a vigorous IgM type antibody response to both soluble and particulate antigens[18] and can slowly reject foreign grafts. Both species have abundant peripheral blood lymphocytes although they possess little organised lymphoid tissue. Indeed, in lower vertebrates in general, with the exception of the thymus, there is no clear demarcation between lymphoid and myeloid tissues; proliferating blood cells are found throughout connective tissues and small foci of lympho-myeloid tissue are present in the digestive tract, in association with the kidneys and somewhat less frequently with the gonads.

The main lympho-myeloid organ in primitive fishes is probably the typhlosole or spiral valve[19]. This is a collection of blood sinusoids and aggregates of lymphoid cells associated with the portal vein and inserted into a fold of intestine. In the absence of haemopoietic bone marrow which first appears in amphibia, the spiral valve is presumably an important source of both lymphocytes and myeloid cells. The thymus probably exists as a separate lymphoid organ in all vertebrates, although there have been some doubts as to its presence in hagfish. However, young specimens of this species have not been examined.

Two distinct molecular classes of antibody are found in some Osteichthyes, notably teleosts, and this is also true for Reptilia and Amphibia. Teleosts are also among the lowest vertebrates to have distinct areas of lymphocytes (white pulp) in spleen. Lymph node-like structures are first found in Amphibia, although they have no capsule and little internal organisation and clearly are rudimentary structures in comparison to mammalian lymph nodes.

The anatomy of the lymphoid system of birds has been the subject of considerable interest in recent years. As mentioned in Section 2.1.2, this is largely because in addition to a thymus, which is concerned with the production and export to other lymphoid tissues of T lymphocytes, birds possess a second major lymphoid organ, the bursa of Fabricius, which produces and exports B lymphocytes. Birds also possess lymphoid tissue in spleen, bone marrow and along the gastro-intestinal tract. However, they lack the highly-organised lymph nodes found in mammals, but instead have small lymphocytic foci situated along lymphatic vessels. Recently, birds have been found to make immunoglobulin resembling mammalian IgA as well as IgM and IgG-like immunoglobulins[20].

Mammals have a highly-developed immunological capacity, not only in terms of the rapidity of foreign graft rejection, but in the elaboration of multiple molecular classes of antibody. In addition to abundant lymphoid tissue associated with the gastro-intestinal tract, in bone marrow and spleen, mammals have highly-organised lymph nodes through which lymphocytes recirculate between blood and lymph[21]. Despite the absence of an obvious counterpart to the bursa of Fabricius, there is substantial evidence that mammals possess T and B lymphocyte classes.

It is uncertain whether separate classes of T and B lymphocytes exist among vertebrates below the level of birds, although in view of the immunological potential of lower vertebrates it seems highly likely that they do. Clearly, if B lymphocytes are present in lower vertebrates, then their maturation must depend on some organ or tissue more primitive than the bursa of Fabricius. Hence, the bursa may be a specialised adaptation of a more basic model of vertebrate B cell maturation; this is an argument which will be taken up further in Section 2.3.3.2.

2.1.5 Immune responses—ancillary cells

The vast amount of new data concerning the role of lymphocytes in immune responses has tended to overshadow the importance of other cell types, e.g. macrophages, eosinophil leucocytes, etc., see 9. However, it would be a mistake to underestimate the importance of these cells, and clear evidence is now available that some cells, especially macrophages, are concerned in the initiation of immune reactions via handling or processing of antigen and also as participants in the effector side of cell mediated responses (see Chapter 3).

2.2 CELLS OF THE LYMPHOID SYSTEM

The lymphoid system, at least as seen in higher vertebrates, is made up of a number of discrete organs and a system of vessels or channels through which lymph (an extracellular fluid rich in lymphocytes) is eventually discharged into the venous system. The organs, thymus, lymph nodes, spleen and gastrointestinal-associated structures, e.g. Peyer's patches, appendix, tonsils; each consist of a fairly dense aggregation of lymphocytes supported by a meshwork of branched reticular cells. In addition, substantial numbers of lymphocytes are contained within haemopoietic bone marrow typifying the close association between lymphoid and myeloid tissue seen throughout vertebrate phylogeny (see Section 2.1.4).

Identification and classification of the various cell types within the lymphoid system has, of necessity, been heavily dependent on morphological considerations. While morphological criteria have been and continue to be of value in formulating any general classification, it is important to remember that this approach suffers from severe limitations; in particular, cells of similar morphology may well be functionally different. Fortunately, methods are now becoming available by which cell types can be distinguished on the basis of surface markers, e.g. antigens, receptors, etc., or on the basis of physical properties, e.g. size, density, adherence, etc. Some of these methods will be discussed in later sections where it will be clear that they have already greatly contributed to current views of the lymphoid system.

2.2.1 Lymphocytes

One of the main distinctive morphological features of lymphocytes is that they are round cells with a high nucleus to cytoplasmic ratio (Figure 2.1). In the light microscope, the nucleus frequently appears to be round, but with the electron microscope most lymphocytes can be shown to possess a nuclear indentation. Their cytoplasm contains a rather variable number of mito-chondria, a small Golgi area and a few lysosomes. In living preparations they show a characteristic polarised mobility which gives them a 'hand mirror' appearance.

Even by morphological criteria, lymphocytes are a heterogenous population varying considerably in size. They have been divided into small, medium and large categories, but this classification is somewhat arbitrary since their size distribution pattern is continuous. They are widely distributed in the body forming a large proportion of cells in blood and peritoneal fluid and the great majority of cells in lymph. They are also the main cellular constituents of the various lymphoid organs. As mentioned in Section 2.1, a major recent advance has been the identification of two classes of lymphocytes—T and B cells. A brief account of how these terms came into use and how they are currently applied is given below.

2.2.1.1 Definition of T and B lymphocytes

Roitt et al.[22] have suggested that the term *T cell* should be applied to those lymphocytes which are derived from the thymus (these cells have also been referred to as 'thymus-processed', 'thymus-derived' or 'thymus-dependent' lymphocytes), while the term *B cell* should be used for those lymphocytes matured under the influence of the bursa of Fabricius of birds (or its equivalent organ/s in mammals). Alternative names are 'thymus independent' or 'marrow-derived cells'. Hence, this terminology classifies lymphocytes according to the 'primary' lymphoid organ from which they are derived. It has proved to be a satisfactory system of classification and has been widely adopted. Some points of confusion have, however, arisen and it is worth attempting to clarify them at this stage.

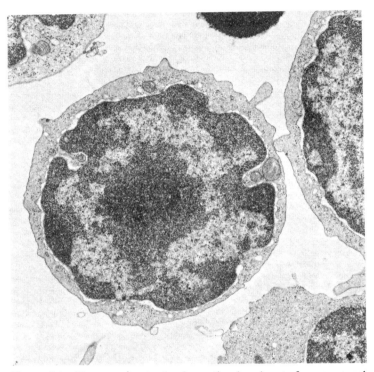

Figure 2.1 Electron micrograph of a resting lymphocyte from a normal mouse spleen. × 25 000

Most lymphocytes *within* 'primary' organs (thymus and bursa) are immature cells and so it seems inappropriate to refer to them as T or B lymphocytes. Rather, these terms should be reserved for cells in peripheral lymphoid organs (lymph nodes, spleen, etc.) which have matured to a stage of 'immunological competence'. Secondly, although a mammalian organ equivalent to the avian bursa of Fabricius has not been identified, there is compelling evidence for the presence of a mammalin population of cells analogous to avian B lymphocytes. It is known that cell precursors of this mammalian population are present in bone marrow; however, there is no conclusive evidence that bone marrow itself is a bursal-equivalent site and even if it were the lymphocytes within it would probably be of the 'immature' type. Hence, mammalian B lymphocytes should not be equated with bone marrow lymphocytes.

Finally, it should be noted that these definitions do not imply that T and B lymphocytes are homogeneous populations, indeed, some evidence is available to the contrary (see Section 2.4.3).

2.2.2 'Blasts' and plasma cells

When lymphocytes are activated either *in vivo* or *in vitro* they enlarge and divide (see Section 2.1.1). At the light microscope level, the cells formed are large 'pyroninophilic' blast cells. Damashek[23] named these cells 'immunoblasts'—this led to some controversy since at the time their immunological role was not known with certainty. However, the term has become increasingly acceptable as knowledge about the functional importance of these cells in immune responses has accumulated. It has also become clear that within the general category 'immunoblasts', there are two subpopulations of T and B 'blasts' corresponding to the respective small lymphocyte classes. With the light microscope, these subpopulations are indistinguishable, but with the electron microscope T immunoblasts are very rich in polyribosomes and contain little or no rough endoplasmic reticulum[24] (Figure 2.2) while B immunoblasts are characterised by the presence of endoplasmic reticulum[25].

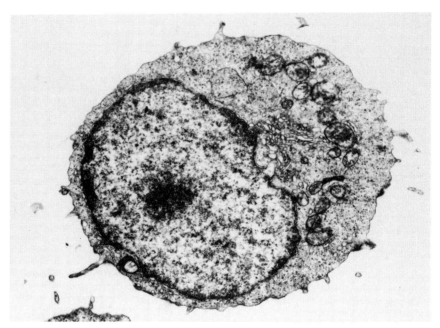

Figure 2.2 Electron micrograph of T 'blast' cell. Note the abundant ribosomes but sparse endoplasmic reticulum. × 25 000 (reduced $\frac{8}{10}$ on reproduction)

(Figure 2.3). These subpopulations can also be separately identified on the basis of surface markers (see Section 2.3.3.1).

There is evidence that the progeny of T immunoblasts are small lymphoid cells, some of which participate in 'cellular immunity'. However, at least a proportion of the progeny of B immunoblasts are classic plasma cells. The

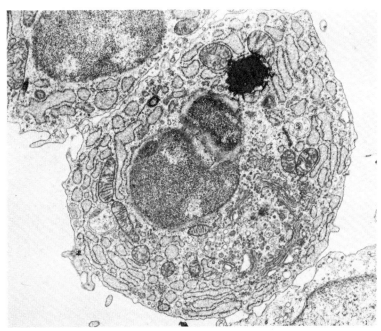

Figure 2.3 Electron micrograph of B 'blast' cell. Note the presence of endoplasmic reticulum (see text). × 36 000 (reduced $\frac{7}{10}$ on reproduction). The black spot is a lipip droplet

experiments of Fagraeus[26] first convincingly demonstrated that plasma cells—cells containing profuse endoplasmic reticulum—are secretors of humoral antibody. These conclusions agree with the notion that B lymphocytes are precursors of the antibody-secreting cell line (see Section 2.2.1.1).

2.2.3 Macrophages

Macrophages are generally large cells with a single round, eccentrically-placed, nucleus and a bulky vacuolated cytoplasm. These cells are usually actively phagocytic (Figure 2.4) and in the electron microscope their cytoplasm usually contains phagosomes, lysosomes and sometimes aggregates of ingested material (Figure 2.5). There has been controversy as to their origin; while it has been claimed that lymphocytes can transform into macrophages, the general consensus of opinion now agrees that tissue macrophages are derived from circulating monocytes, which in turn are derived from precursor cells in bone marrow[27]. It is now possible to grow *in vitro* colonies of monocyte-macrophage cells in semi-solid media; these colonies are thought to be derived from single colony-forming cell (CFC) precursors[28].

Macrophages may well be functionally heterogeneous—in part, this may reflect linear maturational changes in a single monocyte–macrophage line, but it is possible that separate macrophage lines may exist. Thus 'dendritic reticulum cells' found within lymphoid follicles of lymph nodes, spleen, etc. (see Section 2.4.3) seem to be specialised macrophages adapted for long-term retention of antigen on their surfaces (perhaps important for the 'presentation' of antigen to lymphoid cells).

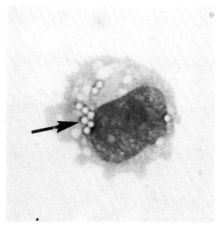

Figure 2.4 Macrophage prepared from a suspension of mouse lymph node cells that had been incubated with polystyrene particles. Note the irregular cell outline and vacuolated cytoplasm containing ingested polystyrene particles. (Cytocentrifuge preparation × 3000)

A great deal of work has been carried out on the role of macrophages in immune responses (see Chapter 3). Certainly, it appears that macrophages are important for the induction of immune responses[29] and it is likely that interactions between sensitised lymphocytes and macrophages (perhaps mediated by soluble factors) are important in the effector side of immune responses (see Chapter 3). This is over and above any general scavenger role macrophages may play. One of the great difficulties in studying macrophage involvement in immune responses is the problem of distinguishing between macrophages (and especially their precursors) and lymphocytes. This is exemplified by the fact that some cells in the peritoneal cavity have a morphology intermediate between monocytes and lymphocytes[30]. While functional methods of separation have become available for tackling this problem, they have not yet been developed to a stage where entirely pure populations of cells can be obtained.

2.2.4 Polymorphonuclear cells

A general description of the various types of polymorphonuclear cells—neutrophils, basophils and eosinophils—may be found in standard histological texts[3]. The functions of these cells are poorly understood. They are able to phagocytose bacteria and have a high content of proteolytic enzymes. Their presence at sites of tissue injury has led to the suggestion that one of their main functions is to remove cellular debris by phagocytosis and digestion. Evidence is also available that they play a part in producing tissue damage

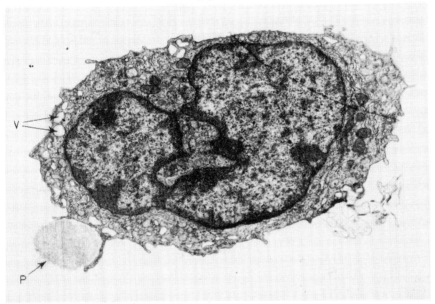

Figure 2.5 Electron micrograph of macrophage. Note cytoplasm contains many vesicles and vacuoles (V). × 5000 (reduced $\frac{8}{10}$ on reproduction). P is a particle which is being phagocytosed

especially in 'allergic' or 'anaphylactic' responses. This damage may be due to release of vasoactive amines (e.g. from basophils) or may be secondary to the deposition of antigen–antibody complexes which fix complement (C′) and release chemotactic factors, which in turn attract polymorphs to the site of deposition (e.g. the kidney glomerulus in certain types of nephritis[31]). Damage is then produced by release of polymorph enzymes or the plugging of glomerular capillaries by polymorphs.

It is likely that in the various immune responses in which they participate, polymorphs act as ancillary cells to sensitised lymphocytes. Indeed, the stimulus for polymorph localisation in sites of immunological reactions may depend upon lymphocyte activation, e.g. the eosinophilia characteristic of macroparasitic infestations may be dependent on T lymphocyte activation[32]. Clearly, much remains to be learned about the roles of these somewhat 'neglected' cell types in immunity as a whole.

2.3 ORIGINS OF LYMPHOCYTE POPULATIONS: PRIMARY LYMPHOID ORGANS

The concept of 'primary' and 'secondary' lymphoid organs has been introduced in Section 2.1.3. Briefly, this is based on the notion that there are primary lymphoid organs which are mainly concerned with the production of lymphocytes, and secondary lymphoid organs which receive lymphocytes from the primary sites of production and in which immune reactions take place. The primary organs themselves are dependent on an inflow of stem cells (lymphocyte precursors) which reach them via the bloodstream. Since this section is concerned with primary lymphoid organs, it is clearly relevant to discuss stem cells first. Avian lymphopoiesis will then be considered since the bursa of Fabricius is of special significance to an understanding of B lymphocyte maturation (see Section 2.3.3.2). Finally, current knowledge of mammalian lymphopoiesis will be reviewed.

2.3.1 Stem cells

The term 'stem cell', although not wholly satisfactory, is useful for defining those cells which are capable of extensive proliferation as well as differentiation to mature 'end' cells[33]. Thus, haemopoietic stem cells are ancestral to the various mature blood cell types. In recent years it has been established that there is a hierarchy of haemopoietic stem cells, each category being defined by its potential for proliferation and differentiation (reviewed by Metcalf and Moore[28]).

First in order is a class of stem cell which is 'multipotential', i.e. can differentiate into any mature blood cell—lymphocyte, erythrocyte, granulocyte or platelet. This stem cell is assayed by its ability to form macroscopic spleen colonies of proliferating myeloid cells when injected into irradiated mice[34]—each colony is derived from a single stem cell which is referred to as the colony-forming unit (or CFU stem cell). The clonal nature of these colonies was shown by the presence of unique, radiation-induced, chromosome markers within them[35]. These markers were also found in lymphocytes indicating a common origin of myeloid and lymphoid cells from CFU stem cells. (Figure 2.6).

Multipotential stem cells give rise to 'line-progenitor' cells, which also possess extensive proliferative capacities, but are restricted in terms of differentiation to particular lines of haemopoietic maturation, e.g. erythroid, granuloid, etc. One of these line-progenitor stem cells can be assayed by its capacity to form colonies of macrophage or granulocyctic cells *in vitro* (*in vitro* colony-forming cells or CFC)[28]. There is some evidence that the crucial factor determining the differentiation of a multipotential stem cell into a particular line-progenitor cell is the 'micro-environment' into which the multipotential stem cell migrates[36, 37]. Thus, while haemopoietic defects due to mutant alleles at the W locus in mice are thought to be due to intrinsic stem cell defects, those due to mutants at the SI locus produce a defect in the 'microenvironment' necessary for stem cell maturation[38]. Humoral factors, e.g. erythropoietin, are thought to govern the further development of line-progenitor cells[28].

In terms of location, the first haemopoietic stem cells are found in the embryo yolk sac. In mammals, haemopoiesis in yolk sac is succeeded and gradually replaced by blood cell formation in foetal liver and spleen, and finally by haemopoiesis in bone marrow where it persists throughout life. This progression gave rise to a controversy as to whether each new site appeared by differentiation of new stem cells *in situ*, or by migration of stem cells from pre-existing sites. Two types of experiment have provided strong support for the latter view. By using the sex chromosomes as cell markers, extensive cross-migration of haemopoietic stem cells has been demonstrated between chick embryos joined by a parabiotic union[39]. This suggests that stem cell

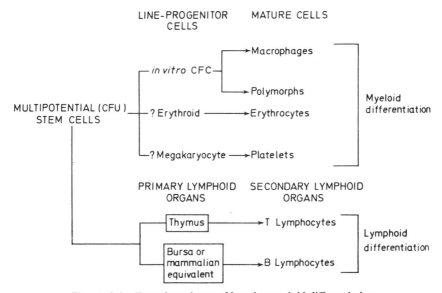

Figure 2.6 Tentative scheme of lympho-myeloid differentiation

migration is a prominent feature of embryonic haemopoiesis. Secondly, developing mouse embryos deprived of yolk sacs and cultured *in vitro* fail to generate haemopoietic cells, whereas embryos cultured under similar conditions with intact yolk sacs develop extensive intraembryonic haemopoiesis[40]. Yolk sac may well be the only *de novo* site of formation of multipotential haemopoietic stem cells—all other cells are derived by migration and self-renewal of stem cells from this site.

The morphological identity of haemopoietic stem cells has proved elusive but recent cell separation techniques based on density and size of CFU cells support the notion, first put forward by Maximow[41], that stem cells of the early embryo are large cells (perhaps the 'haemocytoblasts' of Maximow, cells with prominent nucleoli and basophilic cytoplasm containing abundant free ribosomes[42]). On the other hand, CFU stem cells of the adult are a heterogeneous population of smaller cells; it has been suggested that some of them have a lymphocyte-like morphology.

2.3.2 Avian lymphopoiesis

Two main lymphoid organs develop within the avian embryo, the thymus, and an organ unique to birds, the bursa of Fabricius. Both organs initially are derived from epithelial cells, the thymus from a downgrowth of pharyngeal pouch epithelium and the bursa as an outpouching of cloacal epithelium. Controversy has surrounded the question of the origin of the lymphocyte populations in both organs. Although initially it was thought that they arose by 'transformation' of epithelial cells, the chromosome marker experiments employing parabiosed chick embryos sharing a common circulation (mentioned in Section 2.3.1) have shown that lymphocytes in both organs are derived from stem cells which migrate into the epithelial anlage from the blood stream (see review[43]). The likely origin of these stem cells is the yolk sac, which is the main haemopoietic organ throughout avian embryogenesis. Although the nature of these cells is not known, it is tempting to speculate that they may be multipotential stem cells which differentiate into either T or B lymphocytes depending upon whether they migrate into thymus or bursa respectively.

2.3.2.1 *Thymus—the maturation of T lymphocytes*

The inflow of stem cells into the avian epithelial thymic rudiment begins at 6–7 days' incubation. This is known because if the rudiment is removed at 6 days' incubation and cultured *in vitro*, it fails to generate lymphocytes, whereas if it is removed at later stages and cultured, lymphocytes do develop within it[44]. Large basophilic cells are seen within the thymus for the first time at the 7-day stage which provides evidence, albeit indirect, that they may be stem cells. Certainly, they correspond in morphology to the cells thought to be embryonic haemopoietic stem cells (see Section 2.3.1) and similar cells are also seen in the bursa of Fabricius just before lymphopoiesis begins. The morphological similarity between the cells presumed to be stem cells of thymus and bursa provides some support for the notion of a common lymphoid stem cell.

Thymic morphogenesis proceeds rapidly and by 12 days' incubation the avian thymus contains large numbers of small lymphocytes and well-defined cortical and medullary areas. However, little is known about the timing of functional maturation—cells which bind antigen have been demonstrated at 14 days' incubation[45] which suggests that antigen-recognition receptors may be present at this stage. The nature of T cell receptors is a controversial topic (see Chapter 10) and this is especially so in birds[46] where the lack of data for T cells is in marked contrast to the ample evidence for the presence of immunoglobulin receptors on B cells (see Section 2.3.2.2).

Migration of thymus cells to peripheral lymphoid organs of chickens has been demonstrated by labelling thymus cells with radioisotopes[47]. Since neonatal thymectomy mainly influences 'cell-mediated' immune responses[48], T cells are thought to be essential participants in these reactions (see Section 2.1.2).

2.3.2.2 *Bursa of Fabricius—the maturation of B lymphocytes*

The bursa is already a sac-like structure by 10 days' incubation. On about the 12th day of incubation the lining epithelium grows down as localised swellings or follicles into the underlying mesenchyme and shortly afterwards large basophilic cells (probably stem cells—see Section 2.3.1) penetrate these follicles. By 17 days' incubation, large numbers of lymphocytes are present within the developing follicles. Using radioisotope marker methods, bursal lymphocytes have been shown to migrate to a variety of lymphoid organs, and, perhaps surprisingly in view of its role as a 'primary' organ, to the thymus[49] (see Section 2.1.3).

Studies on the effects of bursectomy, particularly if carried out during embryogenesis, support the view that the bursa controls the maturation of the cell line (B cells) involved in the secretion of immunoglobulin[50]. Thus, bursectomy at 17 days' incubation may result in complete agammaglobulin-aemia thereafter. The manner by which the bursa controls immunoglobulin synthesis has recently been under intensive investigation. Kincade and Cooper[51], using purified goat antibodies to chicken μ, γ and light chains labelled with fluorochromes have shown that immunoglobulin synthesis (IgM) is initiated within bursal cells at 14 days' incubation, i.e. 24–48 h following the arrival of stem cells within bursal follicles. IgG producing cells are present by the time of hatching (21 days' incubation). The question arises as to whether separate lines of maturing stem cells are induced to synthesise either IgM or IgG respectively, or whether cells which initially synthesise IgM later switch to IgG synthesis. Evidence that an IgM to IgG switch takes place within a single cell line has come from the fact that many bursal cells contain both classes of antibody and also that injection of antibodies

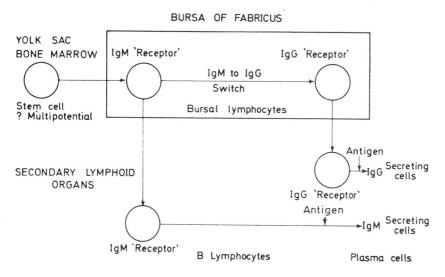

Figure 2.7   Model of avian B lymphocyte maturation as proposed by Cooper *et al.*[53] (see text)

to μ chains beginning on day 13 of embryogenesis suppresses not only IgM synthesis but also IgG[52].

Cooper *et al.*[53] have proposed a general scheme for avian B cell maturation based on these results, whereby antibody variability in terms of both specificity and class is generated following the replication of a multipotential stem cell within the bursa. Further, they propose that heterogeneity of antibody-combining sites emerges during the stage of IgM synthesis, thus avoiding the need to repeat the process during the later stage of IgG synthesis. Because immunoglobulin within the embryonic bursa is seen mainly at cell surfaces rather than within cell cytoplasm, they postulate that immunoglobulins produced by bursal lymphocytes are not secreted but are incorporated into cell membranes as 'receptors' for antigen.

Thus, the basis of this scheme is that the bursa is the site of maturation of stem cells to B lymphocytes which possess surface immunoglobulin receptors. These lymphocytes are committed to class and specificity of antibody which they secrete when they have migrated to peripheral tissues and been stimulated by antigen (Figure 2.7). The scheme is speculative but is an attractive one and provides an acceptable account of bursal function based on current knowledge. Deeper problems such as the nature of the inductive effect of the bursa on lymphopoiesis are entirely unknown.

2.3.3 Mammalian lymphopoiesis

Most of what is known about lymphocyte production in mammals has been gleaned from experimental work in rodents. Although it is questionable how applicable this data may be to other mammalian species, at least the broad principles should be of general relevance. The main lymphoid organ of all mammalian embryos is the thymus. The development of the mouse thymus has been studied in considerable detail and this will be discussed first. Much less is known about the production of B lymphocytes in mammals, but new methods are available for studying this problem, and the current state of knowledge will be discussed.

2.3.3.1 T lymphocyte maturation

(a) *Origins of thymus lymphocytes*—The mammalian thymus, like the avian thymus (see Section 2.3.2), is derived from pharyngeal pouch epithelium. However, as in the chick embryo, lymphocytes of the mammalian thymus are derived from precursor (stem) cells which enter the epithelial organ rudiment from the blood stream. Thus, if the thymic rudiment is dissected from embryos of 10 days' gestation and cultured *in vitro* it fails to generate lymphocytes, but rudiments removed from 11 and 12 day embryos do become lymphoid *in vitro*[44]. These results strongly suggest that stem cells first enter the embryonic mouse thymus sometime between 10 and 11 days' gestation and, interestingly, large basophilic cells can be seen within the thymus for the first time at 11 days (it has already been suggested that these may be embryonic stem cells—see Section 2.3.1). The flow of stem cells to the thymus continues throughout embryogenesis and into adult life[54]—this is to provide replacement for lymphocytes lost by cell death or migration (see Section 2.3.3.1c). The origin of these stem cells follows the progression of haemopoietic sites seen during ontogeny. Thus, initially they are derived from yolk sac and foetal liver, but in the adult animal they are derived from bone marrow[55].

(b) *The differentiation of thymus lymphocytes: surface antigens*—It is now known that each differentiated tissue possesses its own unique array of surface antigens (in addition to antigens common to all tissues, e.g. histocompatibility antigens—see Chapter 9). These tissue-specific antigens have been named 'differentiation antigens' since they result from selective gene expression in particular types of differentiated cell[56]. Differentiation antigens have been studied most extensively on lymphocytes, mainly because of the ease with which viable suspensions of lymphocytes can be obtained for immunisation and for testing by cytotoxicity or fluorescence techniques.

Differentiation antigens may be defined by antisera raised in other species (heteroantisera) or within the same species (alloantisera)[57]. However, heteroantisera need extensive absorption in order to make them specific for a particular tissue and so the best-defined differentiation antigens are alloantigens detected in species where the availability of genetically-homogeneous inbred strains makes the matter of raising and testing antisera a straightforward process. In addition, the genetic basis of alloantigens can be studied in appropriate matings. It is no surprise to find, therefore, that the most extensive use of differentiation antigens has been in mice where a number have been defined (see Ref. 16 for a review).

Some of these differentiation alloantigens are expressed on T but not on B lymphocytes. The thymus-leukaemia (TL) antigens[56] are expressed only on lymphocytes within the thymus and not on peripheral T cells. A remarkable feature of this system is that whereas TL antigens are normally detected in a proportion of mouse strains (the TL positive strains), they can be demonstrated in leukaemias of all strains, including those that are TL negative. This has been taken to suggest that the structural genes coding for TL are present in all mice, but are controlled by another gene which governs expression versus non-expression.

θ antigen is another alloantigen and is expressed on thymus lymphocytes and peripheral T lymphocytes but not on B cells. It is determined by a single genetic locus at which there are two alleles which govern expression in all mouse strains. It has proved, therefore, a very useful marker of mouse T cells[16]. The θ antigen is also present in brain tissue. Other alloantigens have been described on mouse T cells and a number of heteroantigens have been detected on T cells of various species including those of man[58].

In addition to their value as cell markers, surface antigens have also proved useful for studying the differentiation of T lymphocytes. Thus, the maturation of stem cells within the embryonic thymus is accompanied by profound changes in representation of surface antigens. This was demonstrated by dissecting out thymic rudiments of mouse embryos of 14 days' gestation (when θ and TL alloantigens cannot be demonstrated on thymic cells), and culturing them *in vitro* for various periods of time[59]. It was found that in this *in vitro* environment, where no further entry of cells which themselves might be θ or TL positive can occur, the morphological transition from large stem cell to small lymphocyte which takes place over a 4-day period is accompanied by the expression of θ and TL antigens on lymphocyte surfaces. It is very likely that comparable changes take place during the maturation of stem cells in the adult thymus[56].

(c) *Thymus lymphocytes and T lymphocytes: maturation pathways*—Although T lymphocytes in peripheral organs are derived from the thymus[60], there are substantial differences between thymus lymphocytes and peripheral T lymphocytes in terms of both functional parameters and cell surface antigens. Thus, only a minority of thymus lymphocytes ($<10\%$) have been shown to be immunologically responsive and this population, like peripheral T cells, is less sensitive to the cytolytic effects of corticosteroids than the majority of thymus lymphocytes[61].

These observations have established the fact that there are two distinct categories of lymphocyte within the thymus—a majority of cells which seem to be immunologically inert and so have been referred to as the 'immature' population, and a minority which is probably situated in the thymic medulla and which is 'T-like' in many of its properties. This division is further substantiated by the fact that whereas the 'immature'' population is TL positive in some strains, the 'T-like' thymic population as well as T cells in peripheral organs are always TL negative[62]. There are also considerable quantitative differences in the representation of θ and H2 antigens on 'immature' thymus lymphocytes (much more θ, much less H2) as compared to 'T-like' thymic cells and peripheral T cells.

It has been suggested that there are two major steps in the differentiation of T lymphocytes[59]. The first involves the maturation of stem cells to 'immature' thymus lymphocytes and is accompanied by the appearance of θ and TL antigens, while the second step is the change from 'immature' thymus lymphocytes to 'T-like' thymus cells which then migrate to peripheral lymphoid organs. This second step is accompanied by a loss of TL, a reduction in θ and a gain in H2, as well as by the acquisition of functional properties necessary for immunocompetence (e.g. receptors for antigen).

Attractive though this scheme seems to be, there are a number of complicating factors. First, there is no unequivocal evidence that stem cells must pass through the 'immature' thymus lymphocyte stage before maturation to T cells; a quite separate stem cell to T lymphocyte pathway may exist. Second, a number of observations make it unlikely that most peripheral T cells are derived from the 'T-like' population of the thymic medulla. This 'T-like' population is an extremely stable one and persists in the medulla for long periods of time[63], whereas the rate of migration of cells from the thymus is known to be high[64]. It could be argued that most of the migrating cells are 'immature' thymus lymphocytes which die in peripheral organs; only the 'T-like' migrant cells persist. Certainly, the rapidity of turnover of 'immature' thymus lymphocytes suggests that most must die somewhere, but there is nothing to exclude the possibility that some do mature to T cells within peripheral organs (Figure 2.8). Thus, despite recent advances in knowledge of T lymphocyte functions, the precise roles of thymus lymphocytes remain obscure.

(d) *The thymic 'micro-environment'—thymic hormones*—It has generally been accepted that the epithelial cells of the thymus, either by direct contact or by the elaboration of diffusible substances, or perhaps by both, induce the differentiation of stem cells to thymus lymphocytes. Although there is an extensive literature on the effects of thymic extracts on lymphopoiesis[65], reproducible assay systems for demonstrating these effects have only recently been available[66]. If the assay systems can be shown to represent something

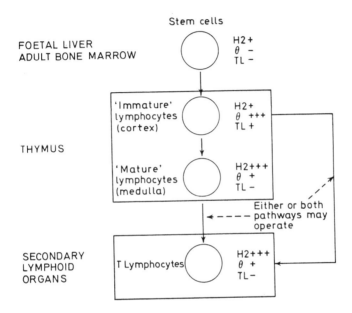

Figure 2.8 Pathways in the maturation of mouse T lymphocytes showing some of the changes which occur in surface antigens (H2, θ and TL—see text) N.B. The possibility that stem cells may mature to T cells without passing through 'immature' thymus lymphocyte stage has not been excluded

which is meaningful in terms of T cell function, then clearly an important advance will have been made. In the meanwhile, the situation can be summarised by saying that there is tentative evidence for the role of thymic hormones in the further maturation of lymphocytes which have already passed through the thymus[67].

2.3.3.2 B lymphocyte maturation

(a) *Stem cells and bursal-equivalent organs*—Mammalian lymphocytes which arise independently of the thymus are usually referred to as B cells on the basis that they are analogus to lymphocytes derived from the avian bursa of Fabricius (see Section 2.1.2). While there is much evidence to support this proposition, it should be remembered that there is no definitive evidence that the two populations are entirely comparable.

Certainly, the search for a mammalian organ which is equivalent to the bursa has been largely unrewarding. Various gastro-intestinal lymphoid organs (appendix, tonsils, Peyer's patches) have been put forward as possible bursal equivalents[68]. However, none of these proposals has been substantiated. Indeed, they are based on a supposed developmental homology with the bursa and on the assumption that from a phylogenetic viewpoint, intestinal epithelial influences on B lymphocyte maturation are to be expected. In fact, the histogenesis of the bursa is very different from that of mammalian intestinal lymphoid organs—in the bursa, lymphopoiesis is initiated *within* epithelial follicles by the differentiation of large basophilic stem cells, whereas in intestinal organs, lymphocyte proliferation is largely found *beneath* epithelium in mesenchymal tissue and even in the neonatal animal many of these lymphocytes are T lymphocytes (see Section 2.3.3.1). The suggestion that Peyer's patches, appendix, etc., are bursal-equivalent organs also largely overlooks the fact that these organs are present in birds.

From a phylogenetic viewpoint, the close association between lymphoid and myeloid tissue in primitive vertebrates suggests that perhaps myeloid tissue (foetal liver and spleen, adult bone marrow) may serve as both sources of stem cells *and* inducers of B lymphocyte maturation. Evidence of this effect has recently been obtained.

(b) *Lymphocyte production in foetal liver and spleen, and adult bone marrow* —Lymphocytes are present in both liver and spleen during foetal development although it has not been shown that they are produced within these sites. Evidence for an *in situ* origin of lymphocytes within adult bone marrow is more convincing and has been obtained using isotopic labelling techniques[69]. However, the nature of bone marrow lymphocytes is not known and it is certainly premature to suggest that they are B lymphocytes. Nonetheless, a recent study, utilising the presence of immunoglobulin on B cells as a marker, demonstrated B cells in all haemopoietic tissues (liver, spleen and bone marrow) during late foetal development in the mouse[70]. This suggests, but does not conclusively prove, that B lymphocyte differentiation is multifocal in mammals, being located in all haemopoietic sites. The implication is that adult bone marrow may be an important source of B cells which, however, may require further maturation in lymph nodes, spleen, Peyer's patches, etc. If this study can be confirmed and extended, the search for a discrete bursal equivalent organ may no longer be worth while, it perhaps being best to think of the bursa as a special revolutionary adaptation confined to birds.

(c) *A model for mammalian B lymphocyte differentiation*—On the basis of evidence for an IgM to IgG switch during the maturation of B lymphocytes in birds (see Section 2.3.2.2), Lawton *et al.*[71] have proposed that during mammalian B lymphocyte differentiation μ, γ and α chain constant region genes are sequentially expressed in each developing clone of B lymphocyte— a clone being defined by the expression of a pair of variable region genes. In order to test their model, they have attempted to interrupt IgM synthesis in newborn mice by multiple injections of anti-μ sera. As predicted, they found a reduction in numbers not only of IgM but also of IgG and IgA bearing

B lymphocytes. The actual location/s where 'switching' might occur in the maturation of B cells is unresolved, but there are certainly no reasons for believing that it is confined to foetal liver and bone marrow, if these are eventually shown to be the primary sites of mammalian B cell development.

(d) *B lymphocyte differentiation: surface antigens*—As mentioned earlier (see Section 2.1.2), there is compelling evidence that mammalian B lymphocytes are precursors of antibody-secreting (plasma) cells. Indeed, the terms B lymphocyte and antibody forming cell precursor (AFCP) can now probably be equated. Further investigation of these problems should be aided by the availability of markers for cells of the B axis. Perhaps, one of the most useful markers for B lymphocytes is the fact that immunoglobulin can be demonstrated on these cells by the use of anti-immunoglobulin sera. Since most B cells have readily demonstrable immunoglobulin on their surface whereas T cells do not[72], under most conditions and probably in most species, surface immunoglobulin can be used as a B cell marker.

B cells of mice can also be recognised by heteroantisera directed against a species specific surface antigen[73] (MBLA—mouse specific B lymphocyte antigen), while antibody secreting (plasma) cells can be recognised by allo-antisera directed against the PC (plasma cell) alloantigen[74] or heteroantisera against a plasma cell heteroantigen[75] (MSPCA—mouse specific plasma cell antigen).

Receptors for complement[76] and for the Fc portion of immunoglobulin[77] are possessed by most B, but not resting T lymphocytes and so provide useful markers in a variety of species.

2.4 SECONDARY LYMPHOID ORGANS

2.4.1 General topographical features

The detailed histology of secondary lymphoid organs, e.g. lymph nodes, spleen, Peyer's patches, etc., can be found in various textbooks[1, 3]. Only a brief summary of the main topography will be presented here.

Lymph nodes are encapsulated organs consisting of a reticular framework packed with lymphocytes. They are served by an afferent lymph vessel which breaks up into a number of branches which empty into a sinus lying beneath the capsule (subcapsular sinus). This sinus drains both directly into the efferent lymph vessel leaving the node, and also into sinuses which penetrate the substance of the node (intermediary sinuses). In turn, these drain into medullary sinuses.

It is usual to divide lymph nodes into two broad geographical regions, cortex and medulla. The cortex is made up of loosely packed areas of lymphocytes (diffuse cortex) and tighter aggregates of lymphocytes (lymphoid follicles). The diffuse cortex itself is sometimes subdivided into superficial, mid and deep zones (the mid and deep zones are also known as the paracortex or intermediate area). An important anatomical feature of the diffuse cortex is the presence of post-capillary venules which are lined by a high cuboidal endothelium and are important in lymphocyte recirculation (see Section 2.4.3) (Figure 2.9). The lymphoid follicles may contain central areas of intense mitotic activity, the germinal centres.

The medulla of lymph nodes is divided into sinuses and cords (Figure 2.10). The medullary cords are structures which penetrate from the diffuse cortex into the medulla where they interdigit between the sinuses. They contain blood vessels, macrophages and a variable number of 'blasts' and plasma cells depending upon the level of antigenic stimulation. Cells can move freely into the medullary sinuses which are lymph-filled spaces lined by macrophages.

Peyer's patches are best regarded as modified lymph nodes situated beneath the epithelium of the small bowel. They contain all of the principal features of lymph nodes—diffuse cortex, lymphoid follicles and germinal centres, and post-capillary venules, etc.

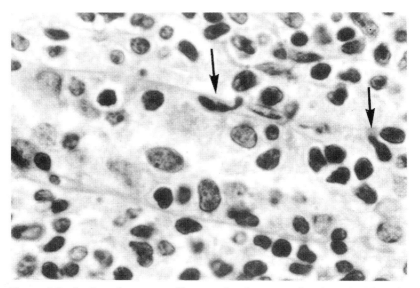

Figure 2.9 Section of a post-capillary venule of a mouse lymph node. The paler nuclei are those of endothelial cells lining the venule; the darker nuclei are those of lymphocytes (Arrows) within the wall of the venule (it is known from marker studies that these lymphocytes are migrating from the venule into the substance of the lymph node—see text). × 3000 (reduced $\frac{8}{10}$ on reproduction)

The spleen differs from lymph nodes in that it is concerned with haemopoiesis and the disposal of effete erythrocytes as well as lymphoid functions. Also, it deals with cells and foreign materials which reach it via the blood rather than via the lymph system. Nonetheless, there are many similarities in terms of the broad organisation of lymph tissue in spleen and nodes. The lymphoid tissue of the spleen (white pulp) follows and indeed surrounds the arterial blood supply, so that a central arteriole can be seen in sections of each white pulp area. The white pulp contains diffuse lymphoid tissue (corresponding to the diffuse cortex of nodes) and lymphoid follicles. It does not contain post-capillary venules. White pulp is separated from red pulp by a marginal sinus and marginal zone.

No structures comparable to lymph node medullary sinuses are present in spleen, but there are cords in the red pulp which contain 'blasts' and plasma cells and correspond to lymph node medullary cords.

2.4.2 T and B areas

One of the most interesting observations with respect to the structure of peripheral lymphoid tissue in recent years has been the recognition of distinct T and B lymphocyte compartments (for a review see Ref. 78). These areas were originally identified by light microscope studies of sections of peripheral lymphoid tissues of neonatally thymectomised rats[79] and mice[80]. Selective

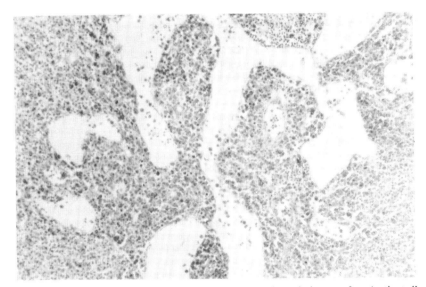

Figure 2.10 Low power view of the medullary cords and sinuses of an 'activated' lymph node draining a tumour induced by murine sarcoma virus. The cords are packed with 'blast'-type cells and the sinuses are very dilated. × 300 (reduced $\frac{8}{10}$ on reproduction)

areas of lymphocyte depletion were seen in the diffuse lymphoid tissue of the splenic white pulp, in the mid and deep areas (paracortex) of lymph nodes and the inter-follicular areas of gastrointestinal lymphoid tissues. These areas were named thymus-dependent (T) areas and the remaining unaffected regions, lymphoid follicles and medulla of lymph nodes, follicles and plasma cells of intestinal lymphoid organs, and the follicles and peripheral areas of splenic white pulp were designated thymus-independent (B) areas. It should be noted that these compartments do not have rigid boundaries and cells can migrate between them.

2.4.3 Lymphocyte recirculation: migratory pathways of T and B lymphocytes

Gowans[21] first demonstrated that a large proportion of lymphocytes recirculate between blood and lymph. The main route of lymphocytes was shown by radioisotope marker methods to be through post-capillary venules of lymph nodes and Peyer's patches[81]. After passing through the substance of

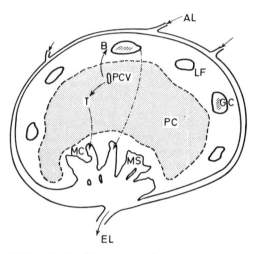

PCV = Postcapillary venule   T Area is shaded
PC = Paracortex   B Area not shaded
LF = Lymphoid follicle   N.B.
GC = Germinal centre   (1) Unbroken arrows are migratory routes of T and B cells from PCV
MC = Medullary cord
MS = Medullary sinus   (2) Broken arrows are tentative routes of passage of T and B cells to efferent lymph
AL = Afferent lymphatic
EL = Efferent lymphatic

Figure 2.11 Topography of lymph node showing T areas and B areas. The migratory pathways of T and B lymphocytes are indicated—in part, at least, these pathways are speculative (see text)

lymph nodes, recirculating lymphocytes enter efferent lymphatics and eventually return to blood via the thoracic duct (transit time is about 14 h)[82] (Figure 2.11).

Lymphocytes are also known to leave the blood in the spleen and enter the white pulp areas (Figure 2.12). They probably do so by migrating from the marginal sinus and after some time in white pulp they return to blood by an unknown route (transit time *ca.* 5 h)[83]. There is evidence that these lymphocytes are part of the same recirculating pool which traverses lymph nodes[83].

The majority of recirculating lymphocytes (at least in rodents) are T cells.

Thus, *ca.* 80% of thoracic duct cells in mice are θ positive (and so T cells). However, B lymphocytes have also been shown to recirculate[84] although the tempo is slower than that of T cells. Both B and T lymphocytes enter lymph nodes via post-capillary venules but T cells, labelled with radioisotopes, migrate into the paracortex (T dependent area)[78, 85], whereas B cells, labelled and injected in the same way, localise in and around lymphoid follicles (B

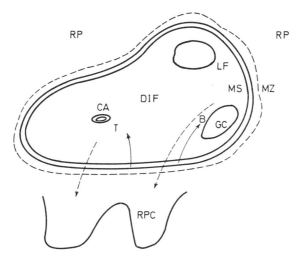

MS = Marginal sinus
MZ = Marginal zone
LF = Lymphoid follicle
GC = Germinal centre
RP = Red pulp
RPC = Red pulp cords
CA = Central arteriole
DIF= Diffuse interfollicular area

N.B. (1) Unbroken arrows are migratory routes of T and B cells from marginal sinus

(2) Broken arrows are tentative routes of return of T and B cells to red pulp cords and to blood

Figure 2.12 Topography of white pulp areas of spleen with tentative migratory pathways (see text)

dependent areas)[85]. Thus, T and B lymphocytes do recognise and, indeed, selectively migrate to their respective compartments. T cells, after passing through the paracortex, reach the medullary sinuses and so efferent lymph, either directly from the paracortex or via intermediary sinuses. The further progress of B cells once they have reached follicular areas is uncertain, but it is reasonable to suppose that some track down to the medulla which is rich in mature cells of the B series, 'blasts' and plasma cells.

Although the precise function of this massive traffic of lymphocytes is not understood, it must be important to immune responses. It certainly would seem to provide an effective means of bringing lymphocytes and antigens together in the induction of immune responses and also for disseminating activated lymphocytes throughout the body. Details of the cellular events which take place during immune responses will be discussed extensively in the following chapter as will the anatomical localisation of antigen in lymphoid tissues (see also Ref. 86). However, it is appropriate to note here that antigens which mainly stimulate 'cell-mediated' immune responses (see Section 2.1.2) produce proliferative changes predominantly in T areas of peripheral lymphoid tissues, whereas those which stimulate 'humoral immunity' cause lymphoid follicle proliferation (and germinal centre formation) and plasma cell production. Of course, most immune responses consist of proliferative changes in both areas, but it is interesting to note that the functional division of the immune system correlates with the broad anatomical division into T and B areas.

Perhaps, it is also worth while mentioning here that a model has been put forward which attempts to relate the antigen-induced differentiation of T (and possibly B) cells in terms of recirculatory properties[87]. The proposal is that virginal T cells (named either T_x or T_1) are non-recirculating sessile lymphocytes located mainly in spleen. When they encounter antigen, they differentiate to memory T_y (or T_2) cells which now recirculate. Following stimulation by antigen, either T_x or T_y cells may secrete a factor which results in non-specific transient trapping of recirculating lymphocytes (mainly T_y) in lymphoid tissues and so results in more T_y cells responding to antigen. The stimulated T_y cells proliferate and differentiate to activated T_z (or T_3) cells which then enter efferent lymph. These T_z cells may largely have lost their ability to recirculate and preferentially migrate to the gut or to sites of inflammation. The model is based on a limited amount of data and certainly is not conclusively proven.

Very little data is available concerning the differentiation of B cells (see Section 2.3.3.2). Considerable interest has centred on the role of lymphoid follicles and especially germinal centres in immune responses and clearly the traffic of B cells to these regions may be relevant. Lymphoid follicles contain a meshwork of dendritic reticular cells on which antigen–antibody complexes are deposited for long periods[88]. It is interesting that B cells, which have already reacted with antigen have been shown to home preferentially to germinal centres and follicular regions[89]. It is tempting to speculate that this 'homing' pattern is consistent with the notion that follicles and germinal centres (perhaps by antigen retained on dendritic cells) are concerned with the further antigen-directed maturation of B cells. However, all of this is speculation and at the moment the eventual fate of lymphocytes within follicles is unknown.

Finally, it will be clear from this discussion that the overlapping distribution of T and B lymphocytes in peripheral lymphoid tissues leaves scope for the types of cell to cell interactions (cell co-operation) discussed in Chapter 3.

2.4.4 The life span of lymphocytes

The life span of a lymphocyte may be defined as the time between two divisions or between a division and cell death. In general, the life span of lymphocytes has been determined by studying the incorporation of the radioactive DNA precursor, tritiated thymidine given *in vivo* either by continuous infusion or as multiple injections. Estimates of life span are based on the persistence of unlabelled cells throughout the thymidine administration—these cells must have arisen prior to the injections (assuming that thymidine is available to all cells). Life span can also be estimated by the fall in proportion of labelled cells after the last injection of isotope although these estimates may be complicated by re-utilisation of radioactive material.

Using these techniques, short-lived (life span less than 2 weeks) and long-lived (life span many months) lymphocytes have been demonstrated in rodents[90], although it should be stressed that there is considerable heterogeneity within these broad groupings. In the past, there was a tendency to try to equate long-lived lymphocytes with T cells and short-lived lymphocytes with B cells. This view is no longer tenable since there are an increasing number of observations which suggest that T and B cell populations contain similar proportions of long- and short-lived lymphocytes. For example, lymphocytes with receptors for complement (B cells)—see Section 2.3.3.2—contain the same proportions of long- and short-lived cells as normal spleen cells[91]. Since immunological memory has been demonstrated in both T and B lines[92] and it is, perhaps, easier to think of memory being carried by non-dividing cells, it is reassuring to find that both T and B cells contain long-lived populations. Finally, it should be noted that a majority of lymphocytes within the thymus are probably short-lived—their high turnover is such that if this were not so the animal would be faced with an overwhelming number of lymphocytes (see Section 2.3.3.1).

2.4.5 General conclusions

An attempt has been made in this chapter to discuss those aspects of lymphoid structure and organisation which are relevant to functional studies of the immune response. The main points which hopefully emerge are the importance of the two main classes of lymphocyte in the various types of immunity, the broad division of the lymphoid system into those organs where lymphocytes are produced and those where immune responses take place, and finally, the correlation between anatomical areas of secondary lymphoid organs and the localisation and migratory pathways of T and B lymphocytes. The methodological approaches which have enabled these conclusions to be made and which should allow further progress in the future have been touched upon.

Acknowledgement

The electron micrographs (Figures 2.1, 2.2, 2.3 and 2.5) were supplied by courtesy of Drs. R. Dourmashkin, George Janossy, Gerald Slavin and Misses Maya Shohat and Susan Whytock.

References

1. Yoffey, J. M. and Courtice, F. C. (1970). *Lymphatics, Lymph and the Lymphomyeloid Complex* (London: Academic Press)
2. Weiss, L. (1971). *The Cells and Tissues of the Immune System: Structure, Functions, Interactions* (A. Osler and L. Weiss, editors) (Prentice Hall: Foundations of Immunology Series)
3. Bloom, W. and Fawcett, D. W. (1968). *A Textbook of Histology*, 9th edn. (Philadelphia: and London: W. B. Saunders)
4. Hungerford, P. A., Donnelly, A. J., Nowell, P. C. and Beck, S. (1959). *Amer. J. Hum. Genet.*, **11**, 215
5. *Transplantation Reviews* (1972). Vol. 11 (Whole issue devoted to mitogens) (G. Möller, editor) (Copenhagen: Munksgaard)
6. Gowans, J. L. and McGregor, D. D. (1965). *Progr. Allergy*, **9**, 1
7. Medawar, P. B. (1958). *Proc. Roy. Soc. (London) B*, **149**, 145
8. Burnett, F. M. (1969). *Cellular Immunology, Books 1 and 2* (Melbourne and Cambridge University Press)
9. Miller, J. F. A. P. (1961). *Lancet*, **ii**, 748
10. Good, R. A., Dalmasso, A. P., Martinez, C., Archer, O. K., Pierce, J. C. and Papermaster, B. W. (1962). *J. Exp. Med.*, **116**, 773
11. Glick, B., Chang, T. G. and Jaap, R. G. (1956). *Poultry Sci.*, **35**, 224
12. Davies, A. J. S., Leuchars, E., Wallis, V., Marchant, R. and Elliott, E. V. (1967). *Transplantation*, **5**, 222
13. Mitchell, G. F. and Miller, J. F. A. P. (1968). *J. Exp. Med.*, **128**, 821
14. Warner, N. L. and Szenberg, A. (1964). *Annu. Rev. Microbiol.*, **18**, 253
15. Cooper, M. D., Peterson, R. D. A., South, M. A. and Good, R. A. (1965). *J. Exp. Med.*, **123**, 75
16. Greaves, M. F., Owen, J. J. T. and Raff, M. C. (1973). *T and B Lymphocytes: Origins, Properties and Roles in Immune Responses* (A.S.P., Elsevier–Excerpta Medica–North Holland: Amsterdam)
17. Cooper, E. L. (1970). *Transpl. Proc.*, **II**, 216
18. Hildemann, W. H. (1970). *Transpl. Proc.*, **II**, 253
19. Kampmeier, O. F. (1969). *Evolution and Comparative Morphology of the Lymphatic System* (Springfield, Illinois: Charles C. Thomas)
20. Bienenstock, J., Perey, D. Y. E., Gauldie, J. and Underdown, B. J. (1972). *J. Immunol.*, **109**, 403
21. Gowans, J. L. (1959). *J. Physiol. London*, **146**, 54
22. Roitt, I. M., Greaves, M. F., Torrigiani, G., Brostoff, J. and Playfair, J. H. L. (1969). *Lancet*, **ii**, 367
23. Damashek, W. (1963). *Blood*, **21**, 243
24. Turk, J. L. and Oort, J. (1970). *Handbuch der Allgemeinen Pathologie*, VII/3, 392 (A. Studer and H. Cottier, editors) (Berlin–Heidelberg–New York: Springer-Verlag)
25. Janossy, G., Shohat, M., Greaves, M. F. and Dourmashkin, R. R. (1973). *Immunology* **24**, 211
26. Fagraeus, A. (1948). *Acta Med. Scand.*, **130** suppl. 204, 1
27. Van Furth, R. (1970). *Mononuclear Phagocytes*, 151 (R. Van Furth, editor) (Oxford: Blackwell Press)
28. Metcalf, D. and Moore, M. A. S. (1971). *Haemopoietic Cells. Frontiers of Biology* Vol. 24 (A. Neuberger and E. L. Tatum, editors) (Amsterdam: North Holland Publishing Co.)
29. Nossal, G. J. V. and Ada, G. L. (1971). *Antigens, Lymphoid cells, and the Immune Response. Immunology. An International Series of Monographs and Treatises* (F. J. Dixon and R. G. Kunkel, editors) (New York and London: Academic Press)
30. Ada, G. L. and Byrt, P. (1969). *Nature (London)*, **222**, 1291
31. Cochrane, C. G. (1971). *J. Exp. Med.*, **134**, 755
32. Walls, R. S., Basten, A., Leuchars, E. and Davies, A. J. S. (1971). *Brit. Med. J.*, **3**, 157
33. Barnes, D. W. H. and Loutit, J. F. (1967). *Lancet*, **ii**, 1138
34. Till, J. E. and McCulloch, E. A. (1961). *Radiation Res.*, **14**, 213
35. Wu, A. M., Till, J. E., Siminovitch, L. and McCulloch, E. A. (1968). *J. Exp. Med.*, **127**, 455

36. Moore, M. A. S. and Owen, J. J. T. (1967). *Lancet, ii*, 658
37. Wolf, N. S. and Trentin, J. J. (1968). *J. Exp. Med.*, **127**, 205
38. Sutherland, D. J. A., Till, J. E. and McCulloch, E. A. (1970). *J. Cell. Physiol.*, **75**, 267
39. Moore, M. A. S. and Owen, J. J. T. (1965). *Nature (London)*, **208**, 956
40. Moore, M. A. S. and Metcalf, D. (1970). *Brit. J. Haemat.*, **18**, 279
41. Maximow, A. A. (1924). *Physiol. Rev.*, **4**, 533
42. Edmonds, R. H. (1966). *Anat. Rec.*, **154**, 785
43. Owen, J. J. T. (1970). *Handb. D. Allg. Pathologie*, VII/3, 129 (A. Studer and H. Cottier, editors) (Berlin–Heidelberg–New York: Springer-Verlag)
44. Owen, J. J. T. and Ritter, M. A. (1969). *J. Exp. Med.*, **129**, 431
45. Dwyer, J. M. and Warner, N. L. (1971). *Nature New Biol.*, **229**, 210
46. Crone, M., Koch, C. and Simonsen, M. (1972). *Transplantation Revs.*, **10**, 36 (G. Möller, editor) (Copenhagen: Munksgaard)
47. Linna, T. J., Bäck, R. and Hemmingson, E. (1971). In *Morphological and Functional Aspects of Immunity*, 149 (K. Lindahl-Kiessling, G. Alm and M. G. Hanna, editors) (New York–London: Plenum Press)
48. Cooper, M. D., Peterson, R. D. A., South, M. A. and Good, R. A. (1966). *J. Exp. Med.*, **123**, 75
49. Durkin, H. G., Theis, G. A. and Thorbecke, G. J. (1971). In *Morphological and Functional Aspects of Immunity*, 119 (K. Lindahl-Kiessling, G. Alm and M. G. Hanna, editors) (New York–London: Plenum Press)
50. Cooper, M. D., Cain, W. A., Van Alten, P. J. and Good, R. A. (1969). *Int. Arch. Allergy*, **35**, 242
51. Kincade, P. W. and Cooper, M. D. (1971). *J. Immunol.*, **106**, 371
52. Kincade, P. W., Lawton, A. R., Bockman, D. E. and Cooper, M. D. (1970). *Proc. Nat. Acad. Sci. USA*, **67**, 1918
53. Cooper, M. D., Lawton, A. R. and Kincade, P. W. (1972). In *Current Problems in Immunology*, **1**, 33 (M. G. Hanna, editor) (New York: Plenum Press)
54. Harris, J. E. and Ford, C. E. (1964). *Nature (London)*, **201**, 884
55. Ford, C. E. and Micklem, H. S. (1963). *Lancet, i*, 359
56. Boyse, E. A. and Old, L. J. (1969). *Annu. Rev. Genet.*, **3**, 269
57. Raff, M. C. (1971). *Transplantation Reviews*, **6**, 52 (G. Möller, editor) (Copenhagen: Munksgaard)
58. Wortis, H. H., Brown, M. C., Cooper, A. G. and Derby, H. A. (1972). *J. Exp. Med.* (in the press)
59. Owen, J. J. T. and Raff, M. C. (1970). *J. Exp. Med.*, **132**, 1216
60. Davies, A. J. S. (1969). *Transplantation Reviews*, **1**, 43 (G. Möller, editor) (Copenhagen: Munksgaard)
61. Blomgren, H. and Andersson, B. (1971). *Cell. Immunol.*, **1**, 545
62. Aoki, T., Hämmerling, U., De Harven, E., Boyse, E. A. and Old, L. J. (1969). *J. Exp. Med.*, **130**, 979
63. Elliott, E. V. (1973). *Nature New Biol.*, **242**, 150
64. Ernstrom, V. and Sandberg, G. (1970). *Acta Path. Microbiol. Scand.*, **78**, 362
65. Davies, A. J. S. (1969). *Agents and Actions*, **1**, 1
66. Bach, J. F., Dardenne, M., Goldstein, A. L., Guha, A. and White, A. (1971). *Proc. Nat. Acad. Sci. USA*, **68**, 273
67. Stutman, O., Yunis, E. J. and Good, R. A. (1969). *J. Exp. Med.*, **130**, 809
68. Cooper, M. D., Perey, D. Y., McKneally, M. F., Gabrielson, A. E., Sutherland, D. E. R. and Good, R. A. (1966). *Lancet, i*, 1388
69. Everett, N. B. and Caffrey, R. W. (1966). In *The Lymphocyte in Immunology and Haemopoiesis*, 108 (J. M. Yoffrey, editor) (G. Arnold Publ.)
70. Nossal, G. J. V. and Pike, B. L. (1973). *Immunology* (in the press)
71. Lawton, A. R., Asofsky, R. A., Hylton, M. B. and Cooper, M. D. (1972). *J. Exp. Med.*, **135**, 277
72. Raff, M. C. (1970). *Immunology*, **14**, 637
73. Raff, M. C., Nase, S. and Mitchison, N. A. (1971). *Nature (London)*, **230**, 50
74. Takahashi, T., Old, L. J. and Boyse, E. A. (1970). *J. Exp. Med.*, **131**, 1325
75. Takahashi, T., Old, L. J., Chen-Jung, N. and Boyse, E. A. (1972). *Europ. J. Immunol.*, **1**, 478
76. Bianco, C. and Nussenzweig, V. (1971). *Science*, **173**, 154

77. Basten, A., Miller, J. F. A. P., Sprent, J. and Pye, J. (1972). *J. Exp. Med.*, **135**, 610
78. Parrott, D. M. V. and De Sousa, M. A. B. (1971). *Clin. Exp. Immunol.*, **8**, 663
79. Waksman, B. H., Arnason, B. G. and Jankovic, B. D. (1962). *J. Exp. Med.*, **116**, 187
80. Parrott, D. M. V., De Sousa, M. and East, J. (1966). *J. Exp. Med.*, **123**, 191
81. Gowans, J. L. and Knight, E. J. (1964). *Proc. Roy. Soc. (London) B.*, **159**, 257
82. Ford, W. L. and Marchesi, V. T. (1971). In *Progr. Immunol.*, 1159 (B. Amos, editor) (New York: Academic Press)
83. Ford, W. L. (1969). *Brit. J. Exp. Path.*, **50**, 257
84. Howard, J. C. (1972). *J. Exp. Med.*, **125**, 185
85. Howard, J. C., Hunt, S. V. and Gowans, J. L. (1972). *J. Exp. Med.*, **135**, 200
86. Ada, G. L., Parish, C. R., Nossal, G. J. V. and Abbot, A. (1967). *Cold Spring Harbor Symp. Quant. Biol.*, **32**, 381
87. Raff, M. C. and Cantor, H. (1971). In *Progr. Immunol.*, 83 (B. Amos, editor) (New York: Academic Press)
88. White, R. G., French, V. I. and Stark, J. M. (1967). In *Germinal Centres in Immune Responses*, 131 (H. Cottier, N. Odartchenko, R. Schindler and C. C. Congdon, editors) (New York: Springer-Verlag)
89. Mitchell, J. (1972). *Immunology*, **22**, 231
90. Everett, N. B., Caffrey, R. W. and Rieke, W. C. (1964). *Ann. N.Y. Acad. Sci.*, **113**, 887
91. Bianco, C., Patrick, R. and Nussenzweig, V. (1970). *J. Exp. Med.*, **132**, 702
92. Cunningham, A. J. and Sercarz, E. E. (1972). *Europ. J. Immunol.*, **1**, 413

3
The Cellular Basis of Immune Responses

W. L. FORD
University Medical School, Edinburgh

3.1   INTRODUCTION

No one will object to the scheme of the immune response in Figure 3.1 which depicts the organism as a black box. Both the input side of the response (antigen) and the output side, as represented by antibody, have undergone refined biochemical analysis which can be presented within this framework. However, the black-box approach is limited because the immune response involves significant biochemical problems which can only be expressed with reference to intermediate cellular events. This was not always obvious for the instructive theory of antibody production as expounded by Pauling[1] envisaged that antigen entered a particular type of cell which was then capable of synthesising antibody directly on an antigen template. Such a scheme required no major changes in the properties of the cell between the entry of antigen and the production of antibody. From the cell biologist's point of view the only detail of interest was to identify the type of cell in which anti-body was formed.

It is now accepted that certain cellular events of which there is little under-standing at a biochemical level are fundamentally important in immune responses. Firstly, the ability of an animal to produce antibodies of a very large number of specificities is thought to be due to the differentiation during development of a very large number of subpopulations of cells each of which responds to a different antigen. Secondly, there is substantial evidence that some antibody responses require the participation of three distinct cell-types namely macrophages, thymus-derived (T) lymphocytes and thymus-inde-pendent (B) lymphocytes. Thirdly, cells which have responded to antigen undergo a complicated sequence of cell division and maturation which coin-cides with the development of their ability to secrete antibody or implement cell-mediated immunity. These maturational changes involve dramatic transformations in the appearance of the cells and also radical alterations in their physiological properties.

The objective of this chapter is to describe what is known and what is unclear about these intermediate events in cellular terms. For the most part, cells will be discussed as if they were little black boxes although it is realised

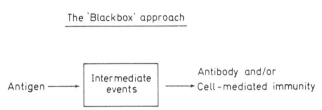

Figure 3.1 A simple model of antibody–formation

that even a final description of immune responses in these terms would only be one stage better than the information imparted in Figure 3.1. Much reliance will be placed on the histological and physiological information set out in the preceding chapter. Several later chapters discuss, in depth, areas which are covered here in outline.

3.2 ANTIBODY RESPONSES AND CELL-MEDIATED IMMUNITY

3.2.1 Basis of the distinction

For several decades it has been conventional to make a primary classification of specific immune responses into humoral immunity, which involves antibody formation and secretion, and cell-mediated immunity, which includes delayed hypersensitivity. Although the findings on which the distinction was based have been frequently confirmed and supplemented, there is still intensive controversy as to the significance of the dichotomy. An extreme point of view is that antibody formation and cell-mediated immunity have evolved independently and that they depend on different molecular and genetic mechanisms for responding to a wide diversity of antigens. The more orthodox viewpoint is that cell-mediated immunity depends on the production of cells which are equipped with a special class of surface bound antibody which enables them to recognise and react against the antigen which stimulated their development. According to this view the difference between the two types of response is comparatively trivial in molecular terms; it depends on whether antibody is secreted or retained on the surface of the cell as a receptor for antigen.

The operative basis of the distinction arose from attempts to produce a state of immunity in animals which had not received antigen by transferring either serum or lymphoid cells from animals which had been immunised (Figure 3.2). The protection afforded by antibody against infection as well as the other consequences of antibody formation can be transferred to a non-immune animal by giving serum from an immune animal (passive immunisation). By contrast delayed hypersensitivity to tuberculin and to simple chemical compounds cannot be transferred with serum but can be transferred by injecting a non-immune animal with intact lymphoid cells from a previously immunised donor[2, 3] (adoptive immunisation).

Adoptive immunisation is believed to be due to the inclusion within the transferred population of cells which can react rapidly on encountering antigen to give rise to the phenomena of delayed hypersensitivity. Therefore, the dichotomy of immune responses has been conceived of as depending crucially on how the response is finally implemented. Antibody is potentially active

Scheme of a transfer experiment

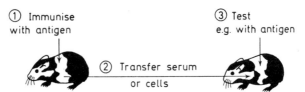

① Immunise
with antigen

③ Test
e.g. with antigen

② Transfer serum
or cells

Figure 3.2 The principle of transfer experiments. Either serum or lymphoid cells are taken from an immunised donor and injected into a recipient which is subsequently challenged. The object is to determine whether the consequences of contact with antigen are passed on to the recipient

at most sites in the body because it is carried by the blood from the relatively immobile cells which produce it. On the other hand, cell-mediated immunity depends on close physical contact between specific 'effector' cells produced as a consequence of immunisation and antigen wherever it may be localised. These specific effector cells must be able to migrate rapidly between the blood and tissues and within the tissues to provide effective protection against microbial infection[4].

The biological value of having two means of implementing specific immune responses is not clear. Cell-mediated immunity provides the most efficient protection against many viral, mycobacterial and fungal diseases whereas antibody is superior in defence against particular bacteria such as pneumococci, streptococci, meningococci, *H. influenzae* and *Pseudomonas aeruginosa*[5].

3.2.2 Example of different means of implementation

The different effector mechanisms of humoral and cell-mediated immunity are well illustrated by a series of experiments which involved immunisation of mice belonging to one inbred strain with cells from mice belonging to a second inbred strain. The immune reaction was against cell-surface antigens which are determined by the complex H-2 locus. Sera from immune mice produced complement-dependent lysis of 'target' cells provided they express the same antigens as do the cells used for immunisation. Antibody-forming cells were identified by layering the immune spleen cells on to the appropriate target cells suspended in gel. A zone of lysed target cells was cleared around each antibody-secreting cell[6]. However, under different experimental conditions the immune population was shown to produce *specific* destruction of target cells which was not complement dependent but which required close contact between the attacking population and the target cells[7]. The latter system was regarded as an *in vitro* model of cell-mediated immunity since the subpopulation responsible for the lysis could be distinguished from the antibody-forming cells in that (a) an anti-theta serum (Chapter 2) abolished its activity[8], and (b) it was inhibited by the addition of specific antibody in the absence of complement[7]. Therefore lymphoid cells from an immune animal include two separable subpopulations each of which can destroy specific target cells; one acts by secreting antibody, the other acts by some other mechanism.

3.2.3 Graft rejection as cell-mediated immunity

The capacity of an animal to reject a skin graft taken from another individual of the same species has been established as an immune response since the work of Medawar[9] which noted that a second skin graft was rejected more quickly than a first skin graft if both grafts were from the same donor. Thus the genetically determined factors which decide whether a graft is rejected came to be regarded as transplantation antigens.

The ability to produce accelerated second-set rejection of skin grafts, i.e. homograft sensitivity, was found to follow the same rules as delayed hypersensitivity; it could not be transferred with serum from an immune animal but could be transferred by inocula of lymphoid cells[10]. Thus skin graft rejection and delayed hypersensitivity are both classified as examples of cell-mediated immunity; 'classical delayed hypersensitivity' is restricted to the local inflammatory response which develops more than 4 h after challenge with an antigen in an immune subject[11]. It is exemplified by the inflammatory response which develops in the skin of a tuberculin sensitive subject after the intradermal injection of tuberculin.

Cell-mediated immunity should not be extended to include a number of effects which are due to antibody secreted by one population of cells becoming attached to the surface of other cells. Examples are the binding of cytophilic antibody to macrophages through a receptor for the F_c fragment[12] and the binding of IgE to mast cells[13] which is responsible for atopic allergic reactions such as hay-fever. In these circumstances the cell to which antibody is bound may show altered reactivity towards a particular antigen—'passive allergisation'[14]. However the cells which implement cell-mediated immunity are 'actively allergised', that is their specific reactivity is an intrinsic property of the cell.

3.3 CELLULAR EVENTS IN ANTIBODY RESPONSES

Niels Jerne[15] has defined perceptively two approaches to the study of antibody responses. Immunochemists have favoured 'trans-immunology' which is to study the product of the response and then to think backwards in time to reconstruct the events which led to that antibody. 'Cis-immunology' is the favoured approach of cellular immunologists. This is to study the events after the injection of antigen which appear to be involved with the initiation of the response. For descriptive purposes, it is convenient to use both approaches by beginning with the question of which cells produce antibody and to work backwards to the role of other cells involved at earlier stages (Section 3.3.2). There follows a description of antibody responses at the level of cell populations and lymphoid organs in the sequence of their occurrence (Section 3.3.2.)

3.3.1 The cells concerned with antibody responses

3.3.1.1 The cell in which antibody is formed

It is well known that antibody is synthesised in, and secreted by, plasma cells but some qualifications of this statement have become necessary. The use of fluorescent antibody according to the sandwich technique[16, 17] confirmed previous evidence[18] that plasma cells produce antibody. A frozen section is made of a tissue which is actively synthesising antibody and treated with a solution of the appropriate antigen. The excess antigen is washed off and replaced by fluorescent antibody which delineates the antibody-containing cells by completing a sandwich of antibody–antigen-fluorescent antibody.

Since then many methods have been developed for detecting antibody production by single cells. The most popular has been the Jerne plaque assay in which lymphoid cells are incubated with sheep erythrocytes which are held in a gel such as agar. In the presence of complement, clear plaques of haemolysis develop around cells forming lytic antibody against the erythrocytes[19]. These haemolysin-forming cells vary in appearance; some are mature plasma cells, but many are large dividing cells while others resemble small lymphocytes. The large cells can be regarded as plasmablasts since their ultrastructure resembles that of mature plasma cells in that they have plentiful endoplasmic reticulum and a prominent Golgi apparatus[20]. Small lymphocytes are seldom found to contain antibody when Coon's technique is applied to tissue sections. Lymphocytes may be over-represented among plaque-forming cells because they go into suspension more readily than do plasma cells. The great majority of small lymphocytes do not secrete large amounts of antibody; this is a function of large dividing plasma cells and, later, of mature plasma cells, which have lost the capacity for further division.

The intracellular sites of antibody synthesis have become amenable to electron-microscopic study by the use of horse-radish peroxidase as an antigen[21, 22]. Antibody is localised by treating ultra-thin sections with a solution of the enzyme, followed by washing. The bound enzyme retains its activity and can be detected histochemically. Early in antibody synthesis, antibody is found in the perinuclear space.[21] In lymphocyte-like cells which

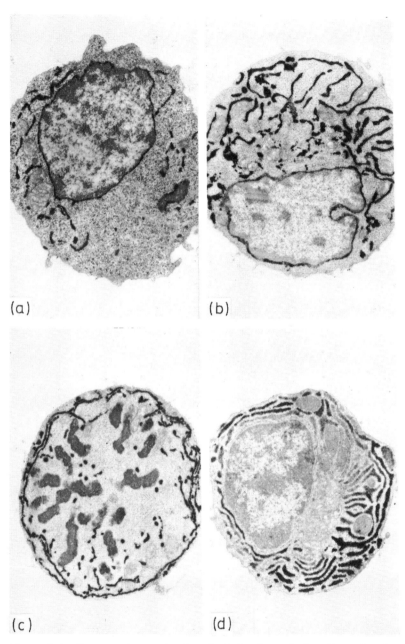

(a)
(b)
(c)
(d)

Figure 3.3 Electron micrograph of antibody-forming cells in efferent lymph from a lymph-node stimulated with horse-radish peroxidase. The dense black material corresponds to the localisation of antibody against peroxidase. (a) and (b), blast cells with antibody in the perivascular space and near the endoplasmic reticulum; (c) cells in mitosis containing antibody; (d) a plasma cell filled with antibody. (By courtesy of B. Morris)

are producing antibody the only site of antibody is perinuclear[22]. Later in the response, plasma cells appear with antibody present between alternate layers of concentric ergastoplasm (Figure 3.3). Antibody is found in plasmablasts during mitosis[22] and appears to be secreted by living cells throughout mitosis[23].

3.3.1.2 The identity of the antibody-forming cell precursor

The origin of plasma cells is a major question in cellular immunology, which in the last few years has been solved to the satisfaction of most workers in this field. There is clear evidence that antibody-forming cell precursors are lymphocytes and, in particular, are restricted to thymus-independent 'B' lymphocytes as defined in the previous chapter.

By the mid-1960s there was no doubt that lymphocytes played some essential role in antibody responses[24]. Much of the evidence came from transfer experiments in which lymphocytes were obtained from one animal and injected into another of the same inbred strain which was then tested by the injection of antigen (Figure 3.2). Animals lacking lymphocytes were deficient in producing antibody and responsiveness was restored by replenishment of the depleted animal with lymphocytes from a normal animal[24] (Figure 3.7).

A second type of transfer experiment involved injecting recipients which had not been immunised with normal lymphocytes from donors which had been immunised with the phage ΦX 174. In normal rats, the response to a second injection of ΦX is much larger than to a first; however, rats produced maximal titres to a first injection if they had been provided with lymphocytes from an immunised donor. This showed that immunological memory is attributable to small lymphocytes presumably because an immune population contains more cells capable of reacting to antigen[25]. A third type of transfer experiment was concerned with immunological tolerance, that is, a state of unresponsiveness towards a particular antigen which is induced by prior administration of that antigen (Chapter 5). Lymphocytes taken from animals which had been made tolerant were unable to restore responsiveness to irradiated recipients unlike lymphocytes from normal donors[26]. Thus lymphocytes are required for primary responses and are responsible for states of specifically-heightened responsiveness, i.e. immunological memory, and specifically diminished responsiveness, i.e. tolerance. The most plausible interpretation of these findings is that small lymphocytes respond to antigen and differentiate to produce antibody-forming cells.

In the last few years more direct and informative evidence has been obtained concerning the role of lymphocytes. An antigenic marker was used to study the origin of antibody-forming cells in irradiated rats which had been replenished with a pure population of lymphocytes. This proved that the precursors of the antibody-forming cells were among the injected lymphocytes and were not radio-resistant host cells[27]. Further evidence is discussed in the following Sections (3.3.1.3 and 3.3.1.4)

3.3.1.3 Different lymphocytes respond to different antigens

The development of methods for studying the binding of labelled antigens to lymphocytes *in vitro* has been responsible for much recent progress[28-30].

Suspensions of lymphocytes were incubated with soluble antigen at $0°C$, washed free of excess antigen and smeared for autoradiography. Only a small minority of lymphocytes bound each antigen whether the animal from which the cells had been obtained had been immunised or not[29, 30]. By using antigen with enough short-range radioactivity to kill selectively the lymphocytes to which it bound, it was found that elimination of the antigen-binding sub-population removed the capacity of the remaining cells to produce the corresponding antibody when transferred to an X-irradiated recipient; other antibody responses were not affected[29]. These results showed not only that small lymphocytes express surface receptors for antigen but also confirmed that different lymphocytes respond to different antigens.

The principle of this experiment—the selective elimination of a subpopulation of antigen sensitive cells—had already been demonstrated by Mishell and Duttons' experiments using a 'hot pulse' of tritiated-thymidine to eliminate the subpopulation which had responded in vitro to sheep erythrocytes to proliferation[31] and by Wigzell and Andersen[32]. The latter attached protein antigens to glass or plastic beads within columns through which lymphoid cells were slowly passed. It was found, by testing the population recovered from the column in the familiar system of transfer to irradiated recipients, that a subpopulation necessary for the appropriate antibody response had been removed but the capacity of the 'passed' population to respond to a different antigen from that on the column had not substantially changed. This system was exploited to show that the subpopulation of cells which were removed possessed immunoglobulin-like receptors presumably on the cell surface[33].

The other side of the coin is selective enrichment—that is the isolation of a subpopulation most or all of which can respond to a given antigen. Enrichment has proved to be technically much more difficult than selective depletion although the use of nylon fibres to which antigen is conjugated as an immuno-absorbent for cells is of particular promise[34].

3.3.1.4 Do antibody-forming cell precursors belong to a particular class of lymphocyte?

Davies and his colleagues produced CBA mice whose spleen and lymph-nodes contain a relatively stable mixture of lymphoid cells—thymus-derived cells with a particular chromosome marker (T6T6) and marrow-derived cells with a distinguishable karyotype. This was achieved by removal of the thymus, whole-body irradiation to destroy most of the host's own lymphocytes, followed by grafting with bone-marrow cells from one donor and thymic fragments from another donor. They found that the origin of lymphoid cells, stimulated to proliferation by antigen, varied dramatically with different antigens; after with some antigens, such as sheep erythrocytes, both populations responded by mitosis[35]. In the same year, Claman and his colleagues reported that marrow cells and thymus cells would together restore a substantial antibody response to irradiated recipients whereas each population transferred alone was very inefficient[36]. Although it seemed a bizarre result this synergy between two populations of lymphocytes has been confirmed repeatedly in mice and rats. The confusion was partly cleared by Miller and his colleagues who showed that in circumstances where synergy between a marrow-derived and a thymus-derived populations was evident, the precursors of the antibody-forming cells belonged exclusively to the marrow-derived population[37].

The implication that thymus-derived lymphocytes do not give rise to antibody-forming cells but play some other role inspired a large number of experiments which have recently been reviewed in depth[37-39]: Some of this work has analysed in terms of T and B lymphocytes, the properties of naturally-mixed lymphocyte populations, e.g. thoracic duct lymphocytes, which had already been established. For example, it was found that immunological memory and immunological tolerance may reflect alterations in the activity of either or both populations; which of the two populations is influenced most by antigen depends on several factors, such as the nature and the dosage of antigen[38-41]. It has also been established that both T and B lymphocytes are capable of binding antigen *in vitro* and that the principle of different subpopulations binding different antigens holds true for both T and B cells. Selective elimination of either the specific T cell or the specific B cell subpopulation prevents an antibody response[42, 43]. However, immuno-absorption of cells to an antigen-coated column is apparently only effective in depleting specifically-reactive B cells[33].

The synergistic activity of B and T lymphocytes has been grafted on to an old immunological problem, the carrier effect[44]. When antibody to a hapten is measured, a small primary response is detected after the injection of the hapten conjugated with a carrier protein. A second administration of hapten is followed by a larger secondary response provided that it is conjugated to the same carrier; if it is conjugated to a different protein another primary response follows. In other words, the capacity of the animal to give an augmented secondary response to the hapten depends on it being immune to the carrier protein on which the hapten is administered; indeed if the animal is tolerant to the carrier protein no primary response to the hapten is detectable[45]. A series of experiments in mice suggested that the capacity to give a secondary antibody response to a hapten depends on the presence of a population of B lymphocytes which is of increased reactivity against the hapten and a population of T lymphocytes which is more reactive than non-immune cells to the carrier[44]. However, this scheme requires modification in order to explain all examples of the carrier effect, such as that found with thymus-independent antigens[45] and in cell-mediated immunity where only T cells are involved[46].

3.3.1.5 The mechanism of co-operation between T lymphocytes and antibody-forming cell precursors

If T lymphocytes are not precursors of antibody-secreting cells but do play a specific role in controlling many antibody responses an obvious problem is by what means do T lymphocytes act? The most significant clue may be that in a few antibody responses T cells are not required and indeed, seem to play no part in the response. It was found that neonatally-thymectomised mice respond normally to pneumococcal polysaccharide despite a deficiency of T cells[47]. This is the most widely studied of the thymus-independent antigens but the list has been extended to include levan, polyvinylpyrrolidine, *E. coli* polysaccharide, polymerised flagellin and others. These substances have two features in common (a) repeated sequences of one antigenic determinant and (b) they persist for long periods *in vivo*[39]. It is not known why only these antigens can activate B cells directly although it has been suggested that multivalent binding of the molecules to antibody-like receptors on the surface of B lymphocytes to produce extensive cross-linking on the surface of the cell may be important[48]. Another unsolved problem is why IgM responses are much less thymus-dependent than IgG responses[39]. As would be expected, none of the thymus-independent antigens elicit delayed hypersensitivity.

Most work on B lymphocyte–T lymphocyte co-operation has been concerned with antibody responses produced by dissociated lymphoid cells *in vitro*. A recently as 1961, it was doubtful whether a primary response had ever been carried through *in vitro* from start to finish[49], but with the development of culture techniques for fastidious lymphoid cells[31,50], *in vitro* antibody responses have become routine. Several groups have described *in vitro* systems in which both T and B lymphocytes are necessary for an antibody response[51-54]. This approach led to an even higher degree of complexity when it was found that a third cell-type is required for an *in vitro* antibody response[55,56]. When lymphoid cells were separated on the basis of their adherance to plastic, the adherent fraction was required as well as B and T lymphocytes, which were both in the non-adherent fraction. As will be described later, macrophages appear to play an essential preliminary role in some antibody responses *in vivo* and macrophages are, in general, adherent. It, therefore, seems likely that the requirement for macrophages and the requirement for adherent cells are one and the same but it is possible to argue against this[51].

Theories of B–T co-operation can be divided into two categories (a) specific—in which reactive T cells exposed to a given antigen can only influence the response of B cells to the same antigen and (b) non-specific in which T cells exposed to an antigen to which they are reactive can influence the response of B cells reacting to a different antigen. If the latter is valid, then the influence of T cells plus antigen is probably very short-range in space and time since the carrier effect, in so far as it is established to be a reflection of B–T co-operation, only occurs if the hapten and carrier determinants are on the same molecule[57], or at least on the same antigenic cell[58].

Both specific and non-specific consequences of T-cell activation have experimental support. The non-specific, augmentative influence of T-cell activation on B-cell function has been assumed to be due to short-range pharmacological mediators which may possibly act as mitogens to increase the number of antibody-forming cells produced from each precursor cell[52,53]. Although immune lymphocytes do produce a mitogenic factor in the presence of the appropriate antigen, its physiological significance has not been established[59]. Recently there has been considerable interest in the 'allogeneic effect'[60] which is the augmentation of an antibody response by the simultaneous induction of an immune response against strong transplantation antigens expressed by a different strain, i.e. allo-antigens. These antigens are responsible for activating an exceptionally high proportion of T lymphocytes in graft-*versus*-host reactions[61] and mixed lymphocytes culture[62] and so the simplest possibility is that the allogeneic effect is due to some non-specific product of T cell activation.

Evidence in the other direction—that the helper function of T cells is specific[44,54] has fired many imaginations. An appealing idea is that T cells capture and concentrate antigen by means of their specific surface receptors. The T cell acts as a matrix for orientating antigenic determinants to form a regular pattern which is particularly effective in engaging the receptors of the antigen-sensitive subpopulation of B lymphocytes. The notion that T cells 'focus' antigen on to the surface of B precursor cells obviously requires at least transient contact between T and B cells with antigen acting as a bridge[57]. This complements the notion that thymus-independent antigens are molecules on which the determinants happen to be arrayed in the repeating pattern necessary for B-cell activation[48].

This antigen-bridge theory is unable to account for the recent finding of Feldmann and Basten that specific B–T cell collaboration can occur when the B and T cells are separated physically by a cell-impermeable membrane[54]. They have also shown that the T helper cells require to have divided in response to antigen before they are capable of collaboration[63] and that the presence of macrophages in the chamber containing the B cells is necessary[64]. Based on this work, and the conclusions of colleagues that immunoglobulin is present on the surface of thymus cells[65], Feldmann and Nossal[66] have proposed a plausible and ingenious scheme for which experimental support is, at present, limited. They suggest that antigens are bound initially by a specific receptor on the surface of immune T cells which consists of monomeric IgM. Complexes of the antigen and the receptor antibody are released by the T cell and become attached non-specifically to macrophages to produce a spatial arrangement of antigenic determinants which is exceptionally efficient at activating responsive B-cells when they come into contact with the antigen-coated surface. In the absence of macrophages B cells which are exposed to the complexes become tolerant[66a]. This model has several advantages which were anticipated on theoretical grounds by Bretscher and Cohn[67,68]. It also has the attraction of explaining the requirement for macrophages at the initiation of immune responses which is the subject of the following section.

3.3.1.6 Macrophages in antibody responses

After the injection of antigen, particulate or soluble, the majority of material localises within macrophages in the anatomical sites described in the following section (3.3.2.1). Despite some reports to the contrary macrophages are not generally believed to produce antibody and indeed the histological sites of antigen localisation and antibody production are distinctly separated[69].

A decade ago it was plausible that the specific events in antibody responses were started by macrophages. The rate at which macrophages phagocytose and digest material is roughly proportional to the 'foreign-ness' of the substance[70]. While macrophages can discriminate between rather similar macromolecules or cells, they only do so by working more or less quickly; they do not react in a specific way to each antigen. The evidence that the specific events of the antibody response are *not* initiated in macrophages is that while isolated lymphocytes reflect specific states of tolerance or immunity in the whole animal, macrophages behave similarly whether they come from normal, tolerant or immune animals[71]. An important proviso is that the activity of macrophages from immune animals may be altered towards a specific antigen by the presence of cell-bound antibody[12] or towards a range of antigens after the interaction of immune lymphocytes and specific antigen[72]. These appear to be secondary effects which do not involve any change in the inherent properties of macrophages.

The contrary idea, that the specific events leading to antibody formation are initiated within macrophages, was supported by the work of Fishman and his colleagues[73] which was very influential during the 1960s. They incubated peritioneal exudate cells with antigen, disrupted the cells and made a phenolic extract of RNA which was added without antigen to a second culture this time of lymph-node cells. Specific antibody synthesis was induced in this culture. This suggested that informational RNA produced by macrophages had been transferred to lymphocytes where it could specify antibody synthesis. This interpretation was opened to question when it was found that this method of extraction produced RNA contaminated by antigenic material. Moreover, such an RNA–antigen complex is more immunogenic than the free antigen[74]. Whether this RNA–protein complexing is of significance in increasing the immunogenicity of antigens remains open but very few now suppose that macrophage RNA plays an informational role in other cells.

Given that the specific events in antibody formation are initiated by the action of antigen on lymphocytes, what is the significance of the uptake of antigen by macrophages? An obvious possibility is that after ingestion by macrophages antigen has no subsequent opportunity to influence lymphocytes and thus plays no part in the antibody response. Thus, macrophages act as an 'antigen sink' and provide a controlling mechanism preventing excessively high concentration of antigen from reaching lymphocytes. This view has been supported by several reports that, in certain circumstances, antibody responses were reduced if macrophages were added to a culture of lymphocytes and antigen[71].

On the other hand there is good evidence that some of the antigen ingested by macrophages remains capable of activating lymphocytes. Some antigens are partially degraded within macrophages and the fragments are either regurgitated or held on the cell surface[75]. The injection of washed macrophages which are loaded with antigen provokes a larger response than the injection of the same amount of antigen alone and removal of the surface-bound antigen with trypsin diminishes the response[76]. Thus immunogenicity of antigens may be improved if they are presented to lymphocytes on the surface of macrophages. This interpretation is not rigorous since the injection of antigen within macrophages produces an abnormal distribution of antigen in favour of lymphoid tissue at the expense of the liver[71].

The necessity for macrophage processing has been supported in experiments with cellular or large macromolecular antigens. For example, sheep erythrocytes were incapable of activating lymphocytes until they had been digested by macrophages[77] but it was later found that a sonicated preparation of sheep erythrocytes could activate lymphocytes without the necessity for macrophage processing[78] suggesting that the role of macrophages is to degrade cellular antigens to a form in which they are capable of binding to lymphocyte receptors. Detailed information on the role of macrophages is lacking but the broad notion that macrophages play a preliminary role in antibody formation by controlling the concentration of antigen to which antigen-sensitive lymphocytes are exposed is likely to prevail. Macrophages can also control the duration for which antigen is accessible to lymphocytes[79].

3.3.2 Antibody responses in terms of cell populations and lymphoid organs

The contributions of four different cell types have now been described working back from antibody-forming cells to their antigen-sensitive precursors (B lymphocytes) and to T lymphocytes and macrophages (summarised in Figure 3.4). The last two cells play a role at the induction of many responses

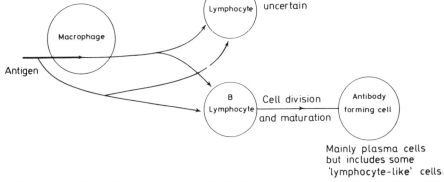

Figure 3.4 The cells involved in antibody–formation. Antibody–forming cells are derived from B lymphocytes. Macrophages may play a non-specific role and T lymphocytes a specific role. For full explanation see text.

which is only partly understood. Whereas macrophages play a non-specific preliminary role the collaborative activity of T cells is specific for each antigen. This information will now be used to give a sequential account of events following the injection of antigen in terms of cell populations and the lymphoid compartments to which they belong.

3.3.2.1 Sites of antigen localisation

Intravenously-injected antigen is mostly taken up by liver macrophages and a substantial minority localises within macrophages of the spleen and bone-marrow. Antigen injected into most other sites, e.g. subcutaneously or intraperitoneally, localises predominantly in the draining lymph-nodes although some is retained locally by macrophages and a variable amount, depending on the nature of the antigen and the dose, spills over into the circulation to reach the liver, spleen and bone-marrow[80]. It is believed that the antigen which localises in the liver plays no part in initiating antibody responses under normal circumstances; the relevant sites of antigen localisation are in the peripheral lymphoid organs, namely the spleen, the lymph nodes and gut-associated lymphoid tissue.

Within the spleen antigen localises in the red pulp, in the marginal zone around the white pulp and in association with dendritic macrophages within germinal centres in the white pulp. Within lymph-nodes antigen localises in medullary macrophages, in macrophages around the subcapsular sinus and again in germinal centres within the superficial cortex[71]. (Figure 3.5). This last

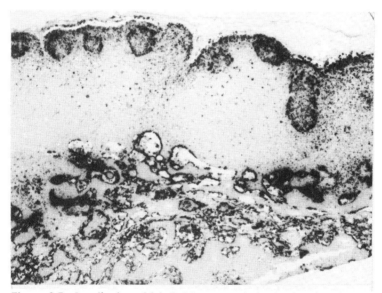

Figure 3.5 Localisation of labelled haemocyanin in the lymph-node of a rabbit. Antigen is present in three sites (a) in sinus-lining macrophages of the medulla (lower half of field); (b) in the superficial part of the lymph-node cortex especially in the subcapsular sinus (near the top of the field); and (c) follicular localisation in germinal centres (circular areas). (By courtesy of J. H. Humphrey and M. Frank)

site is termed follicular localisation (Figure 3.6) and is unique in that it depends on the presence of antibody to hold antigen[81]. Follicular localisation is also distinguished from antigen localisation in other sites in that it is prevented by previous irradiation[82].

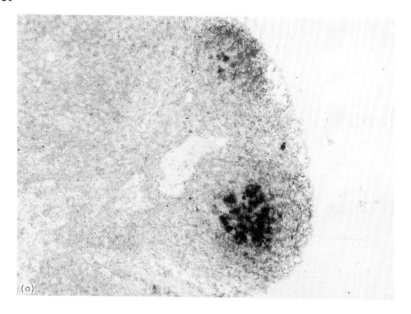

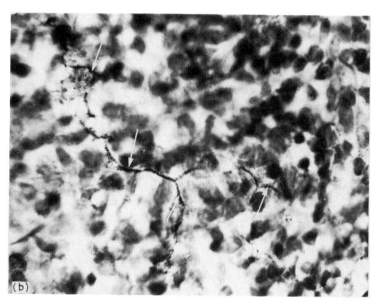

Figure 3.6 Follicular localisation (a) labelled haemocyanin is confined to the germinal centres in the lymph-node of a pre-immunised rabbit. (By courtesy of J. H. Humphrey and M. Frank); (b) Typical lace-like pattern of labelled human serum albumin in germinal centre in the spleen of a guinea-pig. (By courtesy of E. Davidson)

3.3.2.2 The recruitment of lymphocytes

The antigen-specific events in antibody formation are started by the action of antigen on lymphocytes. The precise site in lymphoid tissue where this occurs is not known but at least there is evidence that the minority of lymphocytes which are sensitive to a particular antigen are recruited from the traffic streams of T and B lymphocytes which migrate from the blood through the extravascular spaces of the spleen and lymph nodes and subsequently return to the blood (Chapter 2). This large-scale recirculation of lymphocytes enables an antigen which is localised to a small part of the lymphoid apparatus, say a single lymph-node, to winnow out antigen-sensitive cells from most of the recirculating pool[24]. It has been shown recently that after the arrival of antigen in the spleen the recirculating pool of lymphocytes becomes depleted of a specifically reactive subpopulation[83] and that this depletion involves both hapten-specific and carrier-specific cells—presumably B and T lymphocytes, respectively[84]. Selection of antigen-sensitive cells out of the recirculating pool can account for the depressed response to a second injection of the same antigen injected into a different lymphoid organ from the first[85]. However it does not explain the well-established depression of the response to a different (non-cross-reacting) antigen which is injected a few days after a first antigen. This is called antigenic competition and its mechanism and significance are unknown[86] although saturation of receptors on the macrophage surface for antigen–antibody romplexes is an attractive possibility (see p. 76).

Soon after antigen reaches lymphoid tissue, characteristic histological changes develop and dramatic changes occur in the population of cells released by lymph-nodes into their efferent lymph en route for the blood. Within 24 h of the arrival of antigen large blast cells, rich in ribonucleoprotein, and undergoing rapid proliferation, appear in the periarteriolar sheath of the spleen[87] and the deep zone of the lymph-node cortex[88]. It is now known that most of the cells normally in these areas are T lymphocytes and there is little doubt that this change is a sign of the reaction of T lymphocytes to antigen as described in the following section on cell-mediated immunity. Less obvious changes also occur in the B lymphocyte population within thymus-independent areas. In the lymph-nodes of rabbits which were depleted of T cells the residual lymphocyte population responded to antigen by enlargement and proliferation. This change was first noted in the superficial area of the lymph-node cortex and the proliferating lymphoid cells appeared to migrate towards the medulla[89]. In mice the injection of sheep erythrocytes stimulates some cells in the collar of B lymphocytes surrounding the germinal centres to enter DNA synthesis[90]. It can be concluded that both both B and T small lymphocytes are stimulated by most antigens to enlarge and divide[35]. They do so in their own distinct compartments and, if cell-co-operation depends on the close apposition of B and T lymphocytes, it is likely to occur soon after lymphocytes enter the lymphoid tissue from the blood.

Within one hour of the arrival of antigen at the popliteal lymph-node[91] or the spleen the normally heavy traffic of lymphocytes from these organs into the blood is inhibited. The arrest of lymphocyte migration lasts for a few hours; it may be a mechanism for facilitating the recruitment of a minority of antigen-sensitive cells by slowing down the progress of the majority. Later the flux of cells in efferent lymph from a antigenically-stimulated node rebounds far above the basal level. After *ca.* 72 h the torrent of both large and small lymphocytes reaches a climax[92]. At this time an exceptionally high proportion of the cells are large proliferating cells and many of these are producing specific antibody[22] (Figure 3.3). The fate of these blast cells in efferent lymph is intriguing; no matter which antigen is used to stimulate their production, the majority of these cells localise in the intestine, not only in the gut-associated lymphoid tissue but throughout the lamina propria under the epithelium. Some of these cells develop into plasma cells[93] suggesting that the function of this traffic is the territorial expansion of the site of antibody formation. However, activated T lymphocytes, which do not secrete antibody, localise predominantly in the same site following intravenous injection[94].

3.3.2.3 Cell division in antibody responses

The cellular events between the activation of antigen-sensitive cells and the peak of antibody synthesis have been studied mainly by the Jerne plaque assay which was described as a method for identifying individual cells producing haemolytic antibody to sheep eythrocytes[19]. The technique has been modified for many special purposes including (a) the detection of antibody forming cells (AFC) to chemically-defined antigens by attaching the latter to the surface of sheep erythrocytes; (b) the identification of cells secreting a particular class of antibody. For example, mouse lymphoid cells which secrete IgG antibody can be detected by development with a rabbit antimouse IgG serum[95]; (c) the autoradiography of plaque-forming cells[96] and (d) the affinity of the antibody produced by plaque-forming cells can be estimated by adding graded concentrations of free hapten or antigen to the medium in replicate plates. The higher the affinity of the antibody the lower is the concentration of free hapten required to inhibit the lysis of conjugated erythrocytes[97]. The plaque assay was used firstly to study antibody responses which were induced and maintained *in vivo*. Such experiments consist of administering antigen to a series of animals. The stimulated lymphoid organ is removed from animals at intervals after initiation of the response and a cell suspension is prepared and examined for plaque-forming cells. The background of plaque-forming cells present in the lymphoid tissue of unstimulated animals is estimated. After a latent period of 24–48 h, there is a rapid increase in the number of plaque-forming cells with a doubling time of as little as 4–6 h in some experiments (Figure 3.7). The cells secreting each class of antibody have a characteristic tempo of response which may be modified by antigen dosage[95].

Autoradiographic studies of plaque-forming cells confirmed that cell division is an important factor in the generation of AFCs as had long been suspected. At 3 days after the injection of antigen 55% of plaque-forming cells were labelled by an *in vitro* pulse of tritiated thymidine which supported a rapid rate of AFC proliferation[96]. The need for cell division was established by an experiment on the haemolysin response performed wholly *in vitro*. Administration of a sufficient dose of high specific activity [^{3}H]thymidine to kill the cells which incorporated it prevented a response but the remaining population could later respond to another antigen[31]. In the primary response to DNP-poly-1-lysine at least one cell cycle is required for the transformation of an antigen-sensitive precursor into an antibody-formingec ll[98] but the

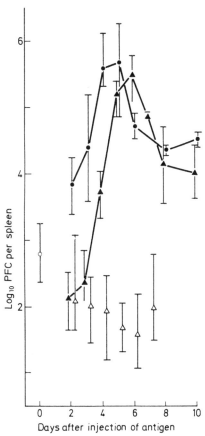

Figure 3.7 Number of cells forming haemolytic plaques to sheep erythrocytes. Plaque-forming cell (PFC) response of normal rats (●). PFCs in rats after 1000 rad (△). PFC response in irradiated rats given 2.5×10^8 lymphocytes prior to antigen (▲). Geometric mean ± range. Background PFC of non-immunised rats ± 1.S.D. (○). (By courtesy of J. C. Howard and J. L. Gowans and the Royal Society)

possibility remains that in response to some antigens antibody formation may precede cell-division.

Cell division is not the only factor responsible for the explosive increase in plaque-forming cell numbers. When a double-label technique was used to measure the cell-cycle time of plaque-forming cells an estimate of 13 h was obtained[99], which is well within conventional cycle times of proliferating cells from adult mammals. The shorter doubling time of plaque-forming cells can be accounted for by (a) variation in the latent period for transformation of antigen-sensitive precursors into antibody producers[100] and (b) asynchronous recruitment of cells from the recirculating lymphocyte pool[101].

It is not known whether the continuous presence of antigen is needed to drive the proliferation of antibody-forming cells and their precursors. A study of lymphocyte activation by anti-allotype antibody showed that the cells must be exposed to the transforming agent for several hours—in fact until the stage of DNA synthesis. Neutralisation of the stimulus during this period is followed by reversal of the morphological changes. However, after the first S phase proliferation is independent of the transforming agent[102].

3.3.2.4 The localisation of antibody-forming cells

The progress of the antibody response may be followed by the detection of cells forming specific antibody in tissue sections obtained at intervals after antigenic stimulation. The proliferation of antibody-forming cells occurs mostly in the red pulp of the spleen, in the medulla of lymph-nodes and in equivalent areas of gut-associated lymphoid tissue. These sites are different from either of the areas in which B and T lymphocytes localise suggesting that after antigenic activation antibody-forming cell-precursors migrate to the areas in which plasma-cells accumulate. It has been reported that the earliest detectable antibody-forming cells in the spleen are found in the white pulp[103] but these are very few and of uncertain significance. Later, after immunisation, some antibody-forming cells are found in germinal centres (see Section 3.5.4).

After prolonged immunisation, antibody-forming cells also appear in the bone-marrow and in non-lymphoid organs, such as the liver and lungs. Antibody-forming cells also occur in many tissues around local deposits of antigen, for example in a subcutaneous granuloma following the injection of antigen in adjuvant[80].

3.4 CELLULAR EVENTS IN CELL-MEDIATED IMMUNITY

3.4.1 Non-involvement of B lymphocytes

Delayed hypersensitivity and graft rejection are mediated by thymus derived (T) lymphocytes; no essential role has been assigned to B lymphocytes and their ultimate product, humoral antibody. Several experiments have shown that a lack of B cells is compatible with normal cell-mediated immunity although this does not necessarily mean that they are not involved when they are present. For example, when the bursa of Fabricius was removed from chickens 4 days before hatching, they were deficient in antibody responses but showed normal delayed hypersensitivity reactions and graft rejection[104]. The deficient antibody responses of bursectomised chickens are attributed to the lack of B lymphocytes partly because of evidence that the bursa release lymphocytes which migrate to the spleen[105]. In mammals a selective deficiency of B lymphocytes is very difficult to produce. However, rabbits which are irradiated heavily enough to eliminate their B lymphocytes population, with thymus shielding to allow rapid replenishment of T cells, show defective antibody formation with normal cell-mediated immunity similar to that of bursectomised chickens[89].

3.4.2 The initiation of cell-mediated responses

3.4.2.1 The site at which T lymphocytes meet antigen

At the cellular level the specific events in cell-mediated immune responses are started by the activation of a subpopulation of specifically-reactive T lymphocytes by antigen. As in antibody formation, there are a number of steps preliminary to the activation of lymphocytes to be considered and they depend largely on the circumstances of the antigenic stimulus. The route by which antigen is injected is very important in determining whether antibody formation or cell-mediated immunity is the predominant form of response[106]. A common way of producing delayed hypersensitivity is to paint the skin with a sensitising chemical ('contact sensitivity') and the commonest way to study graft rejection is to perform skin grafting. These are particularly effective ways of raising cell-mediated immunity while the intravenous injection of antigen is particularly ineffective. The reasons underlying this are not understood. When delayed hypersensitivity is induced other than by the dermal route, little is known about possible roles played by other cells prior to T lymphocyte activation.

After either skin grafting or skin painting, blast transformation of lymphocytes is observed in the regional lymph-nodes draining the skin site[88]. Much energy has been expended in trying to decide whether lymphocytes are exposed to antigen in the skin and subsequently migrate via afferent lymphatics to the draining node, i.e. 'peripheral' sensitisation, or whether antigenic material is carried from the skin to the draining node where a much larger population of lymphocytes is available for recruitment, i.e. 'central' sensitisation.

An important empirical observation is that alymphatic grafts are rejected in a much longer time than normal[107] although they are rejected eventually[108]. However, lymphatic drainage could be essential for the normal tempo of rejection either because it allows activated lymphocytes to migrate to the draining lymph-node or because it allows antigenic debris to reach the node. There is little doubt that lymphocytes *can* be activated within a skin graft[108] or at the site of injection of a sensitising chemical[109] but where most lymphocytes effectively encounter antigen is still uncertain.

3.4.2.2 Insight gained from graft-versus-host reactions

A cell-mediated immune response which has proved particularly illuminating is the graft-versus-host reaction produced by the injection of lymphocytes into a susceptible recipient[110]. Graft-versus-host (GVH) reactions occur if three well-known conditions are satisfied. (a) the host must express on its cells a transplantation antigen which is alien to the grafted cells. (b) The graft must include sufficient cells capable of reacting against these transplantation antigens. (c) The normal homograft rejection of the host against the graft must fail to operate for some reason.

The most useful experimental situation in which these conditions are satisfied is when the graft consists of lymphocytes from an inbred strain of rat, mouse or guinea-pig and the host is an F_1 hybrid between that strain and a second strain which expresses different transplantation antigens. (Figure 3.8). Transplantation antigens are determined by co-dominant genes

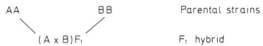

    AA   BB   Parental strains

                    (A x B)F₁   F₁ hybrid

Figure 3.8 A and B represent transplantation antigens determined by alleles at a major histocompatibility locus. Because the F_1 hybrid expresses an antigen which is foreign to each parental strain but the parental strains do not express any antigens foreign to the F^1 hybrid.

F₁ hybrid skin   →Parental host ... graft rejected
Parental skin   →F₁ hybrid host ... graft accepted
F₁ hybrid lymphocytes→Parental host ... graft rejected
Parental lymphocytes →F₁ hybrid host ... graft accepted, host 'rejected'

so that the heterozygous F_1 hybrids express the antigens inherited from both of its homozygous parents. Thus, F_1 hybrids do not recognise parental cells as foreign and parental skin grafts are, therefore, not rejected. A parental lymphocyte graft is also accepted but the graft does not accept the host. In rats an i.v. injection of $50—200 \times 10^6$ parental strain lymphocytes produces a lethal GVH reaction in young F_1 hybrid recipients. For the first week after injection the recipients appear to be normal but they later succumb to a rapidly-developing wasting syndrome.

This reaction can be produced by injecting an F_1 hybrid with an inoculum consisting entirely of parental strain lymphocytes[111]. Indeed, if the large lymphocytes are removed from the injected population, it can be shown that small lymphocytes alone are capable of producing a GVH reaction. Parental strain macrophages are not required for antigen processing; this immune response is started by small lymphocytes reacting directly to the antigens of the recipient.

Parental strain lymphocytes and F_1 hybrid lymphocytes have been cultured together in 'one way' mixed lymphocyte cultures which can be regarded as the *in vitro* equivalent of a GVH reaction. Some of the parental lymphocytes undergo rapid proliferation[62, 112]. The part played by the stimulating cells seems to be passive in that they are equally immunogenic after their capacity to divide is blocked by mitomycin C. Nevertheless, living lymphocytes are the most effective form of stimulation.

A strong case can be made that the small lymphocytes which respond in mixed lymphocyte culture[112] or GVH reactions [113] are almost entirely thymus-derived T lymphocytes. For example, lymphoid populations devoid of B cells respond but populations lacking T cells are inactive[112]. Moreover, there is no evidence for synergy between T lymphocytes and *specifically-reactive* B lymphocytes in GVH reactions as occurs in many antibody responses[114].

3.4.3 Intermediate events in cell-mediated immunity

A second context in which the parental against F_1 hybrid GVH system has produced invaluable data concerns the fate of the T lymphocyte subsequent to activation by antigen. Within 18–36 h of injection, labelled parental-strain small lymphocytes transform in the spleen and lymph-nodes on the F_1 hybrid recipient into a cell with a very different appearance. It is a much larger cell with a basophilic and pyroninophilic cytoplasm associated with a high concentration of ribonucleoprotein. The chromatin pattern of the nucleus is 'open' and the nucleolus is prominent[111]. Electron-microscopic examination of these cells shows that the cytoplasm contains abundant polyribosomes and little or no endoplasmic reticulum so that they are distinguishable from plasma-cell precursors, which have abundant endoplasmic reticulum. This change is called lymphoblastic transformation. It is not confined to GVH reactions, but is also seen in lymph-nodes which drain the site of application of a skin-sensitising chemical, or lymph-nodes reacting to a skin graft[88]. There is no reason to doubt that this transformation is a consequence of T lymphocytes reacting to antigen.

The large pyroninophilic cells into which small lymphocytes transform, enter a DNA synthetic phase and continue into a rapid sequence of several successive cell divisions[111]. The progeny of successive divisions are progressively smaller cells and eventually an expanded clone of small lymphocytes is produced from each small lymphocyte which reacts initially[77, 88, 94]. Whereas the large pyroninophilic cell is fixed in tissues its progeny are mobile cells; they are released into the blood and distributed throughout the body.

This sequence of events has been studied *in vitro* by culturing lymphocytes from an immune subject in the presence of tuberculin[115]. Each lymphocyte which reacted produced 64 daughter cells or more and the generation time varied from 7.5 to 38 h. Lymphoblastic transformation has also been studied *in vitro* using phytohaemagglutamin and other mitogens. Phytohaemagglutamin induces transformation only in T lymphocytes[116] and acts not by virtue of its antigenicity but as a nonspecific mitogen presumably inducing transformation in cells which react to many different antigens. Phytohaemagglutamin short circuits the normal mechanism of antigenic activation to produce blast cells of identical appearance to those induced by antigen.

3.4.4 The implementation of cell-mediated immunity

3.4.4.1 The role of sensitised lymphocytes

An immune animal gives a delayed hypersensitivity reaction following a challenging injection of antigen into the skin or elsewhere. This reaction is believed to be implemented by a population of lymphocytes which have arisen within lymphoid tissue in response to the original exposure to antigen. These sensitised lymphocytes require to make close contact with the antigen in order to set in train local events which are apparent as an inflammatory or necrotic lesion. The rejection of skin grafts and usually of organ grafts is due similarly to the production of a population of sensitised lymphocytes. Accelerated second-set rejection of a graft occurs if the recipient already possesses a population of sensitised lymphocytes.

Two general approaches to the study of these events have been pursued. Firstly, *in vitro* 'models' of cell-mediated immunity have been set up, in which cells from an immune animal have been exposed to antigen and consequences have been observed which are thought to be relevant to delayed hypersensitivity or graft rejection. Secondly, the origin of the cells which infiltrate a delayed hypersensitivity lesion or a skin graft prior to rejection have been studied *in vivo*. Naturally, *in vitro* systems permit a more detailed analysis of events but there is a major difficulty in assessing the relevance of *in vitro* phenomena to complicated processes in the whole animal.

3.4.4.2 In vitro *experiments*

A simple method for measuring the rate of migration of peritoneal exudate cells *in vitro* was developed by George and Vaughan[117]. They confirmed previous work which suggested that the movement of lymphoid cells from an immune guinea-pig was slowed down in the presence of the antigen to which the animal had been sensitised[118]. Later it was found that, whereas most of the cells which were immobilised were macrophages, this was consequent upon the interaction of antigen with sensitised lymphocytes in the peritoneal exudate population[119]. This led to the isolation of a soluble protein from cultures of immune lymphocytes and antigen which would inhibit the migration of any macrophages. This protein, migration inhibition factor (MIF), was found to be less effective in the absence of specific antigen[120]. Thus, macrophage migration is influenced by the combined action of MIF and antigen; in this respect MIF resembles the T cell product which is believed to underlie the co-operation of T lymphocytes, B lymphocytes and macrophages in antibody responses[66] (Section 3.3.1.5).

Soluble factors which are released when immune lymphocytes meet antigen ('lymphokines') have been shown to have many other activities of which a mitogenic influence on other lymphocytes[59] and a cytoxic action are arguably the most interesting. In delayed hypersensitivity to tuberculin, the cytotoxic factor is active against 'innocent bystanders', that is, cells which do not contain and are not coated with the antigen[121]. It is supposed that the cytotoxic factor may be responsible for the necrosis occurring in delayed hypersensitivity and that MIF may be instrumental in inducing macrophages to accumulate. However, evidence that these substances do in fact play a significant role is lacking.

Experiments on the cytotoxic activity of lymphocytes immune to the transplantation antigens of target cells have already been described[6-8] (Section 3.2.2). The cytotoxic activity was inhibited by an anti-theta serum which is good evidence that the cells are thymus-derived. It is almost certain that these cytotoxic cells are the progeny of the T lymphocytes which transformed in lymphoid tissue in response to the primary injection of antigen, although this has not been proved rigorously except in a GVH system[94,138].

3.4.4.3 In vivo *experiments*

Histological examination of a delayed hypersensitivity lesion or a graft undergoing rejection shows a heavy cellular infiltrate consisting predominantly of mononuclear cells. Some of these are typical small lymphocytes but usually most are larger cells which in this situation are difficult to classify as macrophages or large lymphocytes. Most of the mononuclear cells enter the lesion from the blood and have been produced by division of precursors in the bone marrow within the previous few days[122]. Thus, thymus-derived small lymphocytes do not make a dominant contribution to the infiltrate. Experiments in which immune lymphoid populations are labelled and followed into skin grafts have suggested that such cells enter grafts indiscriminately, that is, regardless of its antigenic constitution[123, 124]. This raises a difficult paradox in that it is well established that the transfer of sensitised lymphocytes to a previously non-immune animal brings about accelerated second-set rejection[10]. Furthermore, when primary rejection is long delayed by grafting on to an alymphatic bed, the transfer of sensitised lymphocytes is followed by prompt second-set rejection[108]. How do sensitised lymphocytes bring about rejection if most of them do not enter the graft? The paradox is usually resolved by supposing that a small minority of lymphocytes in the cellular infiltrate which are specifically reactive against the relevant antigens are capable of initiating the lesion[125]; the infiltration of other cells is a consequence of this. There is recent evidence that there is a slight accumulation of specifically-reactive cells in skin grafts[126]. However, the part played by the majority of mononuclear cells, which are not specifically reactive, is unclear. There has been much speculation that the recruitment of macrophages may be important in reinforcing the attack of lymphocytes on target cells. However it is equally plausible that macrophages play no essential role in the destructive process but merely dispose of the cell debris which has resulted from the aggressive activity of sensitised lymphocytes.

3.4.5 Anomalous aspects of cell-mediated immunity to strong transplantation antigens

The rejection of tissue grafts is governed by genetically-determined antigens. In the few species which have been studied thoroughly, multiple independently-segregating genes determine the rejection of skin grafts. However, in each species a major locus has been identified, e.g. H-2 in the mouse and HL-A in the human. The immune response to the 'strong' antigens determined by a major locus is in several important respects different to the immune response to the 'weak' antigens determined by the other minor loci. (Chapter 9)[127].
  Experiments on the cytotoxic action of immune lymphocytes on target

cells bearing a complex of several antigenic specificities, which were all determined by genes within the H-2 locus, have revealed several differences from the *in vitro* systems of delayed hypersensitivity, for example, to tuberculin. When a mixture of specific and non-specific target cells are exposed to immune lymphocytes the 'innocent bystanders' are unharmed, so target cell lysis is a consequence of direct contact by the attacking cells; there is no evidence of a cytotoxic factor in this system[7]. A more disturbing and heterodox conclusion is based on the detailed results of Brondz[128]. Using a range of inbred strains he immunised mice with one set of H-2 antigens and tested their lymphoid cells for cytotoxicity against either the same set of H-2 antigens or a different but overlapping set. In general the target cells were attacked only when the immunising set of antigens and the target cell set were the same or nearly the same. Brondz concludes that the immune cells recognised not single antigenic specificities but a certain pattern of specificities on the surface of target cells and he cites an impressive body of evidence in support of this. One difficulty in interpretation is that the antigens which are recognised serologically as belonging to the H-2 locus may be different from the antigens which are recognised by immune T lymphocytes and are therefore relevant to cytotoxicity studies. The H-2 locus includes *ca.* 200 cistrons of which several determine established H-2 specificities and others determine antigens which are perhaps only recognised by T-cells[128a].

A second anomaly is the high proportion of T lymphocytes from a non-immune animal which respond to the antigen or antigens determined by the major locus by blastic transformation and cell division. Three groups working on either mixed lymphocyte culture (MLC)[62] or GVH reactions[61, 129] in different species have produced estimates of responders which are between 1 in 10 and 1 in 10^2. This is several orders higher than the proportion of non-immune cells thought to be capable of responding to other antigens, for example 1 in 10^5 to sheep erythrocytes[130] or 1 in 10^6 to flagellin[131]. Although such a high proportion of lymphocytes proliferate in GVH reactions and in MLC there is no doubt that different cells respond to different antigens[13, 132] as in responses to other antigens. It is not clear whether an exceptionally high proportion of lymphocytes are responsive to transplantation antigens of *other* species. Lafferty and Jones showed that vigorous GVH activity is usually confined to donor–host combinations belonging to the same species or to closely related species[134] and the MLC response of lymphocytes to antigens of distant species is usually less, but there are some exceptions[135].

The biological significance of the exceptional number of lymphocytes precommitted to respond to strong transplantation antigens is unknown but of several possibilities recently discussed[136] one can now be discounted. The idea that animals are pre-immunised by microbial antigens which cross-react with transplantation antigens has been contradicted by the finding that the lymphocytes of germ-free rats are fully active in both MLC and GVH reactions[137].

Recent experiments on a parental *vs.* F_1 hybrid GVH system have illuminated some points while emphasising the paradoxes. Sprent and Miller injected parental thymus cells into irradiated F_1 hybrid mice of a different H-2 phenotype[93, 113, 138]. Between 3 and 5 days after transfer, a torrent of large and small lymphocytes issued from the lymphoid tissue of the recipient into the thoracic duct. These cells were all derived from the transferred thymus cells which had proliferated in response to the H-2 antigens of the hybrid recipient. These 'activated T.TDL' had substantial cytotoxic activity which was specific for target cells bearing the same antigens as the host in which they had been produced[138]. However, their proliferative activity in GVH or MLC against presumably the same antigens was reduced. The most straightforward interpretation of this is that the cells which react by proliferation are different from those which exert a cytotoxic effect, although rigorous evidence for this has still to be obtained.

An alternative mechanism of specific target-cell destruction has been found in circumstances of cross-species immunisation in which T lymphocytes are not involved. Two cells are required; one secretes specific antibody which adheres to the target cells, the second plays a non-specific role[139]. It is undecided whether the latter is a monocyte or a special class of B lymphocyte. It is not certain that this mechanism is important in graft rejection or even that it is properly classified as cell-mediated immunity.

3.5 IMMUNOLOGICAL MEMORY

3.5.1 Definition

Acquired immunity has come to mean an alteration in the way an animal reacts to antigen and, therefore, in the broad sense, all immune phenomena are examples of memory. However 'immunological memory' is now used in a more restricted sense which is best explained by an example. After a second intravenous injection antigenic material is normally eliminated more rapidly because of antibody remaining from the first response; this is not regarded as immunological memory. The second administration of antigen also leads to a new (secondary) antibody response which begins earlier and usually achieves higher titres. Moreover the affinity of the antibody is, as a rule, consistently high throughout the secondary response whereas it is low at least at the start of the primary response[140]. The capacity to produce a secondary antibody response is based on changes in the population of antigen-sensitive cells and it is this that is referred to as immunological memory.

In the case of antibody responses, it has been established that antibody-forming cells are not antigen-sensitive precursors in a secondary response[141]. but in cell-mediated immunity the situation is less clear. This is because, instead of residual antibody, there remains sensitised lymphocytes whose activities may be difficult to distinguish from a new response, i.e. a true secondary response in cell-mediated immunity. However, reasons will be given later for supposing that in cell-mediated immunity the sensitised lymphocytes which implement a response are different from the lymphocytes which initiate a new response to a second dose of antigen.

3.5.2 The cellular basis of memory

As described earlier, the ability to give a secondary antibody response can be conferred on a virgin animal by prior injection of recirculating lymphocytes from an immune animal[25], showing that immunological memory is disseminated throughout the body by lymphocyte migration. However, removal of most of the recirculating lymphocytes after priming does not significantly affect a secondary response[142]. The implication that there is a supplementary mechanism for immunological memory has been substantiated recently by experiments in which a primary antigenic stimulus is confined to one footpad. When a second dose of antigen is given into the opposite foot a secondary response is seen in the draining lymph-node (contralateral to the first injection) presumably because of its supply of recirculating lymphocytes. However, a more rapid and more vigorous response occurs if the antigenic challenge is given to the same lymph-node as responded to the first stimulus. After a few weeks the responses of the contralateral and ipsilateral nodes converge but the substantial difference found at first suggests that there is a local form of memory of which the cellular basis is unknown[143, 144].

The size of a primary antigen dose has also been found to be critical for the development of immunological memory. A large dose of sheep erythrocytes which gave maximum antibody titres was ineffective in priming for a secondary response and this was not due to antibody feed-back inhibition. By contrast, very small doses of antigen which produced no detectable primary response did produce immunological memory and the optimum antigen dose for priming is a moderate dose which is much below the optimum for a primary antibody response[145]. Thus, a primary response and priming for the secondary response appear to be competitive. This is explained most easily by supposing that both antibody-forming cells and memory cells are derived from the same virgin precursors.

The model of Sercarz and Coons[146] proposes the existence of a primed antigen-sensitive cell (y-cell) as a necessary intermediate stage between the virgin antigen-sensitive precursor (x-cell) and the antibody-forming cell (z-cell) (Figure 3.9). Only small doses of antigen are required to produce the $x \rightarrow y$ transformation which takes a finite period of perhaps a few days. The $y \rightarrow z$ transformation is produced by persistent antigen or by a second administration of antigen. The basis of immunological memory is a population of y-cells—a type of cell which is absent from the non-immune animal.

An alternative model denies the existence of the y cell (Figure 3.9b). Immunological memory is due to expansion of a selected population of x-cells. Because it is known that the *population* of cells which respond in an immune animal is different from the population which responds to the primary stimulus (apart from simply being expanded), the affinities of the antibody-like receptors must be considered. It is supposed that virgin cells with a wide range of affinities are activated by a primary injection of antigen (Figure 3.9b). This leads at some stage to asymmetric cell division resulting in z-cells plus an expanded population of x-cells identical with the virgins. As the concentration of antigen falls, the high-affinity x-cells have a selective advantage in competing for antigen and proliferate throughout one or more new cycles of asymmetric cell division; the low-affinity x^1-cells are not reactivated. This model is consistent with evidence that the changes in affinity throughout the primary response reflect the change in affinity of the antigen-sensitive cells[147]. It also fits in with the high-affinity antibody produced at the start of a primary response to an exceptionally small dose of antigen[148]. There is also some evidence for asymmetric cell division[99], although it is probably uncommon[149].

The choice between the alternative models hinges on whether there is a qualitative difference between the individual cells (rather than populations) which react in primary and secondary responses. Such a qualitative difference has been suggested by the finding that the primary response to sheep erythrocytes is inhibited specifically by the passive transfer of 7-S antibody but

Theories of immunological memory

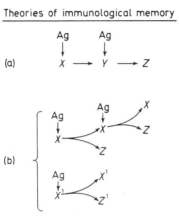

Figure 3.9 Alternative hypothesis of immunological memory. (a) is the X-Y-Z hypothesis of Sercarz and Coons; (b) envisages asymmetric cell division and takes into account precursor cells with receptors of high (x) and low (x^1) affinities. For full explanation see text.

the secondary response is resistant[150]. However, this is not difficult to reconcile with the asymmetric cell division model because the passively-transferred antibody and cell-bound receptor antibody can be thought of as competing for the same antigen. The high-affinity receptors of an immune population will have an advantage compared to the receptors of lower average affinity in an non-immune population.

3.5.3 Memory in cell-mediated immunity

Similar considerations probably apply in cell-mediated immunity. However, while individual antibody-forming cells are now easily distinguishable, individual cytotoxic lymphocytes are not yet identifiable. Therefore, the evidence that the T lymphocytes in an immune population which respond by proliferation (memory cells) are different from the effector (e.g. cytotoxic) lymphocytes is circumstantial and unsatisfactory. In two situations immunisation against strong transplantation antigens brought about a large increase in cytotoxic activity while proliferative activity against the same antigens fell[138, 151]. This is awkward to reconcile with the idea that the cyto-toxic cells in an immune population are the same as those which react by proliferation. It is likely to be analogous to the situation in which a large dose of antigen produces a maximal number of antibody-forming cells but is defective in priming for a secondary response[145]. Also, in patients immunised with brucellin, migration inhibition, presumably an effector cell function, is not correlated with antigen-induced lymphocyte proliferation, presumably a test of memory. This dissociation is seen between the temporal patterns of the two measurements and also in the two measurements between individual patients[152]. It is uncertain whether the helper function of T cells in thymus-dependent antibody responses is attributable to cytotoxic cells, 'memory' cells or to a third population.

3.5.4 Germinal centres and immunological memory

As described in the previous chapter, germinal centres are located in thymus independent areas of peripheral lymphoid organs such as the lymph-nodes and spleen and sometimes in other tissues in response to local antigenic stimulation. They may have nothing to do with immunological memory but the notion that they are involved in the development of memory has been popular for so long that this is a convenient context in which to describe the few facts that are known about them.

The precise structure of germinal centres varies in detail from species to species. A pale spherical mass consisting predominantly of large lymphoid cells is one constant feature. Within this area two types of 'macrophage' may be found (a) tingible-body macrophages which have cytoplasm stuffed with cell debris which is stained by haemotoxylin—hence 'tingible' (Figure 3.10), (b) dendritic cells which have long processes intertwining among the lymphoid cells (Figure 3.6). In mammals there is a collar or mantle of thymus-independent small lymphocytes around the pale centre and the whole structure is called a secondary nodule.

Germinal centres are dependent on antigenic stimulation but they do not begin to appear until after primary antibody response is well developed[153]. There are unquestionably some antibody-forming cells in germinal centres but the bulk of antibody is synthesised elsewhere[154]. Germinal centres expand rapidly, doubling their volume every 10–12 h[153]. Cell division is thought to be mainly responsible for this because a high proportion of the lymphoid cells label after a single injection of [³H]thymidine and mitotic figures are plenti-ful[155]. The life of germinal centres is limited; they regress at about 3 weeks after their appearance[153].

The origin of the lymphoid cells in germinal centres is a subject of confusion. Recirculating T lymphocytes do not localise in these areas[156, 157] but there are reports that a very few B small lymphocytes can enter[158]. Some blast cells injected into the afferent lymph enter germinal centres in the cortex of lymph-nodes[159]. Germinal centres arise in the absence of the thymus and T lympho-cytes, although there is evidence that some thymus-derived cells may be located within them[160].

When labelled antigen is injected, one of several sites of localisation within

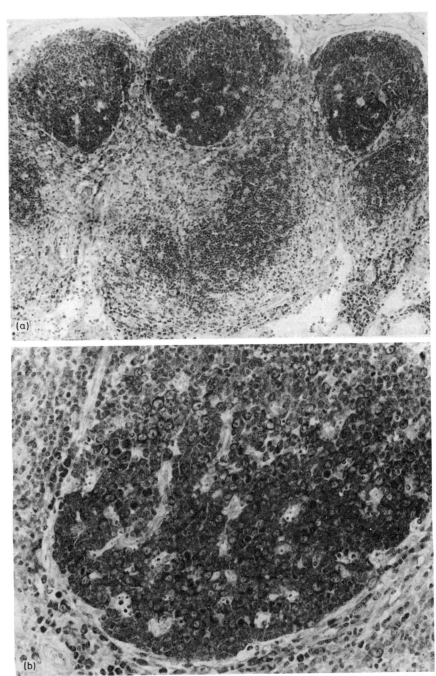

Figure 3.10 Germinal centres in a rabbit lymph-node which was shielded while the animal received whole-body x-irradiation 48 h prior to sacrifice (a) 3 germinal centres are situated in the most superficial part of the lymph-node cortex; (b) a higher power view reveals depletion of the lymphocyte corona which normally surrounds the centre. This is because of redistribution of these cells to lymphoid tissue directly depleted by the irradiation. By contrast the proliferating cells in the germinal centre are unaffected by the irradiation since they are sessile structures. Both mitotic figures and tingible-body macrophages are visible. The latter contains multiple, small, darkly staining (tingible) inclusions. (By courtesy of P. Nieuwenhuis).

lymphoid tissue is on the surface of the dendritic cells within germinal centres as described in Section 3.3.2.1. A recent observation is that two non-cross-reacting antigens will localise in the same follicle[161] which is against the popular image of germinal centres as a specific clone of potential memory cells proliferating in response to an antigen on the surface of dendritic macrophages.

The evidence that germinal centres are involved in immunological memory is only circumstantial. At the height of the germinal-centre formation, small areas of white pulp were dissected out of the spleen. Cell suspensions made from these fragments were highly effective in conferring the ability to give a secondary response when injected into non-immune recipients[162]. The difficulty with interpretation is that while the fragments were rich in germinal centres they were not the only cells transferred. The same workers showed that, when proliferating cells in these spleen fragments were labelled with [³H]thymidine, labelled *small* lymphocytes were later identified in the lymphoid tissue of the recipient[163].

Another approach was to study the lymphocyte population of a thymus-independent area of the rabbit spleen. After whole-body irradiation, this area remained depleted for several weeks but if the appendix was shielded, repopulation occurred more rapidly. However, if the normal antigenic bombardment of the appendix by intestinal flora was prevented, the early repopulation did not occur. Thus the influx of cells into this area of the spleen depended on antigen-induced cell proliferation in the appendix. Most proliferation in the appendix occurs in germinal centres which is further evidence that they produce some B lymphocytes[164]. Thus there is reasonable evidence that some of the recirculating pool of B lymphocytes are produced by cell division within germinal centres. However, most of the small lymphocytes in the collar around a germinal centre are not produced within that particular centre[165]. After four international conferences on the subject[129, 155, 157, 164], the function of germinal centres remains a great enigma.

3.6 INTERACTION BETWEEN ANTIBODY RESPONSES AND CELL-MEDIATED IMMUNITY

3.6.1 Immunological enhancement

When the recipient of a transferable tumour is injected with antiserum against the tumour, the growth of the tumour may be accelerated[166]. The mechanism of this effect, which is called immunological enhancement, is specific inhibition by antibody of the cell-mediated response of the recipient against the tumour. Many examples could be cited of inhibition of the cell-mediated response against tumour grafts, kidney grafts[167] and skin grafts[168] following the transfer of antibody directed against the graft antigens. By contrast, classical delayed hypersensitivity is much more difficult to suppress with antibody[169]. Pretreatment with a moderate dose of antibody against flagellin or sheep erythrocytes did not reduce but increased delayed hypersensitivity while the antibody response was completely suppressed[170]. On the other hand, delayed hypersensitivity to flagellin has been suppressed by a *small* dose of passively-transferred antibody[171]. The inhibitory effect of passive antibody on the antibody response also depends on dosage since pretreatment with small doses of IgM can actually augment the response[171, 172]. In short, both cell-mediated immunity and antibody responses can be suppressed or augmented by pretreatment with antibody but the conditions for each are different.

An analogy is often drawn between immunological enhancement and the feed-back inhibition of passively-transferred antibody on antibody responses[169]. Antibody responses are blocked at the induction stage, as has been confirmed by the recent finding that the recruitment of antigen-sensitive lymphocytes from the recirculating pool is prevented by passively administered antibody[84]. It is natural to suppose that the enhancement of graft survival may be due to blocking of the cell-mediated response at its induction (i.e. afferent inhibition). An alternative mechanism is that the response starts normally, a population of sensitised lymphocytes builds up but they fail to recognise the antigenic target cells in the presence of antibody (i.e. efferent inhibition). Afferent inhibition can be reproduced *in vitro* when a 'one-way' mixed lymphocyte culture is set up (Section 3.4.5). Antibody directed against the 'stimulating' cells prevents the proliferation of the 'responding' cells[173]. Efferent inhibition can also be mimicked *in vitro* since antibody directed against target cells blocks the cytotoxic action of immune lymphocytes[174]. There is a large literature on mechanisms of enhancement *in vivo* which includes evidence in favour of both afferent and efferent inhibition. The analysis of the class of antibody to which enhancing activity belongs has not yet made much progress.

3.6.2 Do humoral and cell-mediated responses compete for T cells?

Although delayed hypersensitivity and antibody formation often occur together, it has been pointed out that anything which increases the one tends to diminish the other. This has recently been highlighted by experiments involving the chemical modification of flagellin by acetoacetylation, which can be graded precisely[175]. Aceto-acetyl flagellin does not produce an antibody response to flagellin; indeed it tends to produce antibody tolerance. On the other hand, it does induce marked delayed hypersensitivity to unmodified flagellin. Because of this and other findings, Parish argues that the antagonism between antibody formation and delayed hypersensitivity has a deeper significance than antibody feed-back inhibition. His hypothesis is based on the premise that the same subpopulation of T cells may either implement delayed hypersensitivity or collaborate with B cells in antibody responses, but cannot do both at the same time. Thus thymus-dependent antibody formation and delayed hypersensitivity somehow compete for reactive T cells[175]. This seems a useful working hypothesis but until the mechanism of T–B collaboration is firmly established any discussion of why T cells may be restricted to either helper cell formation or delayed hypersensitivity would be speculative.

3.7 CONCLUSIONS

If the anatomical details are left aside, the cellular events in immune responses can be boiled down to a rather simple statement as follows. There arises during development a large number of lymphocyte subpopulations each of which is precommitted to respond to only one antigen by virtue of an antibody-like receptor on its surface. Presentation of a sufficient amount of antigen in a suitable form to these receptors activitates lymphocytes to proliferate and differentiate. This gives rise to (a) antibody-forming cells and (b) an expanded population of antigen-sensitive lymphocytes, which is the basis of the larger and earlier secondary response[176].

There are a number of weaknesses and, of course, over-simplifications in this statement, which are dealt with in detail in Chapter 11 but two deserve special emphasis. Selective theories of immunity which envisage that something precommitted to making one specific antibody is selected by antigen have prevailed. There is also good evidence that what is selected by antigen is antigen-sensitive lymphocytes. However, a second stage of selection, at the subcellular level, has not been excluded. The available evidence merely shows that each lymphocyte cannot respond to all or most antigens; it remains possible that each lymphocyte can respond to a very restricted number of antigens. Many experiments show that one antibody-forming cell produces antibody of a single specificity but this does necessarily mean that their antigen-sensitive precursors are similarly unipotential since restriction may follow activation. The obvious experimental approach is to isolate a population all of which can respond to one antigen but this enrichment principle is extremely difficult because exposure of cells to antigen necessary for their separation may inevitably change their properties in relation to a second antigen.

A second uncertainty is how far the statement applies to cell-mediated immunity obviously with the substitution of 'sensitised lymphocyte' for 'antibody-forming cell'. There is no doubt that, as with the B lymphocyte system, different T cells respond to different antigens by virtue of antigen-binding receptors[38, 42, 43, 132, 133]. However, cell-mediated immunity seems to have evolved in invertebrates at a considerably earlier stage than the antibody system which appears in cyclostomes[177]. We have not even begun to understand the evolutionary relationship between the two systems.

References

1. Pauling, L. (1940). *J. Amer. Chem. Soc.*, **62**, 2643
2. Landsteiner, K. and Chase, M. W. (1942). *Proc. Soc. Exp. Biol. Med.*, **49**, 688
3. Bloom, B. R. and Chase, M. W. (1967). *Progr. Allergy*, **10**, 151
4. Hall, J. G. (1969). *Lancet*, **i**, 25
5. Good, R. A., Biggar, W. D. and Park, B. Y. (1971). *Progress in Immunology*, 699 (New York: Academic Press)
6. Nordin, A. A., Cerottini, J. C. and Brunner, K. T. (1971). *Europ. J. Immunol.*, **1**, 55
7. Brunner, K. T. and Cerottini, J. C. (1971). *Progress in Immunology*, 365, (New York: Academic Press)
8. Mauel, J., Rudolf, H., Chapius, B. and Brunner, K. T. (1970). *Immunology*, **18**, 517
9. Medawar, P. B. (1958). *Proc. Roy. Soc. (London), B.*, **149**, 145

10. Billingham, R. E., Brent, L. and Medawar, P. B. (1954). *Proc. Roy. Soc. (London) B.*, **143**, 58
11. Uhr, J. W. (1966). *Phys. Rev.*, **46**, 359
12. Boyden, S. V. (1963) in Cell Bound Antibodies, 7 (B. Amos and H. Koprowski editors) (Philadelphia: Wister Institute Press)
13. Ishizaka, K. and Ishizaka, T. (1971). *Progress in Immunology*, 859 (New York: Academic Press)
14. Coombs, R. R. A. and Gell, P. G. H. (1968). *Clinical Aspects of Immunology*, 2nd edition, 575 (Gell, P. G. H. and Coombs, R. R. A., editors) (Oxford: Blackwell)
15. Jerne, N. K. (1968). *Cold Spring Harbor Symp. Quant. Biol.*, **32**, 591
16. Coons, A. H., Leduc, E. H. and Connolly, J. M. (1955). *J. Exp. Med.*, **102**, 49
17. Leduc, E. H., Coons, A. H. and Connolly, J. M. (1955). *J. Exp. Med.*, **102**, 61
18. Fagraeus, A. (1948). *Acta Med. Scand.*, **Suppl. 204**, 1
19. Jerne, N. K. and Nordin, A. A. (1963). *Science*, **140**, 405
20. Harris, T. N., Hummelerk, K. and Harris, S. (1966). *J. Exp. Med.*, **123**, 161
21. Leduc, E. H., Avrameas, S. and Bouteille, M. (1968). *J. Exp. Med.*, **127**, 109
22. Hay, J. B., Murphy, M. J., Morris, B. and Bessis, M. C. (1972). *Amer. J. Path.*, **66**, 1
23. Claflin, A. J. and Smithies, O. (1967). *Science*, **157**, 1561
24. Gowans, J. L. and McGregor, D. D. (1965). *Progr. Allergy*, **9**, 1
25. Gowans, J. L. and Uhr, J. W. (1966). *J. Exp. Med.*, **124**, 1017
26. McGregor, D. D., McCullagh, P. J. and Gowans, J. L. (1967). *Proc. Roy. Soc. (London) B.*, **168**, 229
27. Ellis, S. T., Gowans, J. L. and Howard, J. C. (1969). *Antibiot. et Chemother. (Basel)*, **15**, 40
28. Naor, D. and Sulitzeanu, D. (1967). *Nature (London)*, **214**, 687
29. Ada, G. L., Byrt, P., Mandel, T. and Warner, N. (1970). *Developmental Aspects of Antibody Structure and Function*, 503 (J. Sterzl and I. Riha editors) (New York: Academic Press)
30. Humphrey, J. H. and Keller, H. U. (1970). *Developmental Aspects of Antibody Formation and Structure*, 485 (J. Sterzl and M. Riha, editors) (New York: Academic Press)
31. Dutton, R. W. and Mishell, R. I. (1967). *J. Exp. Med.*, **126**, 443
32. Wigzell, H. and Andersson, B. (1969). *J. Exp. Med.*, **129**, 23
33. Wigzell, H. (1970). *Transplant Rev.*, **5**, 76
34. Rutihauser, U., Millette, C. F. and Edelman, G. M. (1972). *Proc. Nat. Acad. Sci. (U.S.A.)*, **69**, 1596
35. Davies, A. J. S., Leuchars, E., Wallis, V. and Koller, P. C. (1966). *Transplant*, **4**, 438
36. Claman, H. N., Chaperon, E. A. and Triplett, R. F. (1966). *J. Immunol.*, **97**, 828
37. Miller, J. F. A. P. and Mitchell, G. F. (1969). *Transplant Rev.*, **1**, 3
38. Greaves, M. F., Owen, J. J. T. and Raff, M. C. (1973). *T and B Lymphocytes: Origins, properties and roles in immune responses*, in the press (Amsterdam: A.S.P.Elsevier-Excerpta Medica–North Holland)
39. Mitchell, G. F. (1973). *Contemporary Topics in Immunobiology*, **3**. In the press
40. Mitchell, G. F., Mishell, R. I. and Herzenberg, L. A. (1971). *Progress in Immunology*, 324. (New York: Academic Press)
41. Nossal, G. J. V. (1971). *Progress in Immunology*, 665, (New York: Academic Press)
42. Basten, A., Miller, J. F. A. P., Warner, N. L. and Pye, J. (1971). *Nature New Biol*, **231**, 104
43. Roelants, G. E. and Askonas, B. A. (1971). *Europ. J. Immunol.*, **1**, 151
44. Mitchison, N. A. (1971). *Europ. J. Immunol.*, **1**, 68
45. del Guerico, P. and Leuchars, E. (1972). *J. Immunol.*, **109**, 951
46. Paul, W. E. (1970). *Transplant Rev.*, **5**, 130
47. Humphrey, J. H., Parrott, D. M. V. and East, J. (1964). *Immunology*, **7**, 419
48. Miller, J. F. A. P., Basten, A., Sprent, J. and Cheers, C. (1971). *Cell Immunol.*, **2**, 469
49. Stavitsky, A. B. (1961). *Advan. Immunol.*, **1**, 211
50. Marbrook, J. (1967). *Lancet*, **ii**, 1279
51. Dutton, R. W., McCarthy, M. M., Mishell, R. I. and Raidt, D. J. (1970). *Cell. Immunol* **1**, 196
52. Hartmann, K. U. (1970). *J. Exp. Med.*, **132**, 1267
53. Schimpl, A. and Wecker, E. (1971). *Europ. J. Immunol.*, **1**, 304

54. Feldmann, M. and Basten, A. (1972). *J. Exp. Med.*, **136**, 49
55. Mosier, D. E. (1967). *Science*, **158**, 1575
56. Codenza, H., Lozerman, L. D. and Rowley, D. A. (1971). *J. Immunol.*, **107**, 414
57. Mitchison, N. A., Rajewsky, K. and Taylor, R. B. (1970). *Developmental Aspects of Antibody Structure and Function*, 547 (J. Sterzl and I. Riha, editors) (New York: Academic Press)
58. Schierman, L. W. and McBride, R. A. (1967). *Science*, **156**, 658
59. Vischer, T. L. (1972). *J. Immunol.*, **109**, 401
60. Osborne, D. F. and Katz, D. M. (1972). *J. Exp. Med.*, **136**, 439
61. Nisbet, N. W., Simonsen, M. and Zaleski, M. (1969). *J. Exp. Med.*, **129**, 459
62. Wilson, D. B. Blyth, J. L. and Nowell, P. C. (1968). *J. Exp. Med.*, **128**, 1157
63. Feldmann, M. and Basten, A. (1972). *Europ. J. Immunol.*, **2**, 213
64. Feldmann, M. and Basten, A. (1972). *J. Exp. Med.*, **136**, 722
65. Marchalonis, J. J., Cone, R. E. and Atwell, J. L. (1972). *J. Exp. Med.*, **135**, 956
66. Feldman, M. and Nossal, G. J. V. (1972). *Transplant. Rev.*, in the press
66a. Feldman, M. (1972). *J. Exp. Med.*, **136**, 737
67. Bretscher, P. A. and Cohn, M. (1970). *Science*, **169**, 1042
68. Cohn, M. (1972). *Cell Immunol.*, **5**, 1
69. McDevitt, H. O., Askonas, B. A., Humphrey, J. H., Schechter, I. and Sela, M. (1966). *Immunology*, **11**, 337
70. Rabinovitch, M. (1970). *Mononuclear Phagocytes*, 299 (R. Van Furth, editor) (Oxford: Blackwell)
71. Nossal, G. J. V. and Ada, G. L. (1971). *Antigens, Lymphoid Cells and the Immune Response*, 154 (New York: Academic Press)
72. Mackaness, G. B. and Blanden, R. V. (1967). *Progr. Allergy*, **11**, 89
73. Fishman, M. and Adler, F. L. (1967). *Cold Spring Harbor Symp. Quant. Biol.*, **32**, 343
74. Askonas, B. A. and Rhodes, J. M. (1965). *Nature (London)*, **205**, 470
75. Unanue, E. R. and Askonas, B. A. (1968). *J. Exp. Med.*, **127**, 915
76. Unanue, E. R. and Cerottini, J. C. (1970). *J. Exp. Med.*, **131**, 711
77. Ford, W. L., Gowans, J. L. and McCullagh, P. J. (1966). in *Ciba Found. Symp.* on *The Thymus*, 58, (G. E. W. Wolstenholme and R. Porter editors) (London: Churchill)
78. Shortman, K. and Palmer, J. (1971). *Cell Immunol.*, **2**, 399
79. Askonas, B. A. and Jaroskova, L. (1971). *Developmental Aspects of Antibody Formation and Structure*, Vol. 2., (J. Sterzl and M. Riha editors) (Prague: Publ. House of the Czech Acad. Sci.)
80. Roberts, K. B. and Gowans, J. L. (1970). *General Pathology*, 4th edn., 998 (Lord Florey editor) (London: Lloyd-Luke)
81. Humphrey, J. H. (1969). *Antibiot. et Chemother.*, **15**, 7
82. Hunter, R. L., Wissler, R. W. and Fitch, F. W. (1969). *Advan. Exp. Biol. Med.*, **5**, 101
83. Sprent, J., Miller, J. F. A. P. and Mitchell, G. F. (1971). *Cell Immunol.* **2**, 171
84. Rowley, D. A., Gowans, J. L., Atkins, R. C., Ford, W. L. and Smith, M. E. (1972). *J. Exp. Med.*, **136**, 499
85. O'Toole, C. M. and Davies, A. J. S. (1972). *Nature (London)*, **230**, 187
86. Kerbel, R. S. and Eidinger, D. (1971). *J. Exp. Med.*, **133**, 1043
87. Langevoort, H. L. (1963). *Lab. Invest.*, **12**, 106
88. Turk, J. L. (1967). *Brit. Med. Bull*, **23**, 1
89. Veldman, J. (1970). *Histophysiology and Electron Microscopy of the Immune Response* Thesis (Groningen: Wolters-Noordhoff)
90. Pelc, S. R., Harris, G. and Caldwell, I. (1972). *Immunology*, **23**, 183
91. Hall, J. G. and Morris, B. (1965). *Brit. J. Exp. Path.*, **46**, 450
92. Hall, J. G., Morris, B., Moreno, G. D. and Bessis, M. C. (1967). *J. Exp. Med.*, **125**, 91
93. Hall, J. G. and Smith, M. E. (1970). *Nature (London)*, **226**, 262
94. Sprent, J. and Miller, J. F. A. P. (1972). *Cell Immunol.*, **3**, 385
95. Wortis, H. H., Taylor, R. B. and Dresser, D. W. (1966). *Immunology*, **11**, 603
96. Koros, A. M. C., Mazur, J. M. and Mowery, M. J. (1968). *J. Exp. Med.*, **128**, 235
97. Davie, J. M. and Paul, W. E. (1972). *J. Exp. Med.*, **135**, 660
98. Nakamura, I., Segal, S., Globerson, A. and Feldman, M. (1972). *Cell Immunol.*, **4**, 351
99. Tannenberg, W. J. K., and Malaviya, A. N. (1968). *J. Exp. Med.*, **128**, 895
100. Sterzl, J., Vesely, J., Jilek, M. and Mandel, M. (1965). Molecular and Cellular Basis of Antibody Formation. (J'. Sterzl, editor) 463 (Prague: Czech. Academy of Sciences)

101. Ford, W. L. (1968). *Immunology*, **15**, 609
102. Sell, S., Lowe, J. A. and Gell, P. G. H. (1972). *J. Immunol.*, **108**, 674
103. Ellis, S. T., Gowans, J. L. and Howard, J. C. (1967). *Cold Spring Harbor Symp. Quant. Biol.*, **32**, 395
104. Cooper, M. D., Cain, W. A., Van Alten, P. J. and Good, R. A. (1969). *Internat. Arch. Allergy Appl. Immunol.*, **35**, 242
105. Durkin, H. G., Thesis, G. A. and Thorbecke, G. J. (1971). *Advan. Exp. Med. Biol.*, **12**, 119
106. Pappenheimer, A. M. and Freund, J. (1969). *Cellular and Humoral Aspects of the Hypersensitive State*, 67 (H. Sherwood Lawrence, editor) (London: Cassell)
107. Barker, C. F. and Billingham, R. E. (1968). *J. Exp. Med.*, **128**, 197
108. Tilney, N. L. and Gowans, J. L. (1971). *J. Exp. Med.*, **133**, 951
109. Macher, E. and Chase, M. W. ((1969). *J. Exp. Med.*, **129**, 103
110. Elkins, W. L. (1972). *Progr. Allergy*, **15**, 70
111. Gowans, J. L. (1962). *Ann. N.Y. Acad. Sci.*, **99**, 432
112. Johnston, J. M. and Wilson, D. B. (1970). *Cell Immunol.*, **1**, 430
113. Sprent, J. and Miller, J. F. A. P. (1972). *Cell Immunol.*, **3**, 361
114. Hilgard, H. R. (1970). *J. Exp. Med.*, **132**, 317
115. Marshall, W. H., Valentine, F. T. and Lawrence, H. S. (1969). *J. Exp. Med.*, **130**, 327
116. Doenhoff, M. J., Davies, A. J. S., Leuchars, E. and Wallis, V. (1970). *Proc. Roy. Soc. (London) B.*, **176**, 69
117. George, M. and Vaughan, J. H. (1962). *Proc. Soc. Exp. Biol. Med.*, **111**, 514
118. Rich, A. R. and Lewis, M. R. (1932). *Bull John Hopkins Hosp.*, **50**, 115
119. Bloom, B. R. and Bennett, B. (1966). *Science*, **153**, 80
120. Amos, H. E. and Lachman, P. J. (1970). *Immunology*, **18**, 269
121. Ruddle, N. H. and Waksman, B. H. (1968). *J. Exp. Med.*, **128**, 1267
122. Lubaroff, D. M. and Waksman, B. H. (1968). *J. Exp. Med.*, **128**, 1437
123. Prendergast, R. A. (1964). *J. Exp. Med.*, **119**, 337
124. Hall, J. G. (1967). *J. Exp. Med.*, **125**, 737
125. McCluskey, R. T., Benacerraf, B. and McClusky, J. W. (1963). *J. Immunol.*, **90**, 466
126. Lance, E. M. and Cooper, S. (1972). *Cell Immunol.*, **5**, 66
127. Simonsen, M. (1970). *Transplant. Rev*, **3**, 22
128. Brondz, B. D. (1972). *Transplant Rev.*, **10**, 112
128a. Yunis, E. J. and Amos, D. B. (1971). *Proc. Nat. Acad. Sci. (USA)*, **68**, 3031
129. Ford, W. L. and Atkins, R. C. (1973). *Microenvironmental Aspects of Immunity*. p. 255 (B. Jankovic, editor) (New York: Plenum Press)
130. Kennedy, J. C., Till, J. E., Siminovitch, L. and McCulloch, E. A. (1966). *J. Immunol.*, **96**, 973
131. Armstrong, W. D. and Diener, E. (1968). *J. Exp. Med.*, **129**, 371
132. Zoschke, D. C. and Bach, F. H. (1971). *Science*, **172**, 1350
133. Ford, W. L. and Atkins, R. C. (1971). *Nature New Biol.*, **234**, 178
134. Lafferty, K. J. and Jones, M. A. S. (1969). *Aust. J. Exp. Biol. Med. Sci.*, **47**, 17
135. Widmer, M. B. and Bach, F. M. (1972). *J. Exp. Med.*, **135**, 1204
136. Discussion on 'Theories of Immune Surveillance' (1970). in *Immune Surveillance*, 363 (R. T. Smith and M. Landy, editors) (New York: Academic Press)
137. Nielsen, H. E. (1972). *J. Exp. Med.*, **136**, 417
138. Sprent, J. and Miller, J. F. A. P. (1972). *Cell Immunol.*, **3**, 213
139. McLennan, I. C. M. (1972) *Transplant Rev.*, **13**, 67
140. Steiner, L. A. and Eisen, H. N. (1967). *J. Exp. Med.*, **126**, 1185
141. Cunningham, A. J. (1969). *Immunology*, **17**, 333
142. McGregor, D. D. and Gowans, J. L. (1963). *J. Exp. Med.*, **117**, 303
143. Smith, J. B., Cunningham, A. J., Lafferty, K. J. and Morris, B. (1970). *Aust. J. Exp. Biol. Med. Sci.*, **48**, 57
144. Jacobsen, E. B. and Thorbecke, G. J. (1969). *J. Exp. Med.*, **130**, 287
145. Sterzl, J., Sima, P., Medlin, J., Tlaskalova, H., Mandel, L. and Nordin, A. (1970). *Developmental Aspects of Antibody Formation and Structure*, 865 (J. Sterzl and I. Riha, editors) (New York: Academic Press)
146. Sercarz, E. and Coons, A. M. (1962). *Mechanisms of Immunological Tolerance* 73 (M. Hasek, A. Lengerova and M. Vojtiskova, editors) (Prague: Publ. House of the Czech Acad. Sci.)

147. Siskind, G. W. and Benacerraf, B. (1969). *Advan. Immunol.*, **10**, 1
148. Paul, W. E., Siskind, G. W. and Benacerraf, B. (1967). *J. Exp. Med.*, **127**, 25
149. Nossal, G. J. V. and Lewis, H. (1971). *Immunology*, **20**, 739
150. Rowley, D. A. and Fitch, F. W. (1964). *J. Exp. Med.*, **120**, 987
151. Ford, W. L. and Simonsen, M. (1971). *J. Exp. Med.*, **133**, 938
152. Søberg, M., Andersen, V. and Sørensen, S. F. (1971). *Acta Path. Microbiol. Scand. Section B*, **79**, 495
153. Laissue, J., Cottier, M., Hess, M. W. and Stoner, R. D. (1971). *J. Immunol.*, **107**, 822
154. Sordat, B., Sordat, M., Hess, M. W., Stoner, R. D. and Cottier, M. (1970). *J. Exp. Med.*, **131**, 77
155. Nieuwenhuis, P. (1969). *Advan Exp. Med. Biol.*, **5**, 113
156. Gowans, J. L. and Knight, E. J. (1964). *Proc. Roy. Soc. (London) B.*, **159**, 257
157. Parrot, D. M. V. (1967). *Germinal Centres in Immune Responses*, 168 (H. Cottier *et al.*, editors) (Berlin: Springer Verlag)
158. Mitchell, J. (1972). *Immunology*, **22**, 231
159. Kelly, R. M. (1970). *Nature (London)*, **227**, 510
160. Gutman, G. A. and Weissman, I. L. (1972). *Immunology*, **23**, 465
161. Van Rooijen, N. (1972). *Immunology*, **22**, 757
162. Wakefield, J. D. and Thorbecke, G. J. (1968). *J. Exp. Med.*, **128**, 171
163. Wakefield, J. D. and Thorbecke, G. J. (1968). *J. Exp. Med.*, **128**, 153
164. Nieuwenhuis, P. (1971). *Advan. Exp. Med. Biol.*, **12**, 25
165. Fliedner, T. M., Kesse, M., Cronkite, E. P. and Robertson, J. S. (1964). *Ann N.Y. Acad. Sci.*, **113**, 578
166. Kaliss, N. (1962). *Ann N.Y. Acad. Sci.*, **101**, 64
167. French, M. E. and Batchelor, J. R. (1969). *Lancet*, **ii**, 1103
168. Zimmerman, B. and Feldman, J. D. (1969). *J. Immunol.*, **102**, 507
169. Uhr, J. W. and Moller, G. (1968). *Advan. Immunol.*, **8**, 81
170. Liew, F. Y. and Parish, C. R. (1972). *Cell Immunol.*, **4**, 66
171. Liew, F. Y. and Parish, C. R. (1972). *Cell Immunol.*, **5**, 499
172. Henry, C. and Jerne, N. K. (1968). *J. Exp. Med.*, **128**, 133
173. Gordon, R. O., Stinson, E. B., Souther, S. G. and Oppenheim, J. J. (1971). *Transplant.* **12**, 484
174. Brunner, K. T. and Cerottini, J. C. (1971). *Immunological Tolerance to Tissue Antigens*, 31 (N. W. Nisbet and M. W. Elves, editors) (Oswestry, England: Orthopaedic Hospital)
175. Parish, C. R. (1972). *Transplant Rev.*, **13**, 35
176. Mitchison, N. A. (1972). *Immunogenicity* (Neuberger and Tatum, editors). *North Holland Research Monographs, Frontiers of Biology*, **25**, 87
177. Warner, N. L. (1972). *Immunogenicity* (Neuberger and Tatum, editors). *North Holland Research Monographs, Frontiers of Biology*, **25**, 467

4
Immunological Tolerance and Immunosuppression

J. G. HOWARD

Wellcome Research Laboratories, Beckenham, Kent

Abbreviations

BSA and HSA   = bovine and human serum albumins.
BGG and HGG   = bovine and human gamma globulins.
DNP, DNP-BSA and
    DNP-POL = dinitrophenyl (hapten alone or conjugated with BSA or polymerised flagellin).

4.1 IMMUNOLOGICAL TOLERANCE

4.1.1 Introduction

Immunological tolerance may be defined as acquisition by a lymphocyte population of non-reactivity to specific antigenic determinant(s) and, as such, represents the converse modality of response from immunity. This central deletion of reactivity has been traditionally regarded as (a) antigen-mediated and (b) a transferable property of tolerised lymphoid cells. (Consideration of heterodox views will be deferred.) The nature of the phenomenon remains largely unresolved and its elucidation continues to be sought for reasons of fundamental biological interest and because it represents the most desirable basis for human tissue transplantation. The following account describes the major features of tolerance and what, of necessity, can only be an interim assessment of the cellular mechanisms implicated. More detailed coverage of various aspects will be found in some recent reviews and published symposia[1-7].

4.1.2 Historical

The earliest demonstrations of tolerance following the injection of antigen date from the 1920s, when it was noted that high doses of diphtheria toxoid[8] and pneumococcal polysaccharide[9] suppressed the immune response which could be elicited by smaller quantities and that i.v. injection of guinea-pigs with neoarsphenamine made them unresponsive to its skin-sensitising activity[10]. Both the connecting link between these isolated observations and their biological significance remained unappreciated for two decades, although the phenomenon was more intensively studied with regard to polysaccharides by Felton[11] and to chemical allergens by Chase[12]. A landmark in the development of the 'tolerance' concept was the discovery in 1945 by Owen[13] that dizygotic cattle twins which had exchanged embryonic blood as a result of placental fusion, became permanent stable chimaeras with regard to their haemopoietic (blood-cell forming) tissue. Such non-identical animals were subsequently found to accept exchange skin allografts[14]. In a classic series of investigations, Billingham, Brent and Medawar[15, 16] next reproduced this phenomenon experimentally by introducing spleen cells from an unrelated strain into embryonic or neonatal mice. Independently, Hasek[17] also induced cross-tolerance between chick embryos by fusing blood vessels of the chorioallantoic membrane. These findings seemingly fulfilled the prediction of Burnet and Fenner[18] that exposure to 'non-self' before the period of immunological maturity would lead to permanent deletion of responsiveness to the foreign antigens. On this basis, tolerance of histocompatibility antigens acquired before or soon after birth seemed to differ qualitatively from unresponsiveness produced by high doses of other antigens in adults. This distinction was progressively eroded by demonstrations that both immunity and tolerance to all antigens could be produced according to dosage in immature and adult animals alike (e.g. Refs.[19, 20]). By 1961, the unifying concept of 'tolerance' as enunciated in the Introduction had gained widespread acceptance. This view has been challenged recently by a variety of evidence which implies that tolerance may be a multi-component phenomenon. In view of divergent opinions held by workers in the area, personal bias cannot be wholly avoided in presenting this survey.

4.1.3 Nomenclature

The term 'tolerance' was originally applied to the tissue transplantation model. 'Immunological paralysis' and 'specific unresponsiveness' are frequently used pseudonyms, although they were originally restricted to polysaccharide and protein antigens respectively. Some workers still favour the maintenance of these nomenclatural distinctions.

4.1.4 General characteristics of tolerance

4.1.4.1 Nature of the antigen

Immunogenicity and tolerogenicity are inversely correlated attributes of an antigen. It is usually difficult to induce tolerance of highly-immunogenic antigens without application of some additional immunosuppressive measure. Conversely, weak immunogens like heterologous serum proteins are effective tolerogens. The case that a naturally-occurring antigen can be entirely non-immunogenic and fully capable of inducing tolerance has been made decisively with the capsular polypeptide of *Bacillus anthracis*[21], a homopolymer of D-glutamic acid (average mol. wt 33 500). 'Non-immunogenic' forms of antigen will immunise when administered in Freund's adjuvant and this provides the test for prior induction of tolerance.

This inverse association has been exploited experimentally by modifying antigens such that the usual dominance of immunogenicity over tolerogenicity can be reversed. Two main approaches have proved fruitful:

(a) *Reduction in 'size' of antigen*—Dresser[22] found that removal of aggregates from solutions of bovine γ-globulin by centrifugation eliminated its immunising property for mice and left the major fraction of antigen in highly tolerogenic form. A similar separation can sometimes be achieved by what has been termed '*in vivo* screening', whereby the immunogenic particles are rapidly phagocytosed by the reticuloendothelial system (R.E.S.), whereas tolerogenic antigen persists in the circulation for several days[23].

A similar change is associated with reduction in molecular size of an antigen when this can be accomplished without loss of specificity. Polymerised flagellin (the flagellar protein from *Salmonella adelaide*), monomeric flagellin and the fragment A derived from it have respective mol. wts. of 10^7, 40 000 and 18 000, and it is the smallest of these that is the most potent tolerogen and feeblest immunogen. The effects of step-wise depolymerisation have been studied with polyvinylpyrrolidone[24], dextran[25] and levan[26] and a progressively reducing immunogenic capacity was finally extinguished in all three cases with mol. wt. *ca.* 10 000. The non-immunising levan fraction retained strong tolerance-inducing activity. One notable exception to the general rule is type 3 pneumococcal polysaccharide (SIII), analogous depolymerisation of which incurs parallel loss of both immunogenicity and tolerogenicity[27]. This need not create difficulties for the present argument, as the cellular bases for tolerance of SIII and levan in B cells are very dissimilar (Section 4.1.5.3).

The minimum molecular size which is required for tolerance induction is uncertain, but is clearly greater than that of an antigenic determinant. Attempts to produce tolerance with unconjugated haptens have been unsuccessful. On the other hand, whilst DNP coupled to autologous mouse serum is a totally non-immunogenic complex, it is a highly effective tolerogen[28]. (The carrier probably serves to cross-link the hapten-cell receptor complexes, see Section 4.1.5.4).

(b) *Chemical modification of the antigen*—The finding that a protein can be extensively substituted without necessarily altering its antigenic specificity has been exploited in an important series of experiments by Parish[29]. The effect on monomeric flagellin of increasing extents of acetoacetylation by diketene was to destroy progressively its antibody-inducing capacity, whereas affinity for antibody diminished more slowly. The most heavily substituted flagellins (16.8 and 17.8 acetoacetyl groups) were non-immunogenic and 1 μg of them rendered adult rats tolerant to unmodified antigen. Lysine and methyl-lysine residues were substituted more easily than hydroxyl groups and appeared not to be closely associated with antigenic determinants. Acetoacetyl substitution and its sequelae could be largely reversed by hydroxylamine.

The potentiality of this approach to tolerance is likely to be explored further in the immediate future (see also Section 4.1.4.7).

4.1.4.2 Persistence of antigen

Tolerance to tissue grafts can be induced by neonatal injection of allogeneic lymphoid cells and may last throughout the animal's entire life span. This is best accomplished with F_1 donors which are genetically tolerant of the recipient, thereby obviating the risk of graft-versus-host disease. Durable unresponsiveness is attributable to the establishment of stable chimaerism ensuring a continuing source of foreign histocompatibility antigens. Although they gradually diminish in proportion, dividing donor cells are still demonstrable by karyotypic analysis in tolerant mice almost 2 years of age[30]. The presence of antigen also appears to be a general prerequisite for maintenance of tolerance induced by non-living materials. With non-metabolisable antigens, such as pneumococcal polysaccharides in mice, a single injection can induce tolerance which will last for more than a year[31]. Other macromolecules which are metabolised (or eliminated) only slowly, such as levan[32] or polymers of D-amino acids[33] are likewise capable of inducing prolonged tolerance. Unresponsiveness to rapidly catabolisable proteins, on the other hand, is altogether briefer, unless its loss is prevented by further administration of antigen. A 'tolerance maintenance' dose may be required at regular intervals if the antigen is rapidly cleared.

Antigen persistence is mandatory for the continuance of unresponsiveness, but where is it located and in what form? Unaltered pneumococcal polysaccharide can be detected in the serum of tolerant animals due to continuous exocytosis from phagocytosed depots. This is not so with metabolisable antigens and a gap of even months may occur between their clearance from the circulation and escape from tolerance[34]. To what extent these antigens or fragments of them are retained within the tissues during this period is uncertain owing to limitations of technique. The failure to detect them using ^{125}I-labelling may be meaningful, however, so that the lag before recovery most probably represents the time required for replacement of reactive cells.

4.1.4.3 Specificity of tolerance

A similar high degree of specificity characterises both the tolerant and immune states. Mice of strain X rendered tolerant of another strain (Y) across a major (H-2) antigenic incompatibility will still react against tissues of a third strain (Z), even when the extent of non-identity between the latter and strain Y is minimal. The prolonged suppression of response induced by high doses of pneumococcal polysaccharide is entirely type specific and does not impair antibody synthesis to serologically unrelated carbohydrates. Specificity is even more impressively demonstrated with antigens which show degrees of cross-reactivity. The immune responses to pneumococcal polysaccharides SIII and SVIII (glucuronic acid–glucose and glucuronic acid–glucose–glucose–galactose polymers, respectively) possess a shared component. Nevertheless, mice rendered tolerant to SIII can be immunised against SVIII and vice versa[35]. A similar level of specificity can be demonstrated with proteins, so that rabbits rendered unresponsive to bovine serum albumin (BSA) will give normal responses to cross-reacting albumins of horse, pig, guinea-pig and human origins[36].

Occasional reports of lack of specificity in tolerance require reassessment in terms of T-B cell collaboration, as illustrated by the following example. Rats rendered tolerant to monomeric flagellin (fg specificity) were found to be unresponsive to the serologically unrelated flagellar specificities i and d[37]. As this is a highly T-dependent antigen, it seems most likely that T lymphocytes had been rendered tolerant of a determinant shared between the different flagellins which was either not recognised by B cells or not expressed by them serologically. Verification of this interpretation is the recent finding that T cells primed against flagellin can be killed by exposure to heavily ^{125}I-labelled homologous *or* serologically unrelated flagellin[38].

4.1.4.4 Effect of tolerance on antibody affinity

Affinity refers to the intrinsic association constant between antibody molecules and the corresponding univalent antigenic determinant.

When partial tolerance (Section 4.1.4.7) is induced in neonatal rabbits with a hapten-protein conjugate, there is a profound diminution in the affinity of anti-hapten antibodies elicited in the animals as adults which is far greater than depression of antibody synthesis itself[39]. Similarly, the avidity of antibody (combining power to form stable complexes formed during spontaneous escape from neonatally-induced tolerance to BSA is initially low and increases slowly[40]. Greater suppression of high affinity antibody has also been found to be associated with tolerance to proteins and haptens induced in adult animals[41, 42]. This implies that precursors of cells capable of synthesising higher affinity antibodies are deleted preferentially during induction of tolerance, and this has been affirmed by studies on antibody-secreting (plaque-forming) cells (PFCs). The higher the affinity of antibody formed, the lower is the concentration of antigen needed to inhibit these cells in gels *in vitro*. Precursors of high affinity PFCs have been shown by this technique to be more susceptible to induction of tolerance by BSA or DNP than are those of low affinity[41, 43]. Clearly the affinity of receptor immunoglobulin on the surface of B lymphocytes and the concentration of tolerance-inducing antigen are both critical factors.

4.1.4.5 Immunological immaturity of the recipient

The view that the ease with which tolerance to histocompatibility antigens could be induced during the late foetal or neonatal stages reflected a qualitatively different reaction from that pertaining to adults was abandoned when it was found that both immunity and tolerance could be obtained according to cell dosage in immature and mature animals alike[19]. The tolerance-inducing dose of soluble antigens, such as BGG and pneumococcal polysaccharide is similar for both neonatal and adult mice when related to body weight[20]. On the other hand, the weight adjusted dose of allogeneic cells required to induce tolerance rises steeply within the first few days after birth[45], corresponding with rapid expansion of the animal's lymphocyte population. The view has prevailed that there is no distinction in principle between tolerance induced in adult or perinatal life and that the facility of the latter merely reflects a relative weakness of the potential immune response at this stage.

Sporadic observations continue to reinforce suspicion that this unifying concept may not represent the whole truth. For example, Parish[46] recently reported that whereas acetoacetylated flagellin induced tolerance in adult rats with regard to humoral but not cellular immunity, it produced unresponsiveness at the level of both in neonatal animals. Again, the preferential suppression of high affinity antibody forming cell precursors in neonatally-induced tolerance described by Siskind and his colleagues[47] was not found by them using analysis of tolerance of the same antigens induced in adults.

4.1.4.6 Low zone tolerance

One practical difficulty envisaged by earlier workers concerned with the future possibility of inducing tolerance in man with purified histocompatibility antigens was the sheer quantity of the latter which would be needed. Tolerance appeared to be exclusively a 'high-dose' phenomenon. This pessimistic view was dispelled by the observation of Dresser[22] that BGG became non-immunogenic for mice following de-aggregation and would with one injection of 100 μg induce tolerance against immunogenic challenge. Mitchison[48] subsequently found that repeated injection of sub-immunogenic amounts of BSA, which is poorly immunogenic in mice, would produce tolerance. This he referred to as 'low zone' as distinct from the usual 'high zone' tolerance which could be produced with the same antigen. 'Low zone' tolerance cannot be produced by highly-immunogenic proteins, such as lysozyme, diphtheria toxoid, ovalbumin or ribonuclease, unless these are administered during the temporary immuno-suppressed period following sublethal (600 rad) irradiation[49]. The most striking feature is that the dose of all these antigens required to induce this tolerant state is remarkably constant, whereas the minimum immunogenic dose is highly variable. It appeared that if the immunogenicity of an antigen or the response to it could be sufficiently reduced, then tolerance could be attained with relatively small doses.

Far smaller amounts of flagellin (10^{-7} μg per g daily for 2 weeks) were found to induce tolerance in neonatal rats[50], described as 'ultra-low zone' tolerance as the molar amounts of antigen involved were six orders of magnitude less than in Mitchison's experiments. Some antigens fail to show these two separate zones of tolerance. For example, HSA is non-immunogenic in rats and produces progressively deeper unresponsiveness over a wide range of increasing doses[51]. Whether or not 'low zone tolerance' is determined by the same cellular events as follow antigen overloading is uncertain, for comparative studies have not been reported. Low zone tolerance has always represented partial, rather than total suppression. Ivanyi and Cerny[52] suggested that different mechanisms might be involved with non-immunogenic and immunogenic antigens, the latter inducing an undetected minimal response of high-affinity antibody which could inhibit B cells by attachment of complexes. A requirement for antibody synthesis, albeit at an undetectable level, may explain the lag period which precedes development of low zone tolerance. The ability of minute amounts of antigen complexed with antibody to induce tolerance *in vitro* is described in Section 4.1.5.1.

Recent elucidation of the co-operative roles of T and B cells has indicated that tolerance of T-dependent antigens can result from inactivation of either population (Section 4.1.5.2.). The postulate that low zone tolerance is sited in T rather than B cells has gained support on the basis of their relatively lower dose threshold. The absence of a low zone effect with the T-independent polysaccharides is consistent with this interpretation. The mechanism and wider significance of what is operationally 'low zone' tolerance and its relationship to specific inactivation of T lymphocytes awaits further study with a wider range of antigens. Its ultimate applicability in transplantation tolerance remains conjectural.

4.1.4.7 Incomplete forms of tolerance

(a) *Partial tolerance*—Response curves to a variety of antigens indicate that increase in dosage beyond the optimal immunising amount progressively diminishes the ensuing immunity to a point where total inhibition results. This zone is referred to as 'partial tolerance' for the animals are incapable of responding further to immunisation. Antibody secretion during partial tolerance is not only reduced in quantity, but characteristically shows impairment of affinity maturation (Section 4.1.4.4). More than one event probably underlies this state of hyporesponsiveness. (i) The requisite tolerance dosage thresholds will differ with complex antigens for the individual determinants. This cannot be the sole explanation, however, as partial tolerance is also demonstrable with polymers composed of identical repeating units. (ii) Increasingly severe partial tolerance, induced with both homopolymers and complex antigens, is correlated with a numerical reduction in antibody-secreting cells. Thus some cells can be suppressed, whereas others are triggered to respond by the same dose of antigen. Whether this reflects differences in micro-environment or in the individual cells is not understood. (iii) A reduced rate of antibody synthesis per cell during partial tolerance induced by SIII has been postulated on the basis of an increased incubation time necessary to detect PFC in gel[53]. This proposal requires assessment with other antigens in view of the special features of tolerance with SIII (Section 4.1.5.3).

Many published investigations on tolerance describe states of reduced responsiveness rather than total deletion of reactivity, which needs to be stressed when their practical and theoretical implications are being evaluated.

(b) *Split tolerance*—Establishment of haemopoietic and lymphoid cell chimaerism does not invariably lead to tolerance of all the antigenic determinants possessed by donor cells. For example, A strain mice, injected neonatally with (CBA × C57BL)F$_1$ spleen cells, become fully tolerant with respect to CBA skin grafts, but at best only weakly so for C57BL grafts, in spite of their being demonstrably chimaeric with F_1 cells[54]. Again, the neonatal injection of C57BL♀ mice with low doses of CBA or A ♂ cells leads to durable tolerance in terms of skin graft survival of the male-specific, but not of the foreign H_2 alloantigens[55]. In both models the non-tolerated determinants represent the 'stronger' antigenic differences. This phenomenon has never been explained unequivocally, although the likelihood is that non-tolerated determinants on persisting donor cells are reversibly suppressed, either by serum blocking antibody or non-expression on the surface membrane.

Another kind of split tolerance may also be demonstrated with respect to two determinants on the same molecule. Using rabbit IgG as antigen, Taussig[56] found that 10 times more was required to obtain tolerance in mice to the Fc-sited determinants than for those on the Fab portion.

(c) *Tissue specific lack of tolerance*—Incomplete tolerance also exists at the level of the tissues transplanted, for chimaeras will sometimes reject skin allografts taken from the original cell donors. This is now thought to be due to the possession by epidermal cells of differentiation antigens, not expressed on the tolerance-inducing haemopoietic or lymphoid cells, which are capable of exciting skin graft rejection[57]. The locus controlling these alloantigens in the mouse has been designated SK and at least two alleles are involved. The possible existence of other tissue specific differentiation antigens is clearly important in relation to attempts to induce 'transplantation' tolerance in man.

(d) *Tolerance affecting different categories of immune responsiveness*—Prior injection of an antigen in saline may suppress later development of the cell-mediated immunity which would otherwise follow its administration in complete Freund's adjuvant. As this phenomenon does not incur impairment of humoral response to the same determinants, it has been considered to be distinct from tolerance and referred to as 'immune deviation'[58]. Its significance has been heightened by the recent finding of Parish[29, 46, 59] that tolerance may be induced selectively at the level of either antibody or cell-mediated responses by chemical modification of an antigen. Subjection of flagellin to increasing degrees of acetoacetylation was found to reduce its affinity for homologous antibody without loss of specificity. This was accompanied by (i) progressive loss of the capacity to initiate antibody formation, (ii) increasing tolerogenicity and (iii) augmentation of the antigen's ability to induce cell-mediated immunity. A cyanogen bromide digest of flagellin also retained specificity and produced antibody tolerance with both high and low dose zones. Cell-mediated immunity was amplified at either level, but was correspondingly suppressed when antibody formation was stimulated by intermediate dosages.

An inverse relationship between these two types of response is not a general characteristic of antigens. Parish's experiments are, nevertheless, of great theoretical importance in demonstrating that chemical manipulation of an antigen can modulate the class of immune response and of tolerance which it will evoke. This may turn out to be especially relevant to the transplantation model, where attempts to induce tolerance with isolated histocompatibility antigens have been largely unsuccessful. Daily injection of mice with H_2 antigen from the day of birth onwards was recently reported to result in deletion of the humoral response (haemagglutinating, cytotoxic and enhancing antibodies), whilst the cell mediated capacity to reject skin grafts remained unimpaired[60]. As the antibody response to H_2 antigens is highly dependent on T cell co-operation, the cellular basis for this effect is unclear, unless tolerance has been induced in B cells alone which is contrary to current dogma (Section 4.1.5.2). This experiment is discouraging in relation to controlled induction of transplantation tolerance in man, so that chemical manipulation of histocompatibility antigens might prove fruitful in this respect.

All classes of immunoglobulin may not be equally suppressed during tolerance. This is well illustrated by the recent finding of Liacopoulos and his colleagues[61] that the tolerising dose of DNP-BSA was at least one order higher with respect to the IgG_1 response than for either the IgM or IgG_2 components.

The aforementioned examples of incomplete tolerance point to the need for application of a variety of different methods in assessing quantitatively and qualitatively the extent of unresponsiveness. *Total* deletion of specific immune reactivity is more difficult to obtain than is sometimes conceded.

4.1.5 Cellular aspects of induction and loss of tolerance

4.1.5.1 Tolerance in vitro

New insight into the nature of tolerance has been gained by recent studies on its induction *in vitro*. One approach is to incubate lymphoid cells with antigens and measure their responsiveness to challenge following transfer into lethally-irradiated syngeneic recipients. Substantial degrees of tolerance have been produced in this way with the polymeric antigens *E. coli* lipopolysaccharide[62] and native levan[63], whereas similar attempts with serum proteins have been unsuccessful[64]. Greater importance currently centres around the incisive series of experiments performed by Diener and Feldmann[65-69] who have studied the induction of tolerance to flagellin by its effect on the antibody forming cell response measured wholly *in vitro* by a modification of the Marbrook technique. Their principle findings are as follows.

Total, specific suppression could be induced by increasing the concentration of polymerised flagellin (POL) to 10 times that giving an optimum immune response. This 'high zone' tolerance, which was nearly maximal following incubation of spleen cells for 3 h, was attributed to binding of antigen to cell membrane receptors, as it could be inhibited by prior treatment with either anti-immunoglobulin serum or trypsin. Especially provocative was the finding that monomeric flagellin (MON) was less tolerogenic, and the even smaller fragment A totally inactive (in sharp contrast with its potent tolerogenicity *in vivo*). Whilst immunogenicity and tolerogenicity of flagellins with different molecular weights are *inversely* correlated attributes *in vivo*, it appears that they are correlated *directly in vitro*. Diener and Feldmann explained this anomaly in the following way. The sole factor responsible for tolerisation with POL is the dose of antigen used, and by virtue of its multi-determinant structure it is able to achieve cross-linkage of the receptors on the cell surface. If this is sufficiently extensive, a state of surface immobilisation could result. The failure of MON and fragment A (as well as serum proteins) to tolerise *in vitro* was attributed to the absence of polymeric linkage of determinants. They envisaged that combination with antibody *in vivo* could provide the necessary lattice for the monomeric forms of antigen, thereby achieving the same end result (Figure 4.1) and leading to induction

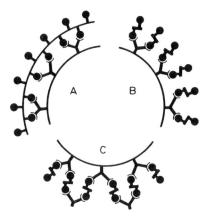

Figure 4.1 Proposed interaction of antigens with recognition sites (immunoglobulins) on the surface of B lymphocytes. (A) Polymeric antigen. (B) Monomeric antigen. (C) Monomeric antigen in the presence of specific antibody. The recognition sites can become extensively cross-linked in situations A and C only, both of which would lead to tolerance. (From Diener and Feldmann[69], by courtesy of Munksgaard)

of tolerance. Compelling support has been provided by other *in vitro* experiments to substantiate their hypothesis: (a) Tolerance to DNP could be induced by DNP-POL conjugates, but only when the number of hapten groups per monomer was relatively high[70], suggesting a requirement for closely spaced determinants on the polymeric carrier to cross-link receptors. (b) An otherwise immunogenic concentration of POL would induce tolerance when a critical amount of antibody was present. The fact that bivalent fragment $F(ab^1)_2$, but not univalent Fab^1, was also effective argues forcibly in support of the cross-linkage concept. (c) Both fragment A and subimmunogenic doses of MON were found to induce tolerance in the presence of an appropriate amount of antibody. (d) Complex-mediated tolerance is not peculiar to the flagellins. The addition of defined amounts of antibody also enabled Diener and Feldmann to induce unresponsiveness with solubilised sheep erythrocytes and chicken γ-globulin[69]. (e) These states of tolerance were also exhibited by the cells following their transfer into irradiated recipients.

The experiments on antigen–antibody mediated tolerance have not been reproduced *in vivo*, which is scarcely surprising in view of additional influences which operate in the intact animal. This should in no way detract from the important theoretical implications of these *in vitro* experiments (Section 4.1.5.4).

4.1.5.2 Characteristics of tolerance in T and B lymphocytes

Recent investigations with a variety of thymus-dependent antigens—serum proteins, hapten-protein conjugates and heterologous erythrocytes—have established that tolerance can be induced in both major classes of lymphocyte[71-76]. Analyses have been carried out either by repopulating irradiated hosts with mixtures of T and B cells from tolerant or normal donors or alternatively by re-equipping tolerant animals with normal cells of either category. Specific unresponsiveness in the intact animal will result from suppression in only T or B cells alone. In general, tolerance can be induced with far greater facility in the T lymphocytes, which (a) may be rendered unresponsive by 100 to 1000-fold less antigen than B cells, (b) require a much briefer induction period (<24 h compared with up to 3 weeks) and (c) remain unreactive for much longer. The second and third of these points are well illustrated in Figure 4.2.

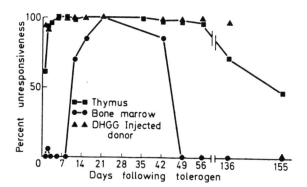

Figure 4.2 Kinetics of the induction and loss of tolerance to deaggregated human gamma globulin (DHGG) in mouse thymus and bone marrow cells as examples of T and B lymphocytes. Cells were taken at various times after injection of the tolerogen and transferred to irradiated recipients together with normal cells of the other category, and the cooperative response to HGG studied. Note much briefer induction period and greater duration of tolerance in T cells. The unresponsive state of the tolerant group of cell donors is also shown. (From Weigle[114] by courtesy of Blackwells)

The difficulty of tolerising B cells has perhaps been overstressed, to the extent that some authors originally denied that it could be accomplished. One problem has been the use of thymus and bone marrow cells as convenient, but not wholly representative, sources of T and B lymphocytes. More information is required about the analogous behaviour of purified populations from lymph nodes and spleen. Thus, a repeat of the experiment shown in Figure 4.2 using spleen rather than bone marrow revealed that tolerance of HGG was induced in these B cells within 3 days, rather than 3 weeks. Again the nature of the antigen studied influences the outcome much more with B than with T lymphocytes. Foreign gammaglobulins are clearly more tolerogenic for the former than are serum albumins, and even more so are the T-independent polymeric antigens (SIII and levan) which will suppress the PFC response in doses of 1 mg or less[26, 77]. Levan is especially striking in that it can induce complete tolerance in B cells within 24 h *in vivo* or partial suppression after only 2 h *in vitro*. This rapidity of onset is comparable with the kinetics pertaining to T cells, so that the relative difficulty which has been experienced in tolerising B lymphocytes may reflect a mechanistic obstacle rather than a more fundamental difference. For example, although it is difficult to induce tolerance to polymerised flagellin *in vivo*, B cells are readily suppressed by it *in vitro*[69, 78].

Mechanisms underlying unresponsiveness in the two classes of lymphocyte are discussed further in the following sections.

4.1.5.3 Reversibly and irreversibly tolerant cells

The central enigma of tolerance at the cellular level has been whether specific lymphocyte inactivation represents an irreversible or reversible process. These alternatives have been conceived as reflecting either cell death or the existence of tolerant cells. The former has been generally favoured, particularly as the delay in recovery of responsiveness following transfer of cells from protein-tolerant donors has been commensurate with a process of cell renewal rather than the reversibility of inactivated cells in an antigen-free environment (e.g. Refs. 51, 79). Until recently, evidence for 'tolerant cells' has been circumstantial, such as the loss of unresponsiveness to sheep erythrocytes following incubation *in vitro* of tolerant lymphocyte populations[80] or induction of graft-versus-host reaction in the intact animal[81]. Most probably in these instances, B cells had not been rendered tolerant and were stimulated by a T cell by-pass mechanism. Early reversibility of tolerance induced *in vitro* following trypsinisation or antigen withdrawal merely implies the existence of a transient reversible stage[69, 82].

A re-evaluation in terms of T and B cells has proved revealing. Support for tolerance in T lymphocytes being due to functional or physical elimination of reactive cells is impressive. In particular, impairment of recovery of responsiveness from protein tolerance by adult thymectomy[83, 84] is strong evidence in favour of a requirement to regenerate new mature T cells. No early recovery of reactivity to T-dependent antigens has been found in irradiated mice repopulated with mixtures of tolerant T and normal B lymphocyte populations. A similar conclusion has been reached by an ingenious approach with regard to histocompatibility antigens[85]. Tolerance induced in neonatal rats by F_1 cells could later be broken by injection of normal host strain lymphocytes. GVH reactive (T) cells of original host origin were detectable (by a chromosome marker) 6 weeks later, but their reappearance was precluded by thymectomy. A strong case for reversibly tolerant T cells has yet to be made, although oblique findings such as the reversibility of their non-reactivity to high doses of the mitogen concanavalin A[86] and the apparent ability of T cells from tolerant mice to co-operate with primed B cells[87], ensure that the last word has yet to be said.

B lymphocytes, however, can clearly be inactivated irreversibly or reversibly according to the antigen studied. Bursectomy of 2-week-old chickens interferes with recovery from tolerance of HSA[88], implying a specific loss of cells as the Bursa of Fabricius is required for maturation of new B lymphocytes. Levan produces complete tolerance in B cells within 24 h *in vivo*. Recovery of reactivity to this T-independent polymer following transfer of tolerised spleen cells to irradiated recipients is only detectable after 50–80 days, again indicating the need for cell renewal[26]. The polysaccharide SIII, however, behaves quite differently. Following a transient immune phase it induces unresponsiveness which will last a year or more, with profound suppression of PFC (although raised numbers of antigen binding cells). Transfer of spleen or bone marrow cells from these mice causes their reactivity to return within a day or so and large numbers of PFC appear in the recipients[89]. Similar findings have been made with *Esch. coli* lipopolysaccharide, although the tolerance it induces is more transient[90]. The mechanism with SIII implies an antigen-mediated, reversible suppression of initially triggered cells[91]. A possible explanation for the surprising dissimilarity between levan and SIII is discussed in the next section.

4.1.5.4 Molecular events in tolerance induction

There seems little point today in adhering to the proposal that contact of antigen with cell receptors can generate distinct immunogenic and tolerogenic molecular signals. The alternative interpretation that the modality of response is determined solely by events at the cell surface has much recent experimental support. An extreme degree of cross-linkage of determinant bound receptors which are immobilised by lattice formation (Section 4.1.5.1) seems the most likely molecular mechanism to be implicated in tolerance. Immunising doses of antigen induce the migration of receptors across the cell membrane to one pole (the phenomenon of 'capping'[92]) and this is quickly followed by appearance of more receptors in greater density. Tolerogenic doses, on the other hand, cause rapid impairment of cap formation[93]. It would appear that immunisation leads to aggregation of receptors by a degree of cross-linking which triggers the differentiation sequence leading to antibody synthesis, whereas tolerance represents immobilisation of receptors by excessive inter-linkage producing a 'frozen state'. Tolerance induction would thus be influenced by two main factors: the dose of antigen and the intensity of surface binding (the latter being determined by the size of antigen and its determinant density together with the affinity of receptors).

This interpretation not only accords well with various characteristics of tolerance, such as the preferential elimination of high affinity precursor cells, but also forms a plausible explanation for the demonstration of irreversibly and reversibly tolerant cells with levan and SIII. Although receptors for polysaccharides are generally of low affinity, levan achieves strong surface binding, presumably by virtue of its heavily branched, multi-site flexible molecule which could also contribute to immobilising lattice formation. In comparison, SIII binds poorly, possibly because its rigid linear structure does not enable it to attach to enough weak receptors. Reversibly tolerant cells may thus represent the continuous dissociation of antigen, such that excessive lattice formation cannot occur. With a persistent antigen like SIII, a state of 'treadmill neutralisation' would exist at the cell surface. The degree of potential reversibility on this basis should increase the lower the affinity of the precursor cell.

What happens to irreversibly suppressed, antigen-coated lymphocytes? The likelihood is that they will be eliminated as effete cells by conventional pathways, such as phagocytosis. A case has been made out for the participation of complement in tolerance induction[94, 95], but the relevant data are not particularly compelling and it seems unlikely to be involved in more than a secondary role facilitating cell elimination.

The aforegoing considerations are experimentally and conceptually concerned with B cells. Whether they are applicable to T cells, which have greater susceptibility to tolerance despite low receptor density, is speculative*. Little progress can be anticipated until the identity and characteristics of T cell receptors have been finally established.

4.1.5.5 Analysis of escape from tolerance

Tolerance is lost spontaneously when antigen is eliminated or, if it is non-metabolisable, falls below a critical level. The lag frequently found before recovery of responsiveness is consistent with a process of recruitment of fresh lymphocytes, although 'reversible' suppression of B cells is produced by some T-independent antigens (Section 4.1.5.3). Tolerance of thymus-dependent antigens is frequently sited in T cells alone, which can explain the following examples of experimentally promoted loss of unresponsiveness. Rabbits can be made fully tolerant to BSA by a course of antigen injections commenced in the neonatal period. However, they will make a quantitatively and qualitatively normal anti-BSA response following injection of various serum albumins which cross-react serologically with BSA[36, 96]. The explanation appears to be as follows. BSA-specific T cells, but not B cells, are rendered unresponsive, so that cross-reacting albumins can interact with T cells specific for unrelated determinants, which then function as necessary 'helper cells' for BSA-specific B cells capable of responding to shared determinants. Tolerance attributable to T cell suppression alone may also be sometimes overcome by 'by-pass' mechanisms which can circumvent the absence of 'specific help' function. Thus, a non-specific B cell stimulant formed by T cells during the proliferative stage of graft-versus-host reaction[97] could explain its capacity to break tolerance of sheep erythrocytes[81]. The ability of a B cell mitogen, lipopolysaccharide, to promote an immune response to HGG in tolerant mice when only the T cells are unresponsive is another example[98].

*See 'Note added in proof'

4.1.6   Is the tolerant state a multi-component phenomenon ?

4.1.6.1   Treadmill neutralisation

A state of tolerance may be simulated in conditions where secreted antibody is continuously neutralised by retained antigen, but this is only pronounced when the latter is, like SIII, non-catabolisable. Antibodies are suppressed peripherally in this way by higher immunising doses of SIII. Antigen–antibody complexes are continuously phagocytosed and unmodified poly-saccharide leaks back gradually into the circulation by excretion from macro-phages[99]. A dose of SIII which extinguishes haemagglutinating (protective) antibodies is one which elicits the maximum number of antibody-secreting cells (Figure 4.3)[77]. The amount of antigen needed to suppress B cells is

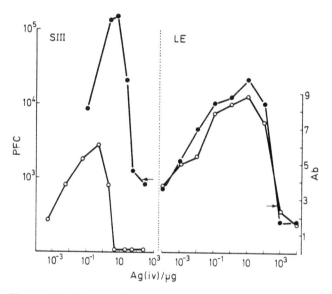

Figure 4.3   A comparison of the plaque-forming cell (PFC) responses in the spleen (●——●) and serum haemagglutinating antibody (Ab) titres (○——○) following different doses of type 3 pneumococcal polysaccharide (SIII) and levan (LE). Arrows indicate background PFC levels. Note extinction of antibody by doses of SIII which elicit maximal PFC responses due to persistence of antigen in serum. This 'treadmill' neutralization phenomenon is not detectable with LE. (From Howard, Miranda, Zola and Christie[166], by courtesy of Plenum Publishing Corporation)

nearly two orders greater than that producing this state of so-called 'tread-mill' neutralisation. Similar masking by persisting antigen also occurs during spontaneous escape from tolerance of SIII, which is first detectable by PFC assay, but not serologically.

At the other extreme, only transient masking occurs with rapidly meta-bolisable antigens. Circulating antigen–antibody complexes are detectable following high immunising doses of serum proteins before the appearance of free antibody[100].

4.1.6.2 Antibody-mediated tolerance and enhancement

Tolerance as an antigen-determined central deletion phenomenon has been generally regarded as clearly distinct from enhancement, a specific blocking effect on cell mediated immunity transferable by serum. (The site of block produced by enhancing sera has been considered to be 'afferent'—deviation of immunising antigen—or 'efferent'—coating of target cells.) A long term dissentient from this conceptual distinction has been G. A. Voisin[101] who has argued that, with regard to the transplantation situation, the two phenomena are causally interrelated. A critical re-evaluation has recently taken place in view of provocative findings uncovered by the Hellströms and their associates[102-104]. Mice rendered putatively tolerant either by neonatal injection with allogeneic cells or by fusion of two embryos at the eight-cell stage (allophenic mice) were found as adults to contain lymphoid cells which were cytotoxic *in vitro* for donor strain target cells. Furthermore, a 'blocking factor' was present in their sera which inhibited expression of this cell-mediated reaction. At least some aspects of conventional tolerance were therefore attributed to serum blocking of concomitant immunity rather than to its central failure.

From the outset, this work did little to shake the cellular foundations of tolerance to proteins and polysaccharides, where central deletion seems an inviolable interpretation[7, 77, 105, 106] with particular regard to the following points: (a) plaque-forming cells are suppressed; (b) tolerance can be transferred by explanted lymphocytes; (c) tolerance can be abrogated by adoptive transfer of normal lymphoctyes which are themselves not inhibited in the 'tolerant environment'. (Recorded difficulties in demonstrating item (c) with some systems are of an operational type, such as antigen persistence or limitations of space for the new cells.)

Disquiet amongst transplantation immunologists, however, concerning the possible *in vivo* implications of the Hellströms' studies, has led to a new series of investigations which have upheld the traditional view, although with a new corollary. Space precludes mention of all recent results in this area, but the following are notable: (a) Cells from tolerant donors cannot induce GVH reaction and, even in vast excess, do not inhibit normal cells from doing so[107, 108]. (b) Tolerance can be broken by transfer of normal syngeneic lymphocytes or by parabiosis with normal syngeneic animals which are not themselves made tolerant[108]. (c) The ability to reject allografts which can be restored to T cell deprived mice by normal lymphoid cells is not prevented by admixture with cells from tolerant donors[109]. (d) Unresponsiveness to histocompatibility (and other) antigens can be induced in neonatally bursectomised, agamma-globulinaemic chickens[110]. No humoral mechanism is arguable on these findings.

The possible *in vivo* significance of 'blocking factor' has emerged from the work of Beverley and his colleagues[111]. Graded doses of F_1 cells were injected into neonatal mice and their immune status as adults was analysed by a variety of approaches. High doses of cells induced classical tolerance and neither blocking factor nor cytotoxic lymphocytes could be found. Lower doses led to states of partial tolerance with low levels of chimaerism coexisting with cytotoxic cells and blocking activity in the sera of some of the animals. It was postulated, therefore, that the humoral type of suppression may thus augment the expression of states of incomplete tolerance.

'Blocking factor' has been considered likely to represent antigen–antibody complexes. The *in vitro* studies of Diener and Feldmann (Section 4.1.5.1) suggest that complexes can induce central tolerance. Although a convincing demonstration of this *in vivo* is still awaited, it seems to provide a likely explanation for low zone tolerance phenomena. Finally, the role of complexes in enhancement itself is currently being explored. Survival of kidney allografts in rats can frequently be greatly extended by enhancing sera and French[112] has produced strong evidence that neither afferent nor efferent blocks are the determining factors. His results indicate that antigen–antibody complexes are released from the kidneys and induce central inhibition. A connection between tolerance and enhancement may possibly lie along these lines.

4.1.6.3 'Infectious' tolerance

This name was applied by Gershon and Kondo[113] to a phenomenon whereby spleen cells from mice rendered tolerant to sheep erythrocytes were found to interfere specifically with the co-operative response to the same antigen by normal T and B cells transferred into thymectomised, irradiated recipients. The effect could not be reproduced in normal animals. The authors attributed their specific immunosuppressive influence to T cell activity, but proof of this and assessment of the wider significance of this interesting observation are currently awaited.

4.1.6.4 'Self' tolerance

What is the current status of the original postulate of Burnet and Fenner[18]—that cells potentially capable of reacting against 'self' antigens would be selectively eliminated during ontogenesis—with regard to more recent insight into the nature of actively acquired tolerance? A highly controversial and relevant observation is that allophenic mice, formed by fusion of two eight-cell embryos, possess lymphocytes cytotoxic for cells of the other lineage and specific factors in their serum which 'block' this activity[103, 104]. The implication that we possess 'blocking' auto-antibodies for every potential specificity in our bodies seems so improbable, that most immunologists are reluctant to accept the allophenic mouse as a model for the normal development of 'self' tolerance.

Nevertheless, the occurrence of auto-antibodies in healthy individuals and their appearance following various experimental manoeuvres in animals have increasingly weighed against a mechanism involving strict clonal deletion of *all* lymphoid cells. A re-evaluation in terms of lymphocyte interactions has produced the interpretation, which is supported by strong circumstantial evidence (see Ref. 114) that the more readily tolerised T cells are suppressed, whereas potentially antihost reactive B cells may not be. Cell-mediated auto-immunity would thus be absent and auto-antibodies only arise under conditions where the lack of specific 'helper' T cells is by-passed. Typical examples are the development in rabbits of haemolytic auto-antibody after immunisation with sheep erythrocytes[115] and of auto-antithyroglobulin following injections of heterologous thyroglobulins[114]. Weigle has argued that this situation is analogous to breaking of acquired tolerance by cross-reacting antigens, where the T cells respond to unrelated determinants (Section 4.1.5.6). The frequency with which auto-immunity develops to certain tissues may result from too low a concentration of antigen in the body fluids to achieve unresponsiveness in B cells.

This explanation is attractive in being reconcilable with observations concerning loss of self-tolerance, whilst avoiding implausibilities inherent in too rigid application of either clonal deletion or 'blocking factor' hypotheses.

4.2 NON-SPECIFIC IMMUNOSUPPRESSION

4.2.1 Introduction

If tolerance had never been discovered, it would undoubtedly have been invented by a science fiction writer as a rational solution to the 'homograft problem' in man. Reality or not, surgeons pioneering human renal trans-plantation 13 years ago were obliged to use and develop non-specific methods of immunosuppression. Many immunologists viewed these early operations as premature and fore-doomed on the grounds that nothing less than tolerance would permit survival of incompatible grafts. In the event, these dire prophe-cies have been proved wrong in relation to the kidney, although experience with other tissues and organs is less satisfactory. The unpredicted, relative success in human transplantation achieved by immunosuppressive methods can, nevertheless, only be regarded as an interim solution. This section briefly summarises immunological features of the main types of suppressives (see Refs. 116, 117), hazards associated with their use and their potential value for facilitating the induction of tolerance.

4.2.2 Characteristics of suppression by various methods

4.2.2.1 Irradiation

A large sub-lethal dose of whole-body irradiation causes massive lysis and impaired mitotic activity of lymphoid cells. The intensity of suppression is radiation dose dependent. The primary antibody response is depressed most effectively when antigen is given 1–2 days after irradiation and the effect may last 50 days or so[118]. 7S antibody formation is more radiosensitive than is 19S[119]. Less suppression occurs when antigen is introduced 12 h before or after irradiation, whilst immunisation 2 days pre-irradiation is little impaired.

The secondary response is relatively radioresistant. Cell-mediated immunity may require slightly higher doses to be totally inhibited, but this varies according to the species studied.

Irradiated animals are extremely susceptible to infection, which is frequently caused by the normal flora of the gut. Although the phagocytic activity of macrophages is a highly radioresistant function, these cells show impairment of digestive activity and ability to kill ingested bacteria after doses as low as 400 rad[120], as well as a reduced ability to participate in the initiation of a response to some antigens[121]. T and B lymphocytes show equivalent radiosensitivity when exposed to various doses of x-rays *in vitro*[122]. On the other hand, several studies have indicated that the helper function of T cells is resistant to the extent of withstanding even 5000 rad[123]. As their proliferative capacity is greatly reduced by 300 rad and abrogated by 500 rad[124], it has been considered that a small residue of non-dividing cells may act as helpers. This radioresistant activity has not been found in all systems examined, so that its cellular basis remains unclear. Antibody secreting plasma cells are highly radioresistant in keeping with the observed minimal effect of irradiation on established antibody synthesis.

4.2.2.2   Corticosteroids—prednisolone

The adrenal cortical hormones are the most widely used clinical immunosuppressants. Prednisolone is particularly valuable for treating transplantation rejection crises and delayed hypersensitivity reactions. Both humoral and cell mediated immunity can be depressed by these compounds and loss of tolerance delayed in experimental animals. The most effective time to commence treatment in relation to exposure to antigen is similar to that described for x-irradiation.

The effects of corticosteroids on cells involved in immune responses now appears to be more selective than was at first appreciated. Macrophages show impairment of both proliferative and digestive capacities. The latter is due to stabilisation of lysosomal membranes, which affects killing of bacteria and solubilisation of particulate antigens. B lymphocytes in the spleen are highly sensitive to corticosteroids, whereas those in bone marrow are more resistant.[125] Whilst the majority of cells in the thymus are sensitive, the resistant 5% are those 'mature' T lymphocytes which have developed GVH reactivity, helper potential and PHA responsiveness[126, 127]. As most peripheral T cells possessing these properties are corticosteroid resistant, why is cell mediated immunity so depressed? It seems likely to be due to a change in cell distribution rather than a lymphotoxic effect, for under the influence of these hormones, peripheral T cells migrate to the bone marrow[128, 129].

4.2.2.3   Alkylating agents—cyclophosphamide

The immunosuppressive activity of nitrogen mustards has been recognised since shortly after World War I, but recent interest has centred around a newer compound—cyclophosphamide (CY) which is both more potent in this respect and less toxic. CY is a transport form of nitrogen mustard which is probably degraded in the liver into an active molecule. It suppresses the proliferation and differentiation of lymphocytes by alkylation of their nucleic acids and probably also possesses some direct lymphotoxic activity. CY is a potent suppressant of humoral antibody formation and whilst most effective when administered before or during the initial stages of the response, it will also reduce established antibody synthesis. Suppression of cell mediated immunity by CY varies greatly with animal species. CY strikingly inhibits rejection of skin, kidney and hemopoietic cell allografts, established GVH reaction and the induction of delayed hypersensitivity and auto-immune encephalomyelitis in mice or rats[130, 132]. Little success has been achieved with dogs.

Two lines of evidence suggest that CY is more active against the B, rather than the T, lymphocyte lineage. First, its administration in adolescent chickens impairs the ontogenic development of the humoral response, although T cell function, assessed by GVH reactivity, remains unimpaired[133]. However, absence of maturation of stem cells resulting from damage to the Bursa of Fabricius, rather than selective suppression of mature B cells, seems to be the explanation of this effect. Secondly, CY preferentially depletes the thymus-independent areas of lymphoid tissue in mice[134] and greatly enriches the proportion of θ-positive (T) cells in lymphocyte populations[135]. In view of these findings, it seems paradoxical that CY is one of the more effective agents available for suppressing GVH and allograft reactions and for establishing cell chimaerism in adult mice.

4.2.2.4 Purine analogues—6-mercaptopurine and azathioprine

6-Mercaptopurine and its imidazole derivative azathioprine (Imuran) are antimetabolites developed by Elion and Hitchings[136] which have become widely used immunosuppressants in clinical practice. Azathroprine is enzymatically converted to an active form in the liver and is now generally preferred as it avoids bone marrow toxicity. The purine analogues are potent inhibitors of the primary humoral response in all animals species tested when given together with antigen, but pre-treatment or delayed administration is ineffective. 7S antibody is far more susceptible to suppression than is 19S. The activity of these drugs on cell-mediated immunity is more variable. In rodents, their effect on skin allograft rejection and GVH reaction is minimal and they do not suppress PHA reactivity. On the other hand, Imuran suppresses human and mouse mixed lymphocyte culture reactions. Their most spectacular effect is in promoting extended survival of kidney grafts in dogs and rabbits and as a result they have been widely adopted for similar use in man.

In spite of the variable activity of azathioprine on cell-mediated responses in the mouse, recent evidence indicates that it acts selectively on T cells[137]. The drug preferentially eliminates those antigen-binding cells which bear the θ-antigen, a marker for T lymphocytes. Why this apparent selectivity is not expressed more dramatically in vivo is unresolved.

4.2.2.5 Folic acid antagonists—amethopterin

Amethopterin (Methotrexate), the methylated analogue of aminopterin, is one of the most potent immunosuppressive compounds known. It functions as a powerful mitotic inhibitor blocking dihydrofolate reductase activity.

Reduced cell-mediated immunity is expressed with delayed hypersensitivity, allograft rejection and experimental auto-immunity models. Both primary and secondary humoral antibody responses are also suppressed, especially when amethopterin is given 1–2 days after antigen, a time when its antiproliferative activity would be most effective. Like the purine analogues, it selectively suppresses 7S antibody more than 19S. Although amethopterin and aminopterin have been used in the treatment of acute leukaemia and chorion-epithelioma, their severe toxicity has precluded adoption as immunosuppressives in man.

4.2.2.6 Antibiotics

Some antimicrobial drugs have immunosuppressant effects which are useful only for studying the regulation of antibody synthesis in vitro[138]. Since they all inhibit protein synthesis they are too non-selective for in vivo use. Actinomycin D is a highly toxic, but potent anti-tumour agent, which limits protein synthesis by inhibiting DNA directed-RNA synthesis. Partial or total inhibition results when the drug is added to cultures of presensitised lymphoid cells at the same time as antigen. Antibody formation in vitro can persist for several days following delayed addition of Actinomycin D, implying that the relevant messenger RNA is relatively stable. Actinomycin D acts correspondingly in intact mice, inhibiting the development of antibody synthesising cells when given with antigen, but failing to suppress pre-sensitised animals[139]. An interesting effect of this drug is its ability to interfere with the induction of tolerance to protein antigens[140].

Chloramphenicol is a depressant of protein synthesis which in mammalian systems inhibits attachment of messenger RNA to ribosomes. High doses depress both the primary humoral response and rejection of skin allografts. The secondary response can be inhibited in vitro when chloramphenicol is added during the inductive but not productive phases. It has been proposed that messenger RNA-ribosome complexes are less vulnerable to the drug once antibody synthesis is established.

Puromycin is a potent inhibitor of protein synthesis which will immediately terminate ongoing antibody synthesis by cells in vitro without killing them. For example, incorporation of puromycin in a gel will inhibit haemolytic plaque formation by sensitised spleen cells. The use of this drug in vivo is precluded by its high toxicity.

4.2.2.7 Antilymphocyte globulin

The immunosuppressive potentiality of antilymphocyte sera (ALS) was only clearly demonstrated in the early 1960s[141, 142], although both the concept and preparation of the reagent were by no means recent. The effect of its repeated injection in the mouse is particularly dramatic. Incompatible skin grafts may be accepted for many months[143], and even skin from other species, including man, may be tolerated for shorter periods. Depression of the humoral response is less marked and more variable depending on the batch of serum used. As a course of ALS produces depletion of recirculating lymphocytes, its effect resembles that resulting from chronic drainage through a thoracic duct fistula. It therefore seemed to offer an advantage chemical over suppressants in being more selective in its spectrum of cellular targets (see Refs. 144, 145).

ALS for use in man has been available for several years, but a critical evaluation of its efficacy is still awaited. The globulin fraction (ALG) is isolated from whole serum to reduce the quantity of foreign protein injected and cross-reactivity with erythrocytes and platelets is abolished by absorption. Nevertheless, the following obstacles remain. (a) It is difficult to standardise the antigen used for immunisation when this is, ideally, human thymus or thoracic duct cells. Accordingly, cultured human lymphoblasts or lyophilised cell membranes are being used increasingly for this purpose. (b) Lack of a wholly satisfactory assay for potency remains a major shortcoming. Immuno-suppressive activity is rarely calibrated on human subjects. Monkeys are used as second best in conjunction with some *in vitro* test which is considered to have predictive value (e.g. rosette-inhibition). (c) A limited investigation in human volunteers has shown that the delay in skin-graft rejection produced by ALG is highly dose dependent. The striking survival of skin allografts which can be obtained in ALS-treated mice requires weight adjusted doses of serum which are far in excess of what could be tolerated in man. (d) Development of antibody to ALG prepared in horses or rabbits can reduce the suppressive activity of later injections due to accelerated clearance. At present ALG is used in conjunction with prednisolone and azathioprine as standard suppressive therapy in transplantation surgery.

ALG selectively inhibits T lymphocytes. Although some batches of serum may contain appreciable anti-B cell activity, this is a variable characteristic. The serum does not appear to act primarily by complement-mediated lysis and immunosuppressive activity is not correlated with cytotoxic titre. It appears to function mainly as an opsonin resulting in the *in vivo* elimination of recirculating lymphocytes by phagocytosis. In certain *in vitro* situations, T cells may be inactivated via steric blocking of their receptors by ALG or its $F(ab^1)_2$ fraction[146].

Entirely monospecific anti-T and anti-B cell sera have been prepared by immunising rabbits with chicken thymus and bursal cells followed by cross-absorption[147]. T or B cell suppression can be achieved selectively by incubating suspensions in the corresponding serum prior to transferring them into irradiated recipients. While such reagents may be of great value for elimina-ting unwanted functions (such as GVH reactivity) from donor cells, they are unlikely to be of much therapeutic value *in vivo* as their post-absorption titres are low.

4.2.3 Hazards of non-specific immunosuppression

The efficacy of long-term immunosuppression has to be continually balanced against hazards associated with the agents used, such as the high toxicity of effective drugs and the risk of foreign protein overloading with ALS, which could produce immunological renal damage or amyloid disease. Other undesirable sequelae are related to a theoretical shortcoming inherent in the basic philosophy of prolonged immunosuppression. Although the selective advantage afforded by the evolution of the vertebrate lymphoid system is poorly understood, it seems likely that some serious dysfunction might result from its functional extirpation. This seems to be borne out by experience with human renal transplantation, which is only undertaken as an attempted life-saving procedure. Susceptibility to infection, especially by viruses and fungi, is greatly increased in suppressed patients. A more controversial illustration is an 80-fold rise in the incidence of neoplasms, particularly of lymphoid tissue, in suppressed transplant patients as compared with the general population[148, 149]. Although a causal association has not been established in man, there are a number of animal experiments which clearly indicate an adverse change in susceptibility. These will be summarised briefly.

Mice suppressed with ALS have shown a greater incidence of tumours induced by both adeno and murine sarcoma viruses[150, 151] and the chemical carcinogen methylcholanthrene[152]. A large series of mice injected wih ALS every 4 days from birth, showed a 42% incidence of tumours, most of which were attributable to polyoma virus[153]. These findings have been associated with failure of cell mediated immunity to either control replication of oncogenic viruses or reject highly immunogenic experimental tumours. Analogous data relevant to the incidence of spontaneous tumours in animals are so far lacking. Thus it is currently uncertain to what extent failure of the postulated 'surveillance' function of T cells to recognise and eliminate mutant, potentially malignant, cells is a real hazard during immunosuppression. Certainly no raised incidence of tumours has been observed following the widespread use of azathropine in non-transplant situations. There is no reason to impute greater risk to ALS than the chemical suppressives, some of which can themselves be carcinogenic under certain conditions. It should be mentioned also that prolonged stimulation of the lymphoid system, by GVH disease for example, can progress to lymphoma development[154].

Because of the undesirable side effects produced by the prolonged use of immunosuppressive agents, such treatments would clearly be superseded if any *specific* alternative could be devised. The potentiality of the short-term application of immunosuppressive agents is considered in the last section.

4.2.4 Use of non-specific immunosuppression for the induction of tolerance

One of the ultimate benefits of some immunosuppressive agents may well turn out to be their use in facilitating the induction of tolerance. If antigen is administered whilst an animal is non-specifically suppressed, it may retain specific non-reactivity long after the general recovery of responsiveness. Thus, an irradiated adult animal can be rendered chimaeric by injection of allogenic bone marrow cells[155]. Mice were found to become tolerant likewise when normally immunogenic doses of protein antigens were administered during the recovery period following 600 rad irradiation[49]. The analogous concept of 'drug-induced tolerance' was established by Schwartz and Dameshek[156, 157] with their demonstration that 6-MP greatly facilitated the induction of tolerance in rabbits by a single injection of heterologous albumins. Following this example, McLaren[158] found that tolerance across a minor histocompatibility barrier could be induced in adult mice by spleen cells together with 6-MP.

Cyclophosphamide has proved to be even more effective, for under its influence tolerance can be induced to highly immunogenic antigens like sheep erythrocytes[159]. Tolerance will result if a normally immunising dose of antigen (but not lower) is given while an animal is suppressed by CY and can be maintained by subsequent doses of antigen alone[160]. CY-induced tolerance to sheep erythrocytes is sited in T cells alone, as evidenced by the behaviour of bone marrow and thymus cells in co-operation experiments and by the inhibitory effect of thymectomy on recovery from tolerance[161, 162]. The inference from all these examples is that tolerance will result from interaction of antigen with T cells whenever the normal triggering sequence is suppressed.

Transplantation tolerance has been successfully induced in mice when modest doses of allogeneic cells were injected during the suppressed phase produced by a course of ALS (e.g. Ref. 163). Permanent chimaerism was not established, however, and its loss preceded recovery of responsiveness. A similar end result was obtained by Brent and his colleagues[164] by injecting a large dose of an allogeneic tissue extract before a course of ALS. Grafts could be accepted permanently when the histo-incompatibility involved was weak. Even more impressive examples of tolerance induction across an H-2 barrier have been produced by injecting allogeneic cells in mice which were transiently immunosuppressed with ALS acting in synergy with methylhydrazine derivatives[165]. Following this manoeuvre, many skin allografts remained viable after six months. Combination of ALS with other suppressive drugs was less effective.

These and many similar experiments suggest one possible direction towards the controlled induction of tolerance in man. The indications are that unless stable chimaerism can be established, only a temporary deletion of responsiveness is likely to occur.

Note added in proof

The induction *in vitro* of tolerance to flagellin in T cells has now been reported by Feldman and Nossal[167]. In view of the fact that both monomeric and polymeric forms of the antigen were equally effective (unlike the outcome with B cells), the mechanisms of tolerisation within these two lymphocyte populations may be dissimilar.

References

1. Landy, M. and Braun, W. (editors) (1969). *Immunological Tolerance* (New York: Academic Press)
2. Nisbet, N. W. and Elves, M. W. (editors) (1971). *Immunological Tolerance to Tissue Antigens* (Oswestry, England: Orthopaedic Hospital)

3. Friedman, H. (editor) (1971). *Immunological Tolerance to Microbial Antigens. Ann. N.Y. Acad. Sci.* **181,** (New York: New York Academy of Sciences)
4. *Immunological Tolerance. Effect of Antigen on Different Cell Populations. Transplant Rev.* **8** (1972). (Copenhagen: Munksgaard)
5. Dresser, D. W. and Mitchison, N. A. (1968). *Advan. Immun.,* **8,** 129
6. Leskowitz, S. (1967). *Annu. Rev. Microbiol.,* **21,** 157
7. Mitchison, N. A. (1971). *Transplant. Proc.,* **3,** 953
8. Glenny, A. T. and Hopkins, B. E. (1924). *J. Hyg., Camb.,* **22,** 208
9. Schiemann, O. and Casper, W. (1927). *Z. Hyg. InfecktKranh.,* **108,** 220
10. Sulzberger, M. B. (1929). *Archs. Derm. Syph.,* **20,** 669
11. Felton, L. D. (1949). *J. Immunol.,* **61,** 107
12. Chase, M. W. (1946). *Proc. Soc. Exp. Biol. Med.,* **61,** 257
13. Owen, R. D. (1945). *Science,* **102,** 400
14. Anderson, D., Billingham, R. E., Lampkin, G. H. and Medawar, P. B. (1951). *Heredity (London),* **5,** 379
15. Billingham, R. E., Brent, L. and Medawar, P. B. (1953). *Nature (London),* **172,** 603
16. Billingham, R. E., Brent, L. and Medawar, P. B. (1956). *Proc. Roy. Soc. (London) B.,* **239,** 357
17. Hasek, M. (1953). *Cslka Biol.,* **2,** 25
18. Burnet, F. M. and Fenner, F. (1949). *The Production of Antibodies* (Melbourne: Macmillan)
19. Howard, J. G., Michie, D. and Woodruff, M. F. A. (1961). *CIBA Symposium on Transplantation, Transplantation Tolerance and Immunity in Relation to Age,* 138 (J. and A. Churchill Ltd. 1962: London)
20. Siskind, G. W., Paterson, P. Y. and Thomas, L. (1960). *J. Immunol.,* **90,** 929
21. Roelants, G. E. and Goodman, J. W. (1970). *Nature (London),* **227,** 175
22. Dresser, D. W. (1962). *Immunology,,* **5,** 378
23. Frei, P. C., Benacerraf, B. and Thorbecke, G. J. (1965). *Proc. Nat. Acad. Sci. USA.,* **53,** 20
24. Andersson, B. (1969). *J. Immunol.,* **102,** 1309
25. Kabat, E. A. and Bezer, A. E. (1958). *Arch. Biochem. Biophys.,* **78,** 306
26. Miranda, J. J., Zola, H. and Howard, J. G. (1972). *Immunology,* **23,** 843
27. Howard, J. G., Zola, H., Christie, G. H. and Courtenay, B. M. (1971). *Immunology,* **21,** 535
28. Borel, Y. (1971). *Nature New Biol.,* **230,** 180
29. Parish, C. R. (1971). *J. Exp. Med.,* **134,** 1
30. Silobrcic, V. (1971). *Europ. J. Immunol.,* **1,** 313
31. Felton, L. D., Kauffman, G., Prescott, B. and Ottinger, B. (1955). *J. Immunol.,* **74,** 17
32. Miranda, J. J. (1972). *Immunology,* **23,** 829
33. Janeway, C. A., Jr. and Humphrey, J. H. (1969). *Israel J. Med. Sci.,* **5,** 185
34. Mitchison, N. A. (1962). *Immunology,* **5,** 359
35. Brooke, M. S. (1966). *J. Immunol.,* **95,** 364
36. Benjamin, D. C. and Weigle, W. O. (1970). *J. Exp. Med.,* **132,** 66
37. Austin, C. M. and Nossal, G. J. V. (1966). *Aust. J. Exp. Biol. Med. Sci.,* **44,** 341
38. Cooper, M. G. and Ada, G. L. (1972). *Scand. J. Immunol.,* **1,** 247
39. Theis, G. A. and Siskind, G. W. (1968). *J. Immunol.,* **100,** 138
40. Dowden, S. J. and Sercarz, E. E. (1968). *J. Immunol.,* **101,** 1308
41. Davie, J. M., Paul, W. E., Katz, D. H. and Benacerraf, B. (1972). *J. Exp. Med.,* **136,** 426
42. Bell, E. B. (1973). *Europ. I. Immunol.* (in the press)
43. Andersson, B. and Wigzell, H. (1971). *Europ. J. Immunol.,* **1,** 384
44. Dresser, D. W. (1962). *Immunology,* **5,** 161
45. Brent, L. and Gowland, G. (1961). *Nature (London),* **192,** 1265
46. Parish, C. R. (1971). *J. Exp. Med.,* **134,** 21
47. Werbling, T. P. and Siskind, G. W. (1972). *Transplant. Rev.,* **8,** 104
48. Mitchison, N. A. (1964). *Proc. Roy. Soc. (London) B.,* **161,** 275
49. Mitchison, N. A. (1968). *Immunology,* **15,** 509
50. Shellam, G. R. and Nossal, G. J. V. (1968). *Immunology,* **14,** 273
51. Bell, E. B. and Shand, F. L. (1973). *Europ. J. Immunol.* (in the press)
52. Ivanyi, J. and Cerny, J. (1969). *Current Topics in Immunol. and Microbiol.,* **49,** 114

53. Baker, P. J., Stashak, P. W., Amsbaugh, D. F. and Prescott, B. (1971). *Immunology*, **20**, 481
54. Brent, L. and Courtenay, T. H. (1961). *Mechanisms of Immunological Tolerance* (*Proc. Symp. Liblice, Prague*), *On the Induction of Split Tolerance*, 113 (1962). (Prague: Publishing House of the Czechoslovak Academy of Sciences)
55. Billingham, R. E. and Silvers, W. (1960). *J. Immunol.*, **85**, 14
56. Taussig, M. J. (1971). *Europ. J. Immunol.*, **1**, 367
57. Lance, E. M. (1971). *Immunological Tolerance to Tissue Antigens*, 291 (N. W. Nisbet and M. W. Elves, editors) (Oswestry, England: Orthopaedic Hospital).
58. Asherson, G. L. (1966). *Immunology*, **10**, 179
59. Parish, C. R. and Liew, F. Y. (1972). *J. Exp. Med.*, **135**, 298
60. Law, L. W., Appella, E., Strober, S., Wright, P. W. and Fishetti, T. (1972). *Proc. Nat. Acad. Sci. USA*, **69**, 1858
61. Liacopoulos, P., Harel, S. and Ben-Efraim, S. (1972). *Transplant. Proc.*, **4**, 390
62. Britton, S. (1969). *J. Exp. Med.*, **129**, 469
63. Kotlarski, I., Courtenay, B. M. and Howard, J. G. *Europ. J. Immunol.* (in the press)
64. Mitchison, N. A. (1968). *Immunology*, **15**, 531
65. Feldmann, M. and Diener, E. (1970). *J. Exp. Med.*, **131**, 247
66. Diener, E. and Feldmann, M. (1970). *J. Exp. Med.*, **132**, 31
67. Feldmann, M. and Diener, E. (1971). *Nature (London)*, **231**, 183
68. Feldmann, M. and Diener, E. (1972). *J. Immunol.*, **108**, 93
69. Diener, E. and Feldmann, M. (1972). *Transplant. Rev.*, **8**, 76
70. Feldmann, M. (1971). *Nature New Biol.*, **231**, 21
71. Chiller, J. M., Habicht, G. S. and Weigle, W. O. (1970). *Proc. Nat. Acad. Sci. (London)*, **65**, 551
72. Chiller, J. M., Habicht, G. S. and Weigle, W. O. (1971). *Science*, **171**, 813
73. Chiller, J. M. and Weigle, W. O. (1971). *J. Immunol.*, **106**, 1647
74. Mitchison, N. A. (1971). *Cell Interactions in Immune Responses*, 249 (O. Mäkelä, A. M. Cross and T. U. Kosunen, editors) (London: Academic Press)
75. Taylor, R. B. (1971). *Immunological Tolerance to Tissue Antigens*, 75 (N. W. Nisbet and M. W. Elves, editors) (Oswestry, England: Orthopaedic Hospital)
76. Rajewsky, K., Brenig, C. and Melchers, I. (1971). *Cell Interactions, 3. Le Petit Symp.*, *Specificity and Suppression in the Helper System*, 196 (L. G. Silvestri, editor) (Amsterdam: North-Holland Publishing Company)
77. Howard, J. G., Christie, G. H. and Courtenay, B. M. (1971). *Proc. Roy. Soc. (London) B.*, **178**, 417
78. Parish, C. R. and Ada, G. L. (1969). *Immunology*, **17**, 153
79. Dietrich, F. M. and Weigle, W. O. (1964). *J. Immunol.*, **92**, 167
80. McCullagh, P. J. and Gowans, J. L. (1966). *The Lymphocyte in Immunology and Haemopoiesis*, 234 (J. M. Yoffry, editor) (London: Edward Arnold (Publishers) Ltd.)
81. McCullagh, P. J. (1970). *J. Exp. Med.*, **132**, 916
82. Byers, V. S. and Sercarz, E. E. (1970). *J. Exp. Med.*, **132**, 845
83. Claman, H. N. and Talmage, D. W. (1963). *Science*, **141**, 1193
84. Taylor, R. B. (1964). *Immunology*, **7**, 595
85. Elkins, W. L. (1972). *Transplant. Proc.* (in the press)
86. Andersson, J., Sjöberg, O. and Möller, G. (1972). *Immunology*, **23**, 637
87. Miller, J. F. A. P., Basten, A., Sprent, J. and Cheers, C. (1971). *Cell. Immunol.*, **2**, 469
88. Ivanyi, J. and Salerno, A. (1972). *Immunology*, **22**, 247
89. Howard, J. G., Christie, G. H. and Courtenay, B. M. (1972). *Proc. Roy. Soc. (London) B.*, **180**, 347
90. Sjöberg, O. (1972). *J. Exp. Med.*, **135**, 850
91. Howard, J. G. (1972). *Transplant. Rev.*, **8**, 50
92. Taylor, R. B., Duffus, P. H., Raff, M. C. and de Petris, S. (1971). *Nature New Biol.*, **233**, 225
93. Diener, E. and Paetkau, V. H. (1972). *Proc. Nat. Acad. Sci. USA*, **69**, 2364
94. Azar, M. M., Yunis, E. J., Pickering, P. H. and Good, R. A. (1968). *Lancet*, **1**, 1279
95. Azar, M. M. and Good, R. A. (1971). *J. Immunol.*, **106**, 241
96. Weigle, W. O. (1961). *J. Exp. Med.*, **114**, 111
97. Katz, D. H., Paul, W. E., Goidl, E. A. and Benacerraf, B. (1971). *J. Exp. Med.*, **133**, 169

98. Chiller, J. M. and Weigle, W. O. (1973). *J. Exp. Med.*, **137**, 740
99. Howard, J. G., Christie, G. H., Jacob, M. J. and Elson, J. (1970). *Clin. Expl. Immunol.*, **7**, 583
100. Ivanyi, J. and Cerny, J. (1965). *Folia Biol., Praha*, **11**, 335
101. Voisin, G. (1971). *Cell. Immunol.*, **2**, 670
102. Hellström, I., Hellström, K. E. and Allison, A. C. (1971). *Nature, London*, **230**, 49
103. Wegmann, T. G., Hellström, I. and Hellström, K. E. (1971). *Proc. Nat. Acad. Sci. USA*, **68**, 1644
104. Phillips, S. M., Martin, W. J., Shaw, A. R. and Wegmann, T. G. (1971). *Nature (London)*, **234**, 146
105. Habicht, G. S., Chiller, J. M. and Weigle, W. O. (1970). *Developmental Aspects of Antibody Formation and Structures*, **2**, 893 (J. Sterzl and I. Riha, editors) (New York: Academic Press)
106. Shellam, G. R. (1971). *Int. Arch. Allergy Appl. Immunol.*, **40**, 507
107. Atkins, R. C. and Ford, W. L. (1972). *Transplantation*, **13**, 442
108. Brent, L., Brooks, C., Lubling, N. and Thomas, A. V. (1972). *Transplantation*, **14**, 382
109. Hamilton, D. N. H. (1973) quoted by Brent, L. and French, M. E. *Transplant Proc.* (in the press)
110. Rouse, B. T. and Warner, N. L. (1972). *Europ. J. Immunol.*, **2**, 102
111. Beverley, P. C. L., Brent, L., Brooks, C., Medawar, P. B. and Simpson, E. (1973). *Transplant. Proc.* (in the press)
112. French, M. E. (1973). *Transplant. Proc.* (in the press)
113. Gershon, R. K. and Kondo, K. (1971). *Immunology*, **21**, 903
114. Weigle, W. O. (1971). *Clin. Exp. Immunol.*, **9**, 437
115. Bussard, A. (1965). *La Greffe des Cellules Hematopoietiques Allogeniques*, 157 (Paris: Centre National de la Recherche Scientifique)
116. Schwartz, R. S. (1965). *Progr. Allergy*, **9**, 246
117. Gabrielsen, A. E. and Good, R. A. (1967). *Advances in Immunology*, **6**, 91 (P. J. Dixon, Jr. and J. H. Humphrey, editors) (New York: Academic Press)
118. Taliaferro, W. H. and Taliaferro, L. G. (1951). *J. Immun.*, **66**, 181
119. Nettesheim, P., Williams, M. L. and Hammons, A. S. (1969). *J. Immunol.*, **103**, 505
120. Nelson, E. L. and Becker, J. R. (1959). *J. Infect. Dis.*, **104**, 20
121. Gallily, R. and Feldman, M. (1967). *Immunology*, **12**, 197
122. Claman, H. N. (1970). *Developmental Aspects of Antibody Formation and Structure*, Vol. 2, 577 (J. Sterzl and I. Riha, editors) (New York: Academic Press)
123. Katz, D. H., Paul, W. E., Goidl, E. A. and Benacerraf, B. (1970). *Science*, **170**, 462
124. Anderson, R. E., Sprent, J. and Miller, J. F. A. P. (1972). *J. Exp. Med.*, **135**, 711
125. Levine, M. A. and Claman, H. N. (1970). *Science*, **167**, 1515
126. Cohen, J. J., Fischbach, M. and Claman, H. N. (1970). *J. Immunol.*, **105**, 1146
127. Cohen, J. J. and Claman, H. N. (1971). *J. Exp. Med.*, **133**, 1026
128. Cohen, J. J. (1972). *Cell Interactions*, 162 (L. G. Silvestri, editor) (Amsterdam: North-Holland Publishing Company)
129. Claman, H. N. and Moorhead, J. W. (1972). *Cell Interactions*, 137 (L. G. Silvestri, editor) (Amsterdam: North-Holland Publishing Company)
130. Shehadeh, I. H., Guttman, R. D. and Lindquist, R. R. (1970). *Transplantation*, **10**, 66
131. Owens, A. H. and Santos, G. W. (1971). *Transplantation*, **11**, 378
132. Glucksberg, H. and Fefer, A. (1972). *Transplantation*, **13**, 300
133. Lerman, S. P. and Weidanz, W. P. (1970). *J. Immunol.*, **105**, 614
134. Turk, J. L. and Poulter, L. W. (1972). *Clin. Exp. Immunol.*, **10**, 285
135. Poulter, L. W. and Turk, J. L. (1972). *Nature New Biol.*, **238**, 17
136. Elion, G. B. and Hitchings, G. H. (1965). *Advan. Chemotherapy*, **2**, 91
137. Bach, J. F. and Dardenne, M. (1972). *Cell Immunol.*, **3**, 11
138. Ambrose, C. T. (1966). *Bact. Rev.*, **30**, 408
139. Jerne, N. K., Nordin, A. A. and Henry, C. (1963). *Cell-bound antibodies*, 109 (Philadelphia: Wistar Institute Press)
140. Claman, H. N. and Bronsky, E. A. (1965). *J. Immunol.*, **95**, 718
141. Waksman, B. H., Arbouys, S. and Arnason, B. G. (1961). *J. Exp. Med.*, **114**, 997
142. Woodruff, M. F. A. and Anderson, N. F. (1963). *Nature (London)*, **200**, 702
143. Levey, R. H. and Medawar, P. B. (1966). *Ann. N.Y. Acad. Sci.*, **129**, 164
144. James, K. (1969). *Progress in Surgery*, **7**, 140

145. *Proceedings of the Conference on Antilymphocyte Serum, Federation Proceedings* (1970), **29,** 97
146. Richie, E. R., Gallagher, M. T., Heim, L. R., South, M. A., and Trentin, J. J. (1972). *Proc. Soc. Exp. Biol. Med.*, **140,** 916
147. Ivanyi, J. and Lydyard, P. M. (1972). *Cell Immunol.*, **5,** 180
148. McKhann, C. F. (1969). *Transplantation*, **8,** 209
149. Penn, I. and Starzl, T. E. (1972). *Transplantation*, **14,** 407
150. Allison, A. C., Berman, L. D. and Levey, R. H. (1967). *Nature (London)*, **215,** 185
151. Law, L. W., Ting, R. C. and Allison, A. C. (1968). *Nature (London)*, **220,** 611
152. Balner, H. and Dersjant, H. (1969). *Nature (London)*, **224,** 376
153. Simpson, E. and Nehlsen, S. L. (1971). *Clin. Exp. Immunol.*, **9,** 79
154. Schwartz, R. S., and Beldotti, L. (1965). *Science*, **149,** 1511
155. Main, J. M. and Prehn, R. T. (1955). *J. Nat. Cancer Inst.*, **15,** 1023
156. Schwartz, R. S. and Dameshek, W. (1959). *Nature (London)*, **183,** 1682
157. Schwartz, R. S. and Dameshek, W. (1963). *J. Immunol.*, **90,** 703
158. McLaren, A. (1961). *Transplant. Bull.*, **28,** 479/99
159. Aisenberg, A. C. (1967). *J. Exp. Med.*, **125,** 833
160. Many, A. and Schwartz, R. S. (1970). *Clin. Exp. Immunol.*, **6,** 87
161. Aisenberg, A. C. and Davis, C., *J. Exp. Med.*, (1968). **128,** 35
162. Many, A. and Schwartz, R. S. (1970). *Proc. Soc. Exp. Biol. (N.Y.)*, **133,** 754
163. Lance, E. M. and Medawar, P. B. (1969). *Proc. Roy. Soc. (London), B.*, **173,** 447
164. Brent, L., Hansen, J. A., Kilshaw, P. J. and Thomas, A. V. (1973). *Transplantation*, **15,** 160
165. Floersheim, G. L. (1971). *Immunological Tolerance to Tissue Antigens*, 257 (N. W. Nisbet and M. W. Elves, editors) (Oswestry, England: Orthopaedic Hospital)
166. Howard, J. G., Miranda, J. J., Zola, H. and Christie, G. H. (1973). *Microenvironmental Aspects of Immunity* (B. D. Jankovic and K. Isakovic, editors) 369, *Characteristics of B cell tolerance induced with T-independent polysaccharides* (in the press) (New York: Plenum Publishing Corporation)
167. Feldmann, M. and Nossal, G. J. V. (1972). *Transplant Rev.*, **13,** 3

5
Antigenicity and Immunogenicity

M. J. CRUMPTON
National Institute for Medical Research, London

5.1 ANTIGENS, HAPTENS AND IMMUNOGENS

The injection of vertebrates with a foreign macromolecule induces the synthesis of antibodies that are bound specifically by discrete areas of the macromolecule called antigenic determinants. Macromolecules that stimulate antibody production are referred to as antigens or immunogens. It is, however, becoming increasingly common to differentiate between the induction of antibody and reaction with antibody by equating immunogen with antibody induction and by using antigen when considering interaction. Thus, whereas immunogenicity describes the capacity of a substance to elicit an antibody response, antigenicity expresses the capacity of the substance to interact with antibody. A considerable body of experimental evidence suggests that the structural requirements for immunogenicity differ from those for antigenicity. For example, simple chemical substances of low molecular weight (e.g. 2,4-dinitrophenol) are not immunogenic, but they will react specifically with antibodies produced by injecting the small molecule attached to a macromolecular carrier, usually a protein. Landsteiner[1] introduced the term hapten to describe these substances. It is evident that in the modern context the terms hapten and antigen share considerable overlap. Antigen is, however, usually reserved for molecules with many determinants whereas hapten is used for molecules or groups corresponding to a single determinant.

Antigens occur naturally as nucleic acids[2, 3], proteins and polysaccharides either as separate molecules or as part of a macromolecular complex such as a virus particle. Most naturally occurring and many synthetic macromolecules (especially synthetic polypeptides[4, 5]) are immunogenic, although proteins are generally better immunogens than polysaccharides and nucleic acids. Lipids are not immunogenic but in some cases can function as haptens[6]. The results of numerous studies indicate that the molecular structure of the immunogen or antigen and its association with other molecules play important roles in determining the capacities of a substance to initiate antibody production and to react with antibody. This chapter will be concerned with defining these relationships.

5.2 ANTIGEN–ANTIBODY INTERACTION

Interaction is characterised by its high order of specificity and has been symbolised with the fitting together of a lock and key[7]. The union between the antigen determinant and the antibody combining site is maintained by non-covalent forces. These forces are identical with those which are primarily responsible for determining protein conformation and comprise four main types: namely, electrostatic interaction, hydrogen bonding, interaction between non-polar side chains caused by the mutual repulsion of solvent and van der Waal's attraction derived from the polarisation of two atoms as they approach each other[8, 9]. Although in most molecular interactions van der Waal's attractions are numerically superior, the contribution made by each type of force to the binding of a particular antigenic determinant will depend on the chemical nature of the antigen. For example, electrostatic bonds cannot play a significant role in the interaction of a neutral polysaccharide with specific antibody.

Non-covalent forces possess two characteristic features which to a considerable extent determine the nature of antigen–antibody interaction. Each force acts over short distances only (e.g. interacting atoms must be less than 6 Å apart before van der Waal's attraction has an appreciable effect), and is weak contributing only between 0 and -4 kcal mol^{-1} to the overall binding energy (association constants for antigen–antibody interaction are usually between 10^4l and 10^{10} mol^{-1}). As a result, the formation of a stable intermolecular complex requires, firstly, that the combining sites approach each other closely otherwise the forces are of insufficient magnitude and, secondly, that the areas of interaction are sufficiently large to counteract the weakness of an individual bond by multiple binding. In other words, the degree of interaction will depend on the relative shapes and sizes of the combining regions.

5.2.1 Effect of a change in shape

The effect of changes in the shape (structure) of lactose on its strength of binding to antibodies against the *p*-azophenyl-*β*-lactoside group are summarised in Table 5.1; alterations in shape were engendered either by a change

Table 5.1 The effect of changes in the structure of lactose on its strength of binding to antibodies raised by immunisation with the *p*-azophenyl-*β*-lactoside group attached to a protein carrier[10]. The strength of binding is expressed as K_{rel} which represents the ratio of the association constant for the analogue relative to that for lactose

Hapten	K_{rel}
Lactose (64 % *β* anomer)	1.00
(4-*O*-*β*-D-galactopyranosyl-D-glucopyranose)	
cellobiose (66 % *β* anomer)	0.0025
(4-*O*-*β*-D-glucopyranosyl-D-glucopyranose)	
methyl *β*-D-galactopyranoside	0.007
methyl *α*-D-galactopyranoside	0.0012

in the spatial distribution of groups or by the substitution of one group by another. The results indicate that a small change in structure is associated with a marked decrease in the strength of binding. For example, cellobiose which differs from lactose only in the configuration of the C-4 hydroxyl group of the galactose residue is bound very much less strongly than lactose. The most rational explanation of this phenomenon is that the change in shape caused a reduction in the closeness of fit and, due to the short-range character of non-covalent forces, a decrease in the number of bonds.

Other dramatic examples of the specificity of antigen–antibody interaction and the effect of small structural changes on specificity are provided by the carbohydrate structures responsible for the Kauffmann–White classification of *Salmonella* strains[11] and for the human blood-group A-, B-, Le[a]- and Le[b]- activities[12-14]. The structural relationships between the various blood-group antigenic determinants are illustrated in Figure 5.1. It is apparent from these studies that the structure of a very small portion of the molecule is of crucial importance in defining the specificity. In the examples quoted this portion corresponds to the non-reducing terminal residue, but in linear unbranched polymers, such as pneumococcal SIII polysaccharide, it coincides with a distinct non-terminal group[15]. Other results suggest that a portion of all antigenic determinants plays a dominant role in determining the specificity, and this portion has been termed the immunodominant group[11].

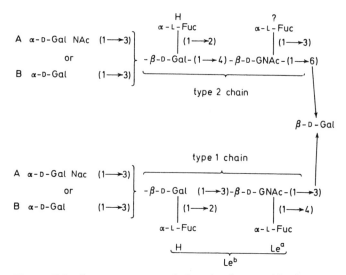

Figure 5.1 Structures proposed for the human blood-group A-, B-, H-, Le[a]- and Le[b]- antigenic determinants (From Lloyd, Kabat and Licerio[13], by courtesy of American Chemical Society).

The figure represents the composite structure for the above determinants and is based on the structures of immunologically active fragments isolated from the respective blood-group specific substances. It is very doubtful whether the highly branched structure shown exists naturally to any extent and certain of the terminal non-reducing residues are missing in the individual blood-group determinants. Thus, A-determinants have terminal N-acetylgalactosamine residues whereas B-determinants have terminal galactose residues, and both A- and B-determinants do not normally possess two fucose residues attached to adjacent sugars of the type 1 and 2 oligosaccharide chains. H- and Le[b]-determinants lack the terminal a-linked N-acetylgalactosamine or galactose residues, whereas the Le[a]-determinants have no fucose linked $a(1{\to}2)$ to the galactose of the type 1 chain. The Le[b]-determinant depends on the presence of two fucose residues attached to adjacent sugars of the type 1 chain. The common galactose-N-acetylglucosamine backbone exists in two forms (type 1 and type 2 chains). A-, B- and H-determinants are associated with both type 1 and 2 chains, but Le[a]- and Le[b]-determinants are based on type 1 chains only. Although fucose may be linked $a(1{\to}3)$ to the N-acetylglucosamine of the type 2 chain, oligosaccharides based on this structure have no Le[a]-, nor Le[b]-activity. Abbreviations: GalNAc = N-acetyl-D-galactosaminopyranosyl; Gal = D-galactopyranosyl; GNAc = N-acetyl-D-glucosaminopyranosyl; Fuc = L-fucopyranosyl

5.2.2 Effect of size

Information on the sizes of antigenic determinants is usually obtained by comparing, on a molar basis, the capacities of fragments of increasing size to inhibit the interaction of the whole antigen with antibody. This approach was initiated by Kabat (reviewed in Ref. 16) who showed for dextran–antibody interaction [dextran is a branched polymer of glucose residues linked mainly $a\,(1{\to}6)$] that the inhibitory capacity of the isomaltose series of oligosaccharides [glucoses linked a $(1\rightarrow6)$] increased with increasing chain length and reached an upper limit at approximately isomaltohexaose. It was concluded that the antigenic determinant of dextran has a well-defined upper limit in size which corresponds to the hexasaccharide. Similar studies have now been carried out with a large variety of natural and synthetic antigens using antisera prepared in various animal species. Some of the results are presented in Table 5.2 together with the size of the fragment which was

Table 5.2   Sizes of antigenic determinants

Immunogen	Determinant	Dimensions (Å)*	Ref.
Dextran	isomaltohexaose	$34 \times 12 \times 7$	17, 18
Silk fibroin	Gly(Gly$_3$ Ala$_3$)Tyr†	29	19
Denatured DNA (Lupus erythematosus serum)	pentanucleotide	$28 \times 10 \times 10$	20
Poly-L-alanine-BSA‡	pentaalanine	$25 \times 11 \times 6.5$	21
Poly-L-lysine + phosphorylated BSA	pentalysine	$27 \times 17 \times 6.5$	22
Poly-γ-D-glutamic acid + methylated BSA	hexaglutamic acid†	$36 \times 10 \times 6$	23, 24
(D-alanyl)$_n$-glycylribonuclease§	tetra-alanine	$20 \times 11 \times 6.5$	25
Sperm-whale metmyoglobin	C-terminal-hepta-peptide	$15 \times 11 \times 9$	26, 27
a-DNP-oligo-L-lysine	DNA-heptalysine		28
Peptidoglycan (antiserum to group A variant Streptococci)	L-Ala-D-Glu-γ-L-Lys-D-Ala-D-Ala	$21 \times 11 \times 6$	29

* The dimensions are those of the most extended conformation except for sperm-whale myoglobin where they correspond to those of the determinant in the native protein
† Larger peptides may, however, be more effective inhibitors
‡ Multichain peptide-protein conjugate prepared by polymerisation with average peptide chain length of ca. 7 residues
§ Peptides of the structure (D-Ala)$_n$-Gly ($N = 1$–4) were coupled to ribonuclease in a one-step synthesis
‖ Drs M. V. Kelemen and H. J. Rogers, personal communication [Kelemen, M. V. and Rogers, H. J. (1972), Proc. Nat. Acad. Sci. USA. 68, 992]

considered to represent the complete determinant. In some cases the interpretation of the data is complicated by a number of factors[25, 30]. Thus, if the determinant possesses a particular conformation which is stabilised by the remainder of the molecule, then increase in inhibitory capacity with increasing size may reflect the stabilisation of the conformation complementary to the antibody combining site rather than the maximum size of the determinant[24, 31]. Additional residues may also non-specifically enhance the binding of the fragment by antibody even without being an integral part of the determinant. For example, the binding of the tripeptide, Ala-Thr-Arg, by antibody to tobacco mosaic virus protein is greatly enhanced by N-octanoylation[32]. This enhancement depends on the increased hydrophobicity of the peptide and, although the mechanism has not been defined, it appears that the octanoyl group either stabilises the peptide conformation which is complementary to the antibody, or more probably, binds non-specifically, in a similar manner to some detergents, to areas topographically distinct from the antibody site, and thus contributes to the overall binding energy of the peptide.

In spite of the above reservations and although the dimensions of the determinants in the complete antigen may differ from those quoted due to folding, this approach has yielded valuable information. The results emphasise that antigenic determinants have a similar maximum size which is independent of their chemical nature and of the animal species in which the antibodies were formed. This concept leads to an important prediction namely, if a hapten attached to a carrier is smaller than the maximum size then the complete determinant will include a portion of the carrier. This prediction has been shown to be correct for a number of haptens. For example, the 2,4-dinitrophenyl group (DNP), which is commonly attached to protein carriers via lysine side chains, is much smaller (*ca.* $7 \times 3.5 \times 2.5$ Å) than the maximum size of antigenic determinants (Table 5.2). The data in Table 5.3

Table 5.3   **Strength of binding of various DNP-haptens to antibodies produced by immunisation with DNP-bovine γ-globulin[33]**

Hapten	Association constant* $(\times 10^{-7} \, \mathrm{l \, mol^{-1}})$
2, 4-Dinitrophenol	0.027
DNP-glycine	0.46
a-DNP-L-alanine	0.88
ε-DNP-L-lysine	2.30
ε-DNP-aminocaproate	2.85

* Association constants were measured by fluorescence quenching at about 30°C in 0.1 M tris–HCl buffer, pH 7.6

show that ε-DNP-L-lysine is bound much more strongly by antibodies to dinitrophenylated proteins than the hapten alone (2,4-dinitrophenol) and indicates that the DNP-determinant includes the lysine side chain[33], whereas more recent results suggest that the determinant extends to the environment beyond the DNP-lysyl group[34]. The importance of the carrier in relation to the determinant is confirmed by the observations that the carrier can contribute up to 30% to the overall strength of binding[35] and that antibodies to a-DNP-L-undecalysine bind seven of the lysyl residues[28].

It is apparent from Table 5.2 that antigenic determinants may be regarded as being made up of a number of residues or subsites[5], similar to those which have been proposed for the active sites of some enzymes (e.g. papain[36]). In this case the overall strength of binding is the sum of the binding strengths of the individual subsites. The contributions made by the individual residues to the overall binding have been assessed for the isomaltohexaose determinant of dextran[37]. The results revealed that the terminal, non-reducing glucose residue contributed *ca.* 40% of the binding energy of the hexasaccharide and that successive glucose residues made decreasing contributions. Various other antigenic determinants have shown similar patterns of behaviour all of which are characterised by one subsite contributing the major portion of the total binding energy. This subsite corresponds to the immunodominant group.

5.2.3 Effect of charge

Electrostatic interactions have frequently been implicated in antigen–antibody interaction and several observations have demonstrated that the net electrical charge of antibodies produced in rabbits is inversely related to the charge of the immunogen. Thus, rabbit antibodies to acidic proteins and synthetic polypeptides are bound less strongly by DEAE-Sephadex and can be separated almost completely by ion-exchange chromatography from antibodies to basic proteins, whereas antibodies to neutral proteins are distributed almost equally between the differently charged fraction[38]. Furthermore, since rabbit antibodies against the same hapten (*p*-azobenzenearsonate group) attached to oppositely charged carriers possessed similar specificities and affinities, the different charges of the antibodies must reflect the overall net charges of the immunogens and are primarily associated with those areas of the antibody molecule other than the combining site[39]. As a result, electrostatic bonds do not necessarily play a predominant role in the interaction between oppositely charged reactants. On the other hand, the inverse charge relationship can be readily understood in terms of the molecules having to approach each other closely before interaction can be established. Recent results suggest that this relationship is mediated at the cellular level by the interaction of the oppositely charged carriers with different lymphocytes[40]. In this case, it is apparent that the complete immunogen (hapten-carrier) initiates antibody synthesis and that degradation does not occur prior to recognition. In contrast to the above results, similar studies carried out in guinea-pigs and sheep have failed to show an inverse relationship between the charges of the antibody and the immunogen[41]. Although the reason for this variation is not known, it may depend on the chemical nature of the immunogen and the nature of the non-covalent forces which are primarily responsible for the union between the combining sites.

5.2.4 Comparison with enzyme–substrate interaction

Antigen–antibody interaction resembles closely the binding of substrate by an enzyme. It appears likely that the points of similarity reflect parameters which determine the efficiency of macromolecular complex formation (i.e. specificity and strength of binding) and which have been selected for during evolution. Figure 5.2 shows the active site of lysozyme occupied by hexa-*N*-acetylchitohexaose[42]. This complex shows the following similarities to antigen–antibody interaction. Firstly, the size of the active site corresponds to a hexasaccharide and is identical with the maximum size of the antibody combining site (cf. Table 5.2); the active sites of papain and carboxypeptidase A show a similar size relationship[36]. Secondly, β-*N*-acetyl-D-glucosamine is bound at subsite C in preference to any one of the other subsites; as a result, it appears that a portion of the substrate is bound preferentially and behaves in a similar manner to the immunodominant group of an antigenic determinant. Thirdly, lysozyme and its natural substrate ($\beta(1\rightarrow4)$-*N*-acetyl-D-glucosamine-$\beta(1\rightarrow4)$-*N*-acetyl-D-muramic acid) show a similar inverse

140

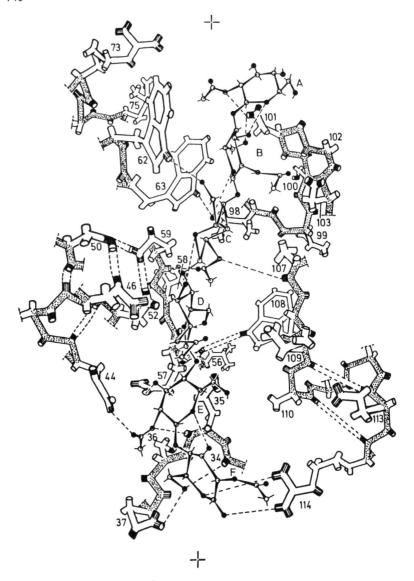

Figure 5.2 Atomic structure of the active site of egg-white lysozyme with a molecule of hexa-*N*-acetylchitohexaose bound to the enzyme (From Blake *et al.*[42], by courtesy of The Royal Society)

The main polypeptide chain is shown speckled, and the N(H) and O atoms are indicated by line and full shading respectively. The locations of sugar residues A, B and C were determined experimentally from the binding of tri-*N*-acetylchito-triose (and *β*-*N*-acetyl-D-glucosamine for residue C). Residues D, E and F occupy positions inferred from model building charge relationship to that between rabbit antibodies and charged immunogens. Moreover, as with antigen–antibody interaction, the charge of lysozyme is primarily associated with those areas of the molecule other than the active site, and electrostatic bonds do not play a dominant role in the binding of substrate. If the analogy between enzyme–substrate and antigen–antibody interactions has reality, then the antibody combining site should resemble the enzyme active site and correspond to a cleft on the surface of the protein. This proposal is consistent with the results of X-ray crystallographic analysis which suggest that the antibody site is represented by a cavity between the H- and L-polypeptide chains[43].

5.2.5 Measurement of interaction

A large number of methods are available for the detection and measurement of antigen–antibody interaction. The different methods vary with respect to a wide variety of parameters but in particular they differ in their applicability and sensitivity. Thus, not all methods are quantitative (e.g. immunodiffusion is primarily a qualitative procedure) and some procedures only are suitable for determining the reaction kinetics and stoichiometry of interaction (e.g. equilibrium dialysis and quenching of antibody fluorescence). As a number of modern comprehensive reviews are available[44-46], individual methods will not be considered in detail. Instead, the more important differences between some of the assays will be emphasised.

Immunochemical methods differ from one another in two important respects which are primarily responsible for their different sensitivities and applicabilities. Firstly, the concentrations of the reactants used can vary over several orders of magnitude (e.g. dilutions of 1:1, 1:10 and 1:250 for quantitative precipitation, macro-complement fixation and micro-complement fixation respectively[47]). Secondly, some assays measure the initial antigen–antibody interaction directly (e.g. fluorescence quenching and direct binding assays such as the Farr test), whereas others rely on the subsequent aggregation of antigen–antibody complexes (e.g. precipitation, agglutination and complement fixation). The exploitation of these differences are illustrated by the following examples.

Numerous studies have revealed that immunochemical methods vary in their capacities to detect differences in reactivity between closely related antigens. For example, a 60% difference between haemoglobins A_1 and S, which differ by one amino acid only, was revealed by micro-complement fixation and a 20% difference was detected by macro-complement fixation, but quantitative precipitation failed to distinguish these proteins[47]. Similarly, as shown in Figure 5.3 chicken, bobwhite quail and turkey lysozymes were readily distinguished by micro-complement fixation whereas little difference was detected by quantitative precipitation[48]. Macro-complement fixation has also been shown to be more sensitive than quantitative precipitation for revealing differences between the Fe^{2+} and Fe^{3+} derivatives of the a-chains of human haemoglobin[49]. The results of these and other comparisons suggest that, in general, micro-complement fixation reveals the largest differences whereas macro-complement fixation, quantitative precipitation, fluorescent titration, antigen binding to an immunoadsorbent and immunodiffusion show increasingly smaller differences. The superiority of micro-complement fixation most probably depends on the low concentrations of reactants used (*ca.* 10^{-10}M antibody), with the result that only the most avid portion of the total antibody population reacts and a small difference in binding affinity between two antigens is amplified into a relatively large difference in reactivity.

The reaction kinetics can be determined only by using those methods that measure the initial phase of the interaction directly. Suitable procedures

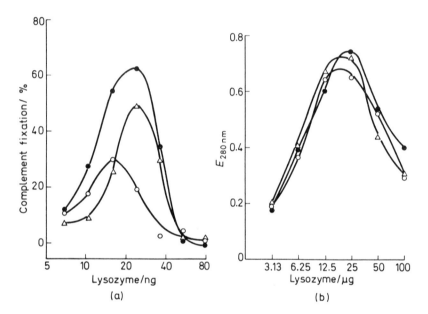

Figure 5.3 Comparison of the immunological reactivities of chicken (●), bob-white quail (△) and turkey (○) lysozymes with an antiserum to chicken lysozyme. The reactivities were measured (a) by micro-complement fixation and (b) by quantitative precipitation (data taken from Ref. 48).

Increasing amounts of lysozyme were added in (a) to 1 ml of a 1:7500 dilution of antiserum and in (b) to 0.15 ml of undiluted antiserum. The immune precipitates in (b) were dissolved in 0.8 ml of 0.5 M NaOH prior to measuring the extinctions of the solutions at 280 nm

include those based on fluorescence (quenching, enhancing and polarisation), equilibrium dialysis and the Farr technique. Each procedure, however, suffers from a number of disadvantages that preclude its general applicability. Thus, fluorescence methods are applicable only to antigens and haptens possessing suitable fluorescent properties (e.g. the DNP group[50] and haemo-globin[51]). Their applicability can, however, be increased by introducing a suitable absorbing group into the antigen, such as by using the 1-(m-nitro-phenyl)flavazole derivatives of the isomaltose oligosaccharides in the dextran–antidextran system[52]. Some of the methods which are suitable for measuring the initial phase of the interaction suffer from the disadvantage that they depend on the availability of purified antibody. This antibody may not, however, be representative of the original total antibody population due to selection during purification[53]. In contrast, the kinetics of the total antibody population can be studied using the Farr technique provided that the antigen or hapten is suitably labelled and is not precipitated by half-saturated ammonium sulphate. The procedure of equilibrium dialysis, in which free hapten distributes equally between two lipid phases whereas antibody-bound hapten is found exclusively in one phase, also suffers from some disadvantages. Thus, the attainment of equilibrium is relatively slow and the pore size of the membranes used does not permit the binding of large molecules to be studied. These disadvantages would, however, be obviated if the recent introduction of two phase aqueous polymer systems[54] proves successful, since these systems are applicable to large molecules and provide almost instantaneous equilibrium.

5.3 MOLECULAR BASIS OF ANTIGENICITY

Knowledge of the structures of the antigenic determinants of polysaccharides, nucleic acids, fibrous proteins, synthetic polypeptides and hapten-carrier complexes has been derived from studies of the capacities of the fragments of the antigen to inhibit the interaction of the whole antigen with antibody. These studies have established that each of the above antigens possesses a number of determinants which collectively express one or a small number of different specificities and which correspond to areas of defined composition, sequence, linkage and size. This approach has also proved applicable to the study of at least some globular proteins[55]. The results emphasise that globular proteins resemble, in general, other antigens but are much more complex in that the capacity to react with antibody is intimately related to the conformation of the whole protein and the determinants of any one molecule express a large number of different specificities.

5.3.1 Location of determinants

Much experimental evidence suggests that the determinants are located in those regions of the antigen that are most exposed to the surrounding environment. This view was based initially on the examination of branched-chain polysaccharides, such as dextran and the blood group substances, whose determinants coincide with the ends of the branches and the terminal residues represent the immunodominant groups. It was also supported by the observation that the majority of the antibodies formed against hapten–protein complexes are directed towards the surface-located haptenic groups. This evidence was, however, not conclusive since no information was available on the conformations of the polymers and the actual spatial arrangements of the determinants. Recently, more direct evidence in favour of the surface localisation of antigenic determinants has come from studies of selected synthetic polypeptides and of globular proteins of known surface structure, such as myoglobin[55]. For example, Sela and his co-workers[4, 5, 56] have shown that whereas antibodies are formed against terminal tyrosine and glutamic acid residues attached to poly-DL-alanine branches linked to a poly-L-lysine backbone (Figure 5.4a), no antibodies are produced when the tyrosyl-glutamyl sequences are coupled directly to the poly-L-lysine backbone and then covered up by the addition of poly-DL-alanine branches (Figure 5.4b). On the other hand, the latter polymer (Figure 5.4b) was immunogenic when the average distance between the branches was increased by interposing blocks of poly-DL-alanine within the poly-L-lysine backbone. Apart from endorsing the general principle that antigenic determinants are readily accessible to the environment, these results also argue strongly in favour of the view that antigens are not degraded *in vivo* prior to the stimulation of the antibody–biosynthetic mechanism.

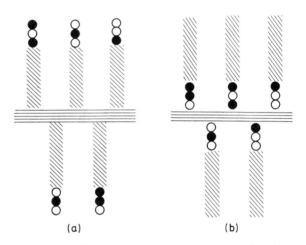

Figure 5.4 Peptides of L-tyrosine (●) and L-glutamic acid (○) were attached in (a) to poly-DL-alanine (diagonal hatching) coupled to poly-L-lysine (horizontal hatching) and in (b) directly to poly-L-lysine and then covered up with poly-DL-alanine (From Sela[5], by courtesy of The American Association for the Advancement of Science)

Although the conclusion that the determinants occupy exposed positions appears to be generally correct, it is apparent that with linear polymers the determinants are not restricted to the ends of the chain but recur at intervals along its length. Thus, pneumococcal SIII polysaccharide, which is a linear polymer of repeating units of [4-*O*-(β-D-glucopyranosyluronic acid)-D-glucose] linked glucosidically β-1,3, has on average one determinant for every ten sugar residues[15]. As noted previously for the determinants of branched-chain polymers, a portion of the determinants of linear polymers contributes a major part of the total binding energy and functions as an immunodominant group. In this case, however, each of the residues comprising the polymer may be immunodominant with the result that populations of antibody molecules with different specificities can be formed against the same portion of the molecule. This situation has been demonstrated to exist for the SIII polysaccharide where both glucose and glucuronic acid may function as the immunodominant group giving rise to two distinct populations of antibody molecules[15].

5.3.2 Role of confomation

The antigenicity of polysaccharides survives heating at 100 °C, whereas that of globular proteins is usually destroyed completely. This dramatic difference in behaviour emphasises the role played by conformation in determining the antigenicity of globular proteins. The importance of this role was recognised early in the development of immunochemistry when it was shown that denatured proteins react poorly, if at all, with antibodies to the native molecule[1]. During recent years the relationship between conformation and antigenicity has been more clearly established by using a number of approaches. Firstly, cleavage of the intramolecular disulphide bridges of proteins under denaturing conditions (e.g. by oxidation with performic acid or by reduction in the presence of urea and subsequent S-carboxymethylation) is invariably associated with significant distortions of their conformations and with a large reduction in their capacities to react with antibodies to the native molecule[57-59]. For instance, Figure 5.5 shows that completely reduced and carboxymethylated bovine serum albumin forms a negligible amount of precipitate with an antiserum to the unreduced protein. The unfolding of proteins by other means is also associated with a reduction in antigenicity, and a recent study[60] using various chemically modified albumins showed that the decrease in antigenic reactivity is directly related to the increase in Stokes radius (Figure 5.6). Secondly, antibodies prepared by immunisation with unfolded polypeptide chains (e.g. reduced and carboxymethylated lysozyme) react to a very much smaller extent with the native protein than the homologous antigen[61]. Thirdly, a more convincing example of the importance of conformation is provided by a comparison of the antigenicities of different conformational states of the same tripeptide (L-tyrosyl-L-alanyl-L-glutamate)[62] that was either polymerised to give an a-helical polymer or was coupled to branches of poly-DL-alanine attached to a backbone of poly-L-lysine in which case the peptide had a random conformation. Antibodies formed against each polypeptide failed to react with the other polymer and the tripeptide inhibited the interaction between the branched-chain polymer and its corresponding antibody only. It is apparent from these results that the specificity of the branched-chain polymer was determined solely by the sequence of amino acids, whereas that of the helical polymer was determined largely by the overall conformation of the molecule. Incidentally, these experiments illustrate the great versatility of synthetic polypeptides in immunochemical studies and the opportunities they provide for tailor-making a molecule to resolve a particular question.

The term, sequential determinant, has been proposed for those determinants of globular proteins whose specificities depend solely on the sequence of amino acids whereas the term, conformational determinant, is used for those determinants whose specificities and spatial arrangements rely on at least a portion of the remainder of the molecule[63]. In view of the very marked decrease in the antigenicity of globular proteins on denaturation, the majority of the determinants must be conformational. Although sequential determinants have been claimed to exist such claims are not very convincing unless supported by knowledge of the three-dimensional structure of the protein in question. On the other hand, it is evident from x-ray crystallographic analyses that short sequences of adjacent amino acids may be exposed on the surface of globular proteins (e.g. see Figure 4.1 in Ref. 64)

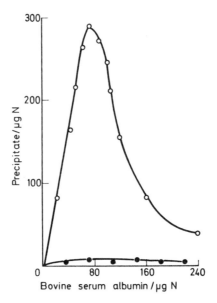

Figure 5.5 Precipitation of native bovine serum albumin (○) and of the completely reduced and carboxymethylated protein (●) with an antiserum prepared by immunisation with the unreduced protein (From Goetzl and Peters[59], by courtesy of Williams and Wilkins)

Complete reduction was achieved by treating a 0.5–1.5% soln. of bovine serum albumin in 8 M urea, pH 7.4, with 0.2 M 2-mercaptoethanol. The thiol groups of the reduced protein were subsequently alkylated using 0.25 M iodoacetic acid. Increasing amounts of albumin were added to a constant volume of the antiserum and the amounts of immune precipitate were estimated by measuring the nitrogen content

and that the potential to form sequential determinants exists. Although such sequences may account for any immunological reactivity that persists after complete denaturation, it seems likely that at least in some experiments the residual antigenicity is due to the persistence of some native structure.

In view of the close relationship between conformation and antigenicity a small conformational alteration would be expected to be expressed as a change in antigenic reactivity. This prediction is supported by the results of numerous studies. Thus, the removal of ferrihaem from metmyoglobin is associated with a small decrease in helical content, an overall swelling or slight increase in asymmetry of the protein and a decrease in reactivity with an antiserum to metmyoglobin[65, 66]. An equally dramatic example of the effect of a small conformational change on antigenicity is provided by oxy- and deoxy-haemoglobin[67]. Figure 5.7 shows that deoxyhaemoglobin reacts less extensively with antibodies against methaemoglobin than does oxyhaemoglobin. This difference is, undoubtedly, related to the change in

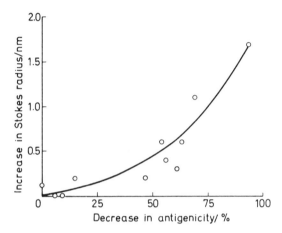

Figure 5.6 Relationship between the increase in Stokes radius of human serum albumin due to various modifications such as acetylation, amidination and carbethoxylation, and the associated decrease in antigenicity with antibodies to the native protein (data adapted from Table 3 of Ref. 60)

The Stokes radius of the chemically modified albumins was estimated by gel-filtration. The decrease in antigenicity was determined by measuring the capacities of the modified proteins to inhibit the binding of ^{131}I-labelled human serum albumin by antibodies to human serum albumin using a modified Farr assay; the results are expressed relative to the inhibition obtained with the native protein

quaternary structure on oxygenation of haemoglobin that arises from the displacement of the atoms in the areas of contact between the subunits by up to 5.7 Å[68]. In contrast to these and many other examples, it would appear that not all conformational alterations have a measurable effect on antigenicity[69].

Comparisons of the antigenic reactivities of globular proteins have also been employed as a probe for conformational similarities. For example, the lack of cross-reactivity between lysozyme and a-lactalbumin has been used as an argument against these proteins having the similar conformations proposed on the basis of their physical and chemical properties[70-72]. The value of this approach is, however, questionable since the absence of reaction may be explicable in terms of specific side chain differences superimposed upon similar conformations for the polypeptide backbone. Thus, although the α- and β-chains of human haemoglobin possess similar conformations, no cross-reactivity between the chains has been detected using their respective antisera[73].

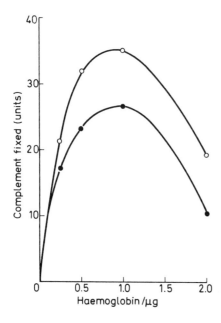

Figure 5.7 Comparison of antigenic reactivities of horse oxyhaemoglobin (○) and of deoxyhaemoglobin (●) by macro-complement fixation using an antiserum prepared by immunisation with horse met-haemoglobin (From Reichlin[67] by courtesy of Academic Press)

Increasing amounts of haemoglobin were added to 9 ml of buffer containing 1.0 ml of a 1 : 80 dilution of antiserum and the extent of reaction was estimated in terms of the number of units of added complement that were fixed (bound) by the immune complex after 14 h at 4 °C; a unit of complement is the amount giving 50% lysis of erythrocytes under standard conditions

5.3.3 Conformational changes induced by antibody

In contrast to the recognition of small conformational changes as differences in antigenicity, the results of a number of studies suggest that specific anti-bodies may induce conformational changes in the antigen[66, 74, 75]. Thus, the activation of defective, mutant enzymes to full enzymic activity by antibodies to the wild-type enzyme (e.g. β-galactosidase[76]) and the enhancement of enzymic activity by certain homologous antisera (e.g. ribonuclease[77]) have been accounted for in terms of an alteration in the conformation of the anti-gen. Conformational changes are most probably also the cause for the release of haem from sperm-whale metmyoglobin by antibodies to the haem-free protein, apomyoglobin[66]. A consideration of the various examples suggests that they comprise two groups that are mediated by two somewhat different, but not mutually exclusive mechanisms. The first group includes those cases in which antibody appears to induce a profound conformational alteration, such as the release of haem from metmyoglobin. Members of the second group comprise those instances where antibody selects and stabilises a pre-existing conformation of the antigen; for example, the increased affinity of ribonuclease S-protein for the S-peptide in the presence of antibodies to the whole enzyme[77] is most probably due to the stabilising effect of the antibodies on the conformation of S-protein that binds the peptide most strongly. The major difference between the two mechanisms is that in the first group the conformation of the antigen when bound by antibody does not pre-exist in equilibrium with other conformations.

A possible mechanism by which specific antibody can promote extensive conformational changes has been proposed previously[66]. It depends on the 'motility' of protein conformation and the assumption that localised areas of the surface of the molecule can undergo small, rapid and reversible fluctuations in shape. In this case, interaction of a localised, transient shape with specific antibody would freeze the conformation of this portion of the surface structure, and the stabilisation of a number of particular, localised conformations would probably promote additional changes elsewhere in the molecule.

If, as has been suggested, antibody can stabilise a pre-existing conformation in equilibrium with other forms, then interaction with antibody should impose a constraint upon the flexibility of antigen molecules. This prediction is supported by the stabilisation by antibody of various enzymes against denaturation (e.g. catalase[78]) and by the observation[79] that the monovalent fragments of antibodies to the helical polymer $(Try-Ala-Glu)_{200}$ promoted a helical conformation in the largely non-helical oligopeptide $(Try-Ala-Glu)_{13}$. The interaction of myoglobin peptides, which possess predominantly random coil conformations, with antibodies against helical portions of native myoglobin[80, 81] is also consistent with this proposal.

5.3.4 Globular proteins as antigens

The localisation and structures of the antigenic determinants of globular proteins have been examined on numerous occasions using various proteins[55, 82-84]. The results of these studies confirm that the structures of the majority of the determinants depend on the overall conformation of the whole molecule. As a result, a complete understanding of the molecular basis of antigenicity can only be derived for those proteins whose three-dimensional structures are known.

Information on the nature of the determinants has been obtained by using two main approaches. Firstly, the isolation and characterisation of immunologically active fragments obtained by enzymic degradation (e.g. myoglobin[85]), chemical degradation (e.g. cleavage of myoglobin at specific amino acid residues[86]), or from mutants with chain-terminating codons (e.g. β-galactosidase[87]). Secondly, the comparison of the antigenicities of proteins differing by one or more amino acid residues and derived either by mutation (e.g. cytochrome C[88] and haemoglobin[89]), or by chemical modification (e.g. lysozyme[69] and myoglobin[90]). Each of these approaches suffers, however, from a number of disadvantages. The first approach appears not to be universally applicable in that it has not proved possible to inhibit the antigenicities of some proteins, especially ribonuclease and cytochrome C, by peptide fragments[88]. Also, the variety of overlapping peptides required to map a determinant completely may not be readily obtained by degradation, although this objection can be overcome by synthesis[91]. The second approach has the disadvantage that change of an amino acid residue, particularly by chemical means, may promote conformational changes remote from the area of modification[92]. Although fairly convincing arguments have been presented in support of the view that the structural effects of single amino acid changes are primarily confined to the local environment[89, 92] unequivocal conclusions concerning the structural basis of a change in immunological reactivity can only be made if the structural changes have been exactly delineated. Conformational alterations are usually monitored by determining the solution properties using conventional procedures[69, 90], but it appears that this method is not ideal and that definitive information can only be achieved by difference Fourier techniques[92]. The above criticism does not, of course, apply in those instances where a change in structure has no effect on antigenicity. For example, reduction of the glutamic acid residues at positions 83 and 85 of myoglobin to the corresponding hydroxy acid failed to give a detectable change in immunological reactivity[90].

In both approaches, the method employed to measure antigenicity is of considerable importance. Thus, differences in activity between modified proteins may not be detected by using certain procedures (see Section 5.2.5). Also, the activities of fragments should be measured relative to that of the native antigen by the technique of hapten-inhibition, since only in this case can knowledge of the surface structure of the antigen be used to derive the structure of the determinant. This is because antisera to the native antigen may contain antibodies against partly denatured forms[58-60] or 'hidden determinants'[93] that react preferentially with fragments of the antigen but fail to bind the native protein. In this case, results obtained by direct measurement of fragment antigenicity (e.g. an eicosapeptide of TMV protein[94]) have questionable relevance to the determinants of the native protein.

In spite of the above criticisms, these approaches have yielded much useful information on the molecular basis of the antigenicity of globular proteins in general, and the nature of the antigenic determinants of sperm-whale myoglobin, egg white lysozome, tobacco mosaic virus protein, cytochrome C and haemoglobin in particular. The major findings of these studies are given in the following summary (see also Figures 5.8 and 5.9).

Firstly, the determinants are restricted to the surface of the protein and do not include buried amino acid residues. The results further suggest that the determinants are preferentially located in the more exposed areas of the surface. Thus, the immunologically active 'loop' peptide (residues No. 64–83) of lysozyme[97, 101] occupies an exposed position (Figure 5.8) and active fragments of myoglobin[85, 100] are adjacent to or include the corners of the folded polypeptide chain (Figure 5.9 and see Figure 5.6, Ref. 90).

Secondly, each protein possesses a finite number of determinants with different specificities. Although the density of determinants has proved difficult to assess, a number of studies suggest about one site per 5000 mol. wt. Direct evidence in support of this suggestion is provided by the observation[51] that haemoglobin binds 6 mol. of Fab fragments per $\alpha\beta$-dimer (mol. wt. 32 000). A similar density (5 sites/$\alpha\beta$-dimer) has been derived from comparisons of mutant haemoglobins[89], whereas myoglobin (mol. wt. 17 800) appears to possess four antigenic regions[86]. In some cases the determinants may not be equally distributed across the surface; for example, a part (fragment A;

mol. wt. 18 000) of flagellin (mol. wt. 40 000) possesses all the determinants (at least 3) of the whole molecule[102].

Thirdly, there is suggestive evidence that a determinant may encompass a larger surface area than that corresponding to the maximum size of the antibody combining site, and that different antisera may recognise overlapping portions of the determinant[94]. If this suggestion is correct, then it may account for the differences in structure reported by different workers for what is apparently the same determinant (e.g. the *C*-terminal determinant of myoglobin[27, 86, 103]).

Fourthly, studies of phylogenetically related and mutant proteins[88, 89] have

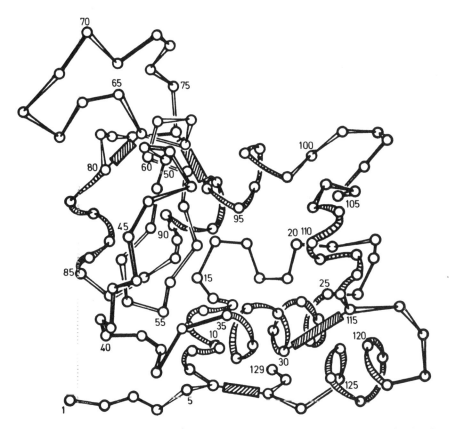

Figure 5.8 A two-dimensional representation of the conformation of a molecule of egg white lysozyme (From Blake *et al.*[95], by courtesy of Macmillan). The amino acid residues are numbered from the *N*- to the *C*-terminii. The cross-hatched portions of the polypeptide chain correspond to α-helical segments and the diagonally hatched rectangles represent disulphide bridges

Immunologically active fragments have been isolated[96, 97] that correspond to two regions of the molecule; firstly, residues No. 1–27 and 122–129 linked by a disulphide bond and secondly, residues No. 57–107 cross-linked by two disulphide bonds but with a break in the peptide chain within the regions 83–86. These areas express different antigenic specificities[98] clearly shown that single amino acid residues can make a decisive contribution to the antigenicity of the whole molecule. For instance, 30–40% of the antibodies to human cytochrome C failed to react with *Macaca mulatta* cytochrome C which differs from the human protein by one amino acid residue only [88]. These studies have also indicated that there is, in general, a direct relationship between the degree of cross-reactivity and the number of amino acid changes (see Figure 6, Ref. 48).

Fifthly, the determinants are primarily associated with the phylogenetically

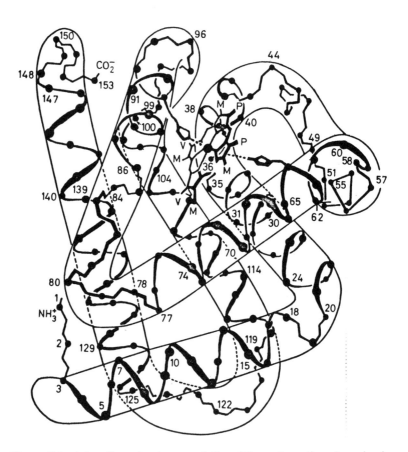

Figure 5.9 A two-dimensional representation of the conformation of a molecule of sperm-whale myoglobin (based on a drawing by Dickerson[99]). The amino acid residues are numbered from the *N*- to the *C*-terminii and are arranged in eight helical segments that are separated by non-helical regions. The polypeptide chain is further folded into a bag-like structure containing a non-polar pocket that is occupied by the haem group, the iron atom of which is linked to histidine residues No. 64 and 93

Immunologically active peptides corresponding to residues No. 15–29, 56–69, 70–76, 77–89, 139–149 and 147–153 were obtained from chymotryptic digests[85], whereas inhibitory fragments corresponding to residues No. 17–31, 79–96, 119–133 and 148–153 were isolated from tryptic digests[100]

non-conserved regions of the polypeptide chain[89, 104]. This concept is consistent with the accepted principle that the immunised animal recognises the structural differences between the antigen and its own corresponding protein.

5.4 MOLECULAR BASIS OF IMMUNOGENICITY

The capacity to induce an immune response represents the product of a complex series of interacting parameters such as the physical state and chemical nature of the immunogen, the species and strain of animal immunised, the degree of dissimilarity in structure between the immunogen and the animal's own molecules, the amount of material injected, the rate of catabolism of the immunogen, etc.[105]. An understanding of the molecular basis of immunogenicity can be achieved only by taking account of all these parameters. It is, also, of considerable importance that the results should be interpreted relative to the cellular aspects of the immune response and especially in the context of the following current theories: (a) the response to a particular determinant is under genetic control[106]; (b) the initiation of antibody production is mediated by the interaction of the antigenic determinant with complementary receptors on the lymphocyte surface[107]. A particular lymphocyte has the capacity to promote the synthesis of antibody of only one specificity which is identical with that of the surface receptor; (c) T- and B-lymphocytes act synergistically in responding to most immunogens[108, 109] and macrophages may also participate in T- and B-cell co-operation[110].

A relationship between the molecular nature of the immunogen, its immunogenicity, and T- and B-cell co-operation can be established if two assumptions are made. Firstly, stimulation of B-lymphocytes depends on the immunogen cross-linking the surface receptors or being bound with a certain minimum affinity[111]. The required degree of binding can be achieved through multivalency either directly for antigens of high molecular weight with repeating determinants of the same specificity (thymus-independent antigens, e.g. polymeric flagellin from *Salmonella adelaide*) or, more usually, indirectly by prior binding to T-lymphocytes (thymus-dependent antigens, e.g. monomeric flagellin). Secondly, interaction of a molecule of the immunogen with T- and B-lymphocytes is mediated by determinants with different structures. In this context a particular globular protein may be regarded as representing a variety of immunogens in that each molecule behaves as if composed of a single antigenic determinant (the hapten) with the remainder of the molecule acting as the carrier. Direct evidence in support of this assumption is available if it is accepted that cellular and humoral immune responses express the prior interaction of the immunogen with T- and B-lymphocytes, respectively. For example, the reaction of glucagon with humoral antibody is mediated by the N-terminus of the polypeptide chain whereas the C-terminus appears to be of primary importance in determining cellular immunity[112]. Also, although reduced and carboxymethylated lysozyme failed to cross-react with humoral antibodies to the native protein, extensive cross-reactivity was observed by cellular immunity[113]. In contrast to the above examples, it is apparent that the same portion of at least some molecules (e.g. the *N*-terminal fragment of oxidised ferredoxin[114]) can elicit both cellular and humoral responses and, consequently, can interact with both T- and B-cells. If the above views are correct then the molecular requirements for immunogenicity include such factors as the number of determinants, whether the determinants possess the same or different specificities and whether they express both hapten and carrier functions, and the spacing or distance between determinants.

5.4.1 Effect of molecular size

Various studies have established that there is a progressive increase in immunogenicity with increasing molecular size and that this relationship is independent of the chemical nature of the immunogen[115-117]. For example, monomeric cytochrome C is a poor immunogen but is converted into a good immunogen by aggregation with glutaraldehyde[118]. Furthermore, the removal of aggregates from bovine immunoglobulin is not only associated with a large reduction in immunogenicity but also with the development of strong tolerance-inducing properties[119]. Similar relationships have been established using flagellin of *Salmonella adelaide* which, due to the availability of various molecular forms, has allowed a more systematic approach. Thus, higher peak antibody titres were obtained with polymeric than monomeric flagellin, although the smallest dose required to produce the peak response showed an inverse relationship (1000 and 10 ng respectively)[115]. Of greater interest are the reports that fragmentation of flagellin with cyanogen bromide or chemical modification with diketene (acetoacetylation) are associated with a marked reduction in immunogenicity and a dramatic increase in tolerogenicity[120, 121]. It appears likely that the basis of these phenomena lies in the molecular requirement for T-B lymphocyte co-operation[122]. Acetoacetylation caused loss of antigenicity (i.e. hapten function) but, in contrast, the capacity to induce cellular immunity (i.e. interaction with T-cells) was promoted[122]. In this case the decrease in humoral antibody production is probably due to the inability to interact with B-lymphocytes, whereas the promotion in tolerogenicity can be explained in terms of the depletion, by binding, of carrier-specific T-cells. It is more difficult to account convincingly for the decrease in immunogenicity and increase in tolerogenicity of fragment A produced by cyanogen bromide cleavage. The slightly reduced affinity of the fragment for humoral antibodies to flagellin[121] suggests, however, that the fragment may not be bound sufficiently strongly by B-lymphocytes to initiate the production of circulating antibodies. Incidentally, the decrease in antigenicity of acetoacetylated flagellin and the associated increase in reactivity with cell-bound antibody parallels the results obtained with partly unfolded lysozyme[113], and argues strongly in favour of the view that the specificity requirements of the T-cell receptor are less stringent than those of the B-cell receptor.

Various attempts have been made to determine the minimum molecular size necessary for immunogenicity. The most definitive study showed, by using a series of *a*-DNP-oligo-L-lysines of increasing size, that the heptamer was the smallest molecule inducing humoral and cell-mediated responses in guinea-pigs[123]. Other studies have demonstrated that low molecular weight oligopeptides such as angiotensin (mol. wt. 1031) are immunogenic[124] and even L-tyrosine-azobenzenearsonate provokes cellular immunity in guinea-pigs[125]. The minimal size required for immunogenicity appears, however, to vary with the chemical nature of the immunogen and is most probably related to the capacity to promote cell co-operation or a high affinity for cell receptors. Thus, the minimal size for polypeptides which depend on T-B co-operation is lower than for polysaccharides with repeating determinants of the same specificity[117]. The importance of size in relation to immunogenicity is emphasised by the recent demonstration that if the *N*- and *C*-terminal antigenic determinants of oxidised ferredoxin were joined by a bridge of five amino acids the molecule was not immunogenic whereas a bridge of ten amino acids conferred strong immunogenicity[114].

5.4.2 Effect of molecular complexity

Numerous results suggest that immunogenicity is directly related to the degree of molecular complexity. For example, synthetic polypeptides composed of 3–4 different amino acids are more immunogenic than homopolymers or polymers containing two different amino acids. Indeed this relationship would be predicted given a requirement for determinants with different specificities for cell co-operation, since the more complex the immunogen the greater the likelihood of different determinants. By analogy, the relatively simple and repetitive structures of polysaccharides and nucleic acids are probably responsible for their poor immunogenicities relative to proteins and also for the profound increase in immunogenicity when coupled to protein. If a high affinity for cell receptors is a prerequisite for good immunogenicity, then molecules with various conformational states in rapid equilibrium would be expected to be poor immunogens. This prediction is supported by some evidence in that the immunogenicity of gelatin was greatly increased by the attachment of short oligopeptides containing tyrosine, which were considered to increase the rigidity of the molecule[127].

5.5 SUMMARY

The order of specificity of antigen–antibody interaction and the size of antigenic determinants reflect the nature of the non-covalent forces responsible for binding. These and some other parameters are shared by other intermolecular complexes, such as enzyme–substrate. Antigens possess a finite number of determinants which correspond to discrete portions of the surface with a well-defined maximal size. A part of the determinant is bound more strongly by antibody than the remainder and is primarily responsible for the specificity. The determinants of a simple polymer with a repetitive structure possess the same or a small number of different specificities, whereas those of a globular protein express a larger variety of specificities the majority of which depend on the conformation of the whole protein. The capacity of a substance to induce antibody formation is determined by its size and chemical nature, and can be accounted for in terms of the number, distribution and specificities of the determinants and their interaction with the antigen receptors of T- and B-lymphocytes.

References

1. Landsteiner, K. (1945). *The specificity of serological reactions*, 2nd edn. (Cambridge, Mass.: Harvard Univ. Press) (reprinted 1962 New York: Dover Publ. Inc.)
2. Plescia, O. J. and Braun, W. (1967). *Advan. Immunol.*, **6**, 231
3. Levine, L. and Stollar, B. D. (1968). *Progr. Allergy*, **12**, 161
4. Sela, M. (1966). *Advan. Immunol.*, **5**, 29
5. Sela, M. (1969). *Science*, **166**, 1365
6. Rapport, M. M. and Graf, L. (1969). *Progr. Allergy*, **13**, 273
7. Ehrlich, P. (1900). *Proc. Roy. Soc. (London)*, **66**, 424
8. Karush, F. (1962). *Advan. Immunol.*, **2**, 1
9. Nemethy, G. (1969). *Ann. N.Y. Acad. Sci.*, **155**, 492
10. Karush, F. (1957). *J. Amer. Chem. Soc.*, **79**, 3380
11. Luderitz, O., Staub, A. M. and Westphal, O. (1966). *Bacteriol. Rev.*, **30**, 192
12. Watkins, W. M. (1966). *Science*, **152**, 172
13. Lloyd, K. O., Kabat, E. A. and Licerio, E. (1968). *Biochemistry*, **7**, 2976
14. Watkins, W. M. (1972). *Glycoproteins*, 2nd edn., 830 (A. Gottschalk, editor) (Amsterdam: Elsevier Publ. Co.)
15. Mage, R. G. and Kabat, E. A. (1963). *Biochemistry*, **2**, 1278
16. Kabat, E. A. (1966). *J. Immunol.*, **97**, 1
17. Kabat, E. A. (1960). *J. Immunol.*, **84**, 82
18. Mage, R. G. and Kabat, E. A. (1963). *J. Immunol.*, **91**, 633
19. Cebra, J. J. (1961). *J. Immunol.*, **86**, 205
20. Stollar, D., Levine, L., Lehrer, H. I. and Van Vunakis, H. (1962). *Proc. Nat. Acad. Sci. USA*, **48**, 874
21. Sage, H. J., Deutsch, G. F., Fasman, G. D. and Levine, L. (1964). *Immunochemistry*, **1**, 133
22. Van Vunakis, H., Kaplan, J., Lehrer, H. and Levine, L. (1966). *Immunochemistry*, **3**, 393
23. Goodman, J. W., Nitecki, D. E. and Stoltenberg, I. M. (1968). *Biochemistry*, **7**, 706
24. Goodman, J. W. (1969). *Immunochemistry*, **6**, 139
25. Schechter, B., Schechter, I. and Sela, M. (1970). *J. Biol. Chem.*, **245**, 1438
26. Crumpton, M. J. (1967). *Nature (London)*, **215**, 17
27. Crumpton, M. J., Law, H. D. and Strong, R. C. (1970). *Biochem. J.*, **116**, 923
28. Levin, H. A., Levine, H. and Schlossman, S. F. (1970). *J. Immunol.*, **104**, 1377
29. Schleifer, K. H. and Krause, R. M. (1971). *J. Biol. Chem.*, **246**, 986
30. Schechter, I., Clerici, E. and Zazepitski, E. (1971). *Europ. J. Biochem.*, **18**, 561
31. Spragg, J., Schroder, E., Steward, J. M., Austen, K. F. and Haber, E. (1967). *Biochemistry*, **6**, 3933
32. Benjamini, E., Shimizu, M., Young, J. D. and Leung, C. Y. (1968). *Biochemistry*, **7**, 1261
33. Eisen, H. N. and Siskind, G. W. (1964). *Biochemistry*, **3**, 996
34. Parker, C. W., Gott, S. M. and Johnson, M. C. (1966). *Biochemistry*, **5**, 2314
35. Paul, W. E., Siskind, G. W. and Benacerraf, B. (1966). *J. Exp. Med.*, **123**, 689
36. Berger, A. and Schechter, I. (1970). *Phil. Trans. Roy. Soc. Lond. B.*, **257**, 249
37. Kabat, E. A. (1956). *J. Immunol.*, **77**, 377
38. Sela, M. and Mozes, E. (1966). *Proc. Nat. Acad. Sci. USA*, **55**, 445
39. Rude, E., Mozes, E. and Sela, M. (1968). *Biochemistry*, **7**, 2971
40. Sela, M., Mozes, E., Shearer, G. M. and Karniely, Y. (1970). *Proc. Nat. Acad. Sci. USA*, **67**, 1288
41. Nussenzweig, V. and Green, I. (1971). *J. Immunol.*, **106**, 1089
42. Blake, C. C. F., Johnson, L. N., Mair, G. A., North, A. C. T., Phillips, D. C. and Sarma, V. R. (1967). *Proc. Roy. Soc. (London) B.*, **167**, 378
43. Poljak, R. T., Amzel, L. M., Avey, H. P., Becka, L. N. and Nisonoff, A. (1972). *Nature New Biol.*, **235**, 137

44. Kabat, E. A. and Mayer, M. M. (1961). *Experimental Immunochemistry*, 2nd edn. (Springfield, I 11: Charles C. Thomas)
45. Williams, C. A. and Chase, M. A. (editors) (1971). *Method Immunology, Immunochemistry* Vol. 3 (New York: Academic Press Inc.)
46. Weir, D. M. (editor) (1973). *Handbook of experimental immunology*, 2nd edn., (Oxford: Blackwell Scientific Publ.)
47. Reichlin, M., Hay, M. and Levine, L. (1964). *Immunochemistry*, **1**, 21
48. Prager, E. M. and Wilson, A. C. (1971). *J. Biol. Chem.*, **246**, 7010
49. Bucci, E. and Fronticelli, C. (1971). *Biochim. Biophys. Acta*, **243**, 170
50. Velick, S. F., Parker, C. W. and Eisen, N. H. (1960). *Proc. Nat. Acad. Sci. USA*, **46**, 1470
51. Nobel, R. W., Reichlin, M. and Gibson, Q. H. (1969). *J. Biol. Chem.*, **244**, 2403
52. Harisdangkul, V. and Kabat, E. A. (1972). *J. Immunol.*, **108**, 1232
53. Stevenson, G. T., Eisen, N. H. and Jones, R. H. (1970). *Biochem. J.*, **116**, 151
54. Desbuquois, B. and Aurbach, G. D. (1972). *Biochem. J.*, **126**, 717
55. Crumpton, M. J. (1967). *Antibodies to Biologically Active Molecules*, 61 (B. Cinader, editor) (Oxford: Pergamon)
56. Sela, M., Fuchs, S. and Arnon, R. (1962). *Biochem. J.*, **85**, 223
57. Brown, R. K., Delaney, R., Levine, L. and Van Vunakis, H. (1959). *J. Biol. Chem.*, **234**, 2043
58. Young, J. D. and Leung, C. Y. (1970). *Biochemistry*, **9**, 2755
59. Goetzl, E. J. and Peters, J. H. (1972). *J. Immunol.*, **108**, 785
60. Jacobsen, C., Funding, L., Moller, N. P. H. and Steensgaard, J. (1972). *Europ. J. Biochem.*, **30**, 392
61. Arnon, R. and Maron, E. (1971). *J. Molec. Biol.*, **61**, 225
62. Schechter, B., Schechter, I., Ramachandran, J., Conway-Jacobs, A. Sela, M., Benjamini, E. and Shimizu, M. (1971). *Europ. J. Biochem.*, **20**, 309
63. Sela, M., Schechter, B., Schechter, I. and Borek, F. (1967). *Cold Spring Harb. Symp. Quant. Biol.*, **32**, 537
64. Hendrickson, W. A. and Love, W. E. (1971). *Nature New. Biol.*, **232**, 197
65. Reichlin, M., Hay, M. and Levine, L. (1963). *Biochemistry*, **2**, 971
66. Crumpton, M. J. (1972). *Protein–protein Interactions*, 395 (R. Jaenicke and E. Helmreich, editors) (Heidelberg: Springer-Verlag)
67. Reichlin, M., Bucci, E., Antonini, E., Wyman, J. and Rossi-Fanelli, A. (1964). *J. Molec. Biol.*, **9**, 785
68. Perutz, M. F., Muirhead, H., Cox, J. M. and Goaman, L. C. G. (1968). *Nature (London)*, **219**, 131
69. Atassi, M. Z., Suliman, A. M. and Habeeb, A. F. S. A. (1972). *Immunochemistry*, **9**, 907
70. Arnon, R. and Maron, E. (1970). *J. Molec. Biol.* **51**, 703
71. Atassi, M. Z., Habeeb, A. F. S. A. and Rydstedt, L. (1970). *Biochim. Biophys. Acta*, **200**, 184
72. Faure, A. and Jolles, P. (1970). *FEBS Lett.*, **10**, 237
73. Reichlin, M., Bucci, E., Fronticelli, C., Wyman, J., Antonini, E., Ioppolo, C. and Rossi-Fanelli, A. (1966). *J. Molec. Biol.*, **17**, 18
74. Celada, F. and Strom, R. (1972). *Quat. Rev. Biophys.*, **5**, 395
75. Melchers, F., Kohler, G. and Messer, W. (1972). *Protein–protein Interactions*, 409 (R. Jaenicke and E. Helmreich, editors) (Heidelberg: Springer-Verlag)
76. Rotman, M. B. and Celada, F. (1968). *Proc. Nat. Acad. Sci. USA*, **60**, 660
77. Cinader, B., Suzuki, T. and Pelichova, H. (1971). *J. Immunol.*, **106**, 1381
78. Feinstein, R. N., Jaroslow, B. N., Howard, J. B. and Faulhaber, J. T. (1971). *J. Immunol.*, **106**, 1316
79. Schechter, B., Conway-Jacobs, A. and Sela, M. (1971). *Europ. J. Biochem.*, **20**, 321
80. Crumpton, M. J. and Small, P. A. (1967). *J. Molec. Biol.*, **26**, 143
81. Atassi, M. Z. and Singhal, R. P. (1970). *J. Biol. Chem.*, **245**, 5122
82. Kaminski, M. (1965). *Progr. Allergy*, **9**, 79
83. Arnon, R. (1971). *Current Topics in Microbiol. Immunol.*, **54**, 47
84. Benjamini, E., Scribienski, R. J. and Thompson, K. (1972). *Contemporary Topics in Immunochem.* Vol. 1, 1 (F. P. Inman, editor) (New York-London: Plenum Press)
85. Crumpton, M. J. and Wilkinson, J. M. (1965). *Biochem. J.*, **94**, 545

86. Atassi, M. Z. and Singhal, R. P. (1970). *Biochemistry*, **9**, 3854
87. Fowler, A. V. and Zabin, I. (1968). *J. Molec. Biol.*, **33**, 35
88. Nisonoff, A., Reichlin, M. and Margoliash, E. (1970). *J. Biol. Chem.*, **245**, 940
89. Reichlin, M. (1972). *J. Molec. Biol.*, **64**, 485
90. Atassi, M. Z. and Perlstein, M. T. (1972). *Biochemistry*, **11**, 3984
91. Young, J. D., Benjamini, E., Steward, J. M. and Leung, C. Y. (1967). *Biochemistry*, **6**, 1455
92. Moffat, J. K. (1971). *J. Molec. Biol.*, **58**, 79
93. Ishizaka, T., Campbell, D. H. and Ishizaka, K. (1960). *Proc. Soc. Exp. Biol. Med.*, **103**, 5
94. Benjamini, E., Shimizu, M., Young, J. D. and Leung, C. Y. (1968). *Biochemistry*, **7**, 1253
95. Blake, C. C. F., Koenig, D. F., Mair, G. A., North, A. C. T., Phillips, D. C. and Sarma, V. R. (1965). *Nature (London)*, **206**, 757
96. Shinka, S., Imanishi, M., Miyagawa, N., Amano, T., Inouye, M. and Tsugita, A. (1967). *Biken. J.*, **10**, 89
97. Fujio, H., Imanishi, M., Nishioka, K. and Amano, T. (1968). *Biken. J.*, **11**, 207
98. Fujio, H., Imanishi, M., Nishioka, K. and Amano, T. (1968). *Biken, J.*, **11**, 219
99. Dickerson, R. E. (1964). *The Proteins*, 2nd edn., Vol. 2, 634 (H. Neurath, editor) (New York: Academic Press Inc.)
100. Atassi, M. Z. and Saplin, B. J. (1968). *Biochemistry*, **7**, 688
101. Arnon, R. and Sela, M. (1969). *Proc. Nat. Acad. Sci. USA*, **62**, 163
102. Parish, C. R. and Ada, G. L. (1972). *Contemporary Topics in Immunochem.* Vol. 1, 77 (F. P. Inman, editor) (New York-London: Plenum Press)
103. Givas, J. K., Sehon, A. H. and Manning, M. (1972). *Biochemistry*, **11**, 1351
104. Byfield, P. G. H., Clark, M. B., Turner, K., Foster, G. V. and MacIntyre, I. (1972). *Biochem. J.*, **127**, 199
105. Borek, F. (editor) (1972). *Immunogenicity* (Amsterdam: North-Holland Publ Co.)
106. Benacerraf, B. and McDevitt, H. O. (1972). *Science*, **175**, 273
107. Mitchison, N. A. (1968). *Symp. Int. Soc. Cell Biol.*, **7**, 29
108. Taylor, R. B. (1969). *Transplant. Rev.*, **1**, 114
109. Paul, W. E. (1970). *Transplant. Rev.*, **5**, 130
110. Feldman, M. (1972). *J. Exp. Med.*, **135**, 1049
111. Klinman, N. R. (1972). *J. Exp. Med.*, **136**, 241
112. Senyk, G., Williams, E. B., Nitecki, D. E. and Goodman, J. W. (1971). *J. Exp. Med.*, **133**, 1294
113. Thompson, K., Harris, M., Benjamini, E., Mitchell, G. and Noble, M. (1972). *Nature New. Biol.*, **238**, 20
114. Levy, J. G., Hull, D., Kelly, B., Kilburn, D. G. and Teather, R. M. (1972). *Cell. Immunol.*, **5**, 87
115. Nossal, G. J. V., Ada, G. L. and Austin, C. M. (1964). *Aust. J. Exp. Biol. Med. Sci.*, **42**, 283
116. Amkraut, A. A., Malley, A. and Begley, D. (1969). *J. Immunol.*, **103**, 1301
117. Howard, J. G., Zola, H., Christie, G. H. and Courtenay, B. M. (1971). *Immunology*, **21**, 535
118. Reichlin, M., Nisonoff, A. and Margoliash, E. (1970). *J. Biol. Chem.*, **245**, 947
119. Dresser, D. W. (1962). *Immunology*, **5**, 378
120. Parish, C. R. and Ada, G. L. (1969). *Immunology*, **17**, 153
121. Parish, C. R. (1971). *J. Exp. Med.*, **134**, 1
122. Parish, C. R. (1971). *J. Exp. Med.*, **134**, 21
123. Schlossman, S. F. and Yaron, A. (1970). *Ann. N.Y. Acad. Sci.*, **169**, 108
124. Sela, M. (1970). *Ann. N.Y. Acad. Sci.*, **169**, 23
125. Alkan, S. S., Williams, E. B., Nitecki, D. E. and Goodman, J. W. (1972). *J. Exp. Med.*, **135**, 1228
126. Richter, W. and Kagedal, L. (1972). *Int. Arch. Allergy*, **42**, 885
127. Sela, M. and Arnon, R. (1960). *Biochem. J.*, **77**, 394

6
Immunoglobulin Structure

R. R. PORTER
University of Oxford

6.1   INTRODUCTION

Immunoglobulins are the proteins which carry antibody activity, that is, which show the power to combine specifically with foreign substances. This antibody activity appears in response to prior entry into the animal, by infection or by other means, of material which is foreign to that animal. The high degree of specificity of the response is an essential feature and implies that each individual animal is capable of synthesising a very wide range of distinct antibody molecules.

This phenomenon is apparently confined to vertebrates but it is probable that a related immune reaction occurs in invertebrates[1], although there is little evidence yet about the molecular mechanism involved.

It is apparent that the immunoglobulins in the blood of any animal must be a highly-complex group of proteins. The resolution of the complexity has depended on the use of a variety of techniques, but particularly on studies of the antigenic specificities of the immunoglobulins. The preparation of antisera able to distinguish between different forms of immunoglobulin in humans has, in turn, depended on the use as antigens of myeloma proteins and Bence–Jones proteins. These are pathological proteins which appear in the blood and urine, respectively, of patients suffering from myelomatosis, a cancer of the lymphoid tissues which synthesise immunoglobulins. The myeloma proteins are each a single molecular species of immunoglobulins. The urinary Bence–Jones proteins are the free light chains of the myeloma proteins present in the blood of the same patient. These pathological proteins are the only known examples of homogeneous immunoglobulins although approximation to homogeneity has been achieved for certain mouse and rabbit antibodies[2].

With the myeloma proteins, it was therefore possible to raise antisera specific to particular kinds of immunoglobulin and use them to distinguish different fractions in the complex mixture of immunoglobulins present in normal serum. Spontaneous cases of myelomatosis are most frequently detected in human patients and, hence, the early work was concerned with the resolution of human immunoglobulins and studies of other immunoglobulins have in most cases followed.

6.2 RESOLUTION OF IMMUNOGLOBULINS

6.2.1 Class

The distinction between high- and low-molecular weight immunoglobulins was made in 1937 when it was shown that horse- anti-pneumococcal antibody occurred in two forms—one of mol. wt. 900 000 and the other 150 000[3]. These two classes are now named immunoglobulin macro, IgM, and immunoglobulin gamma, IgG, respectively. The third major class, immunoglobulin alpha, IgA, was recognised when the technique of immunoelectrophoresis was introduced by Grabar and Williams[4]. It was observed that anti-immunoglobulin antisera would show a third line of precipitation with human serum after separation of the components by electrophoresis. That there were common structural features was apparent from the shared antigenic specificities.

Two minor classes have been identified in human serum after their appearance as myeloma proteins. The first was IgD[5, 6]: it is present in normal serum at concentrations averaging 3 mg $(100 \text{ ml})^{-1}$. The very low concentration is presumably the reason for the difficulty of demonstrating antibody activity in this fraction[6]. Estimates of the mol. wt. of IgD range from 172 000 to 200 000 and particular difficulty arises in isolation and handling due to its exceptional vulnerability to the proteolytic enzymes in the serum.

The second minor class, IgE, has aroused much greater interest because although also present in very low concentrations in serum (<0.1 mg 100 ml^{-1}) it has been identified as the carrier of reaginic antibody activity and is therefore of considerable clinical importance[7, 8]. Again, unequivocal characterisation of the new class of immunoglobulin depended upon the finding of a myeloma protein of this class. Originally named IgND[9], its identity with IgE, the new class of immunoglobulin postulated by Ishizaka and Ishizaka as containing reagins, was shown by the comparison of antigenic specificities and other properties[10]. Homocytotrophic antibodies comparable in biological activity to reaginic antibodies appear to be present in all species in which they have been sought. They are similar in physical properties to IgE from human serum with a sedimentation value of 7 S and a mol. wt. of 190 000.

6.2.2 Subclass

Two of the three major classes of human immunoglobulins have been divided again by antigenic specificity, into subclasses. Thus IgG gives IgG1, 2, 3 and 4 in order of their concentration in the serum and IgA into A1 and A2. The subclasses share the class-specific antigenic determinants but can be further distinguished by subclass-specific antisera. Differences in biological activity have been observed, for example, IgG2 cannot, on intra-dermal injection, give rise to passive cutaneous anaphylaxis on subsequent challenge. It is probably unable to bind to the cell surface. IgG4 does not fix complement[11].

6.2.3 Types

The occurrence of two antigenic types of Bence–Jones proteins and myeloma proteins was reported and these are now known as κ and λ. These specificities are common to all classes and subclasses of immunoglobulins and have since been shown to be due to light chain structures. Though differing substantially in amino acid sequence, the κ and λ light chains are similar in length and apparently perform identical structural and biological roles; no differences have been detected so far. A further subdivision of the λ-chain has been found in both man and mouse immunoglobulins. The κ-chain of rabbit immunoglobulin has also been subdivided.

The term 'isotypic' has been used for all these antigenic specificities of class, subclass, type and subtype as they are found in the immunoglobulins of all individuals of one species[12].

6.2.4 Allotypes

Allotypes are inherited allelic variants detected by differences in antigenic specificity and were first reported in rabbit IgG by Oudin[13], who obtained distinguishing sera by injection of antibody–antigen precipitates from the serum of one rabbit into other rabbits. The use of washed precipitates was an easy method of isolating immunoglobulin and injection of individuals within one species ensured that the only antigenic differences picked up were distinct from the class, subclass and type, which are common to all individuals in one species.

Related individual variations were reported at the same time in human IgG[14] but were recognised in a more complex manner. The serum of rheumatic patients contains high-molecular weight immunoglobulin complexes, rheumatoid factor, which will combine with human IgG. This can be shown by its ability to agglutinate Rh^+ red cells which have been coated with anti-Rh antibody (i.e. with human IgG). Grubb found that the IgG in the serum of different individuals could inhibit the agglutination by competing for binding by the rheumatoid factor. This was true only of the sera of some individuals and was found to be an inherited characteristic.

The same technique of studying the antigenic specificity of immunoglobulin by inhibition of agglutination of coated red cells by anti-immunoglobulin antisera has been extended. Experimentally-produced antisera, rather than rheumatoid factor, have been used to agglutinate and the coating of red cells with immunoglobulins has been done by chemical attachment as well as by using anti-red cell antibodies. It is a rapid technique suitable for screening purposes and has led to the recognition of many antigenic variants of immunoglobulin in human sera and in the sera of other species.

The human allotypic specificities[15] have been named: (a) Gm factors and numbered 1 to 23: these are found on γ-chain; (b) Inv 1–3, found on κ-chain and Isf of uncertain molecular localisation, and (c) Am markers, found on α chains.

Because of the value of genetic markers in attempts to solve the origin of the complexity of immunoglobulins, much effort has been directed to their detection and their molecular localisation in the structure of immunoglobulins from humans, rabbits, mice and other laboratory animals and a full discussion will be found in Chapter 7.

6.2.5 Idiotypes

The last degree of complexity of immunoglobulins to be revealed by the study of antigenic specificity were the idiotypic specificities which were recognised independently in human[16] and in rabbit antibodies[17]. These specificities appear to be unique to antibodies of a given specificity in an individual animal at a given time. Similarly, every myeloma protein from a spontaneously-developed tumour appears to have a unique specificity although in experimentally-induced tumours in mice several examples of apparently identical Bence–Jones proteins have been reported[18, 19].

The idiotypes have been investigated in greatest detail in rabbits where they were first recognised in the following way. The donor rabbit (D) was injected with killed bacteria (*Salmonella typhi*[17] or *Proteus vulgaris*[20]). The anti-bacterial antisera produced were used to agglutinate killed bacteria which after washing and emulsifying with adjuvant were injected into the receptor rabbit (R). Although the response was slow, in most cases antibodies appeared in rabbit R which would precipitate with the antibacterial antibodies in the serum of the donor. Animals D and R had been matched for allotypes as the work originated in a search for new allotypes and the anti-idiotypic serum was found to distinguish between the anti-bacterial antibodies of different donors. That is, the antibodies of each individual had unique antigenic specificities. If, as this suggests, each antibody of a given specific affinity in one animal is unique in structure, as is each myeloma protein, the range of different immunoglobulin molecules is very large indeed.

This classification of the mixture of immunoglobulins into isotype, allotype and idiotype has clarified greatly immunoglobulin complexity. However, this classification bears no relation to the antibody-combining specificities of the molecules with the possible exception of the idiotype. In the latter case there is clearly no simple relationship as antibodies of indistinguishable combining specificity have different idiotypic specificity but it seems likely that the same part of the molecule is involved. The next step was the correlation between primary structure and this classification of the immunoglobulins.

6.3 ISOLATION

Isolation of the immunoglobulins from normal serum has been achieved satisfactorily only for IgG and IgM. IgA, in most animal sera, is in too low a concentration for preparation in fair yields, but it can be isolated rather easily[21] from milk or preferably colostrum where it is the major immunoglobulin component present. Other secretions such as saliva or ascitic fluid have also been used successfully for the isolation of IgA[22].

IgG from serum[23] and IgA from milk and other secretions have been obtained by a combination of ion exchange and exclusion chromatography. IgM is isolated less easily and needs additional steps including euglobulin precipitation and high-speed sedimentation, e.g. from human serum[24] and rat serum[25]. Yields of the three major classes are of the order of 25–50%, but there is the special feature that as all three are heterogeneous with isoelectric points ranging from pH 5 to 8, there is a selection as well as purification during the preparation. In the most commonly used preparation of IgG, for example, serum is passed down an anion-exchange column (e.g. DEAE-cellulose) under conditions in which only IgG passes through unretarded. This, however, gives the most basic fractions and recovery of IgG free from other proteins but with the full range of isoelectric points is not possible[23].

The isolation of myeloma proteins is far easier as concentrations are much higher and pure samples of IgD and IgE have been isolated only from the serum of myelomatosis patients. Such serum may contain 5g (100 ml)$^{-1}$ or more of a single myeloma protein. Considerable enrichment of IgE from normal serum has been achieved by following the activity of the fractions to transfer the reaginic activity, i.e. the capacity to transfer passively immediate type hypersensitivity. Such a concentration of IgE has been reported, for example, from human serum[26] and from rat serum[27] and has been used to prepare specific antiserum.

Immunoabsorbents have become the major method for the isolation of minor components such as IgE or for the isolation of other immunoglobulins on a small scale. For example, rabbit antisera to a human myeloma IgE was prepared and the IgG containing the specific anti-IgE antibody was isolated and polymerised using the ethylchloroformate method. The resulting insoluble absorbent would remove reaginic activity from human serum and some could be dissociated and recovered from the absorbent[28].

Similarly sheep anti-IgE antibodies have been coupled to cyanogen bromide activated Sepharose[8]. This could be used for the binding of myeloma IgE protein for which a 9 ml column had a capacity of 2 mg. It would also bind the reaginic activity from human sera and in both cases the IgE could be recovered from the column by dissociation in acid, in 5 M KI or in 3.5 M NaSCN. Recoveries varied between 30–50% for natural antibodies and 70–90% for the myeloma proteins.

6.4 POLYPEPTIDE CHAIN STRUCTURE

In spite of the obvious complexity of immunoglobulins, whether judged by chemical, physical or biological criteria, it proved possible, before the nature of the complexity was fully understood, to work out the basic polypeptide chain structure.

6.4.1 IgG

The arrangement of the polypeptide chains in rabbit IgG was solved and subsequently shown to be the same for human IgG and that of other species. This early work has been reviewed[29, 30] and it led to the four-chain structure

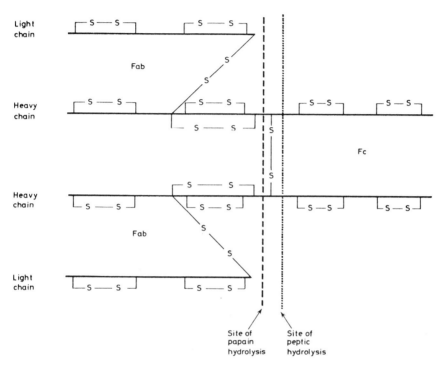

Figure 6.1 Diagrammatic structure of rabbit IgG. Inter- and intra-disulphide bonds are shown. Papain cleavage gives 2 Fab and 1 Fc fragment as shown. Pepsin cleavage gives 1(Fab')₂ fragment held together by the inter-heavy chain disulphide bond and smaller polypeptides derived from the Fc region.

for IgG which is shown in Figure 6.1. All immunoglobulins have the basic structure of two heavy and two light chains. Class and subclass are determined by the heavy chain and type by the light chain (Table 6.1). The positions

Table 6.1 Peptide chains of human immunoglobulins

		Heavy chains	*Light chains*
IgG	...	$\gamma1, \gamma2, \gamma3, \gamma4$	κ or λ
IgM		μ	κ or λ
IgA		$a1, a2$	κ or λ
IgD		δ	κ or λ
IgE		ε	κ or λ

of hydrolysis of the native IgG by papain and pepsin to give Fab, Fc and (Fab')₂ are also shown.

While all IgG molecules from all species examined have the same four polypeptide chain structure, there are striking differences in the numbers and positions of interchain disulphide bonds. This is apparent in the subclasses of human IgG which have been studied in detail by Milstein and colleagues[31] and which are summarised in Figure 6.2. Although a complete amino acid

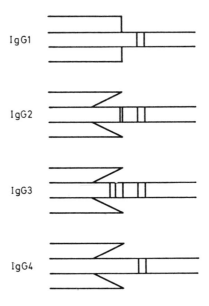

Figure 6.2 The arrangement of the inter-chain disulphide bonds of the four subclasses of human IgG. (From Milstein and Pink[31], by courtesy of Pergamon Press)

sequence is known for only one myeloma protein of the IgG1 subclass[32], the interchain disulphide bonds have been solved for all the human IgG subclasses mainly using the diagonal technique of Brown and Hartley[33] to identify the cystine-containing peptides involved.

In contrast to the marked difference between interchain bonds of the subclasses, the intrachain disulphide bonds are remarkably stable in their positions in all IgG molecules and this led to the postulation of a repeating unit structure of *ca.* 110 residues in both heavy and light chains[32, 34]. Milstein and Svasti[35] have illustrated this point by giving the range in number of amino acid residues within and between intrachain disulphide bonds (Figure 6.3).

This phenomenon of repeating units, which are referred to as homology regions or domains, is a remarkable feature of the immunoglobulin structure. There are two such domains in the light chains, four in the γ-chains and five in the μ-chains[36] and as discussed elsewhere they are believed to have arisen by duplication of a primordial gene coding for a 110 residue section. Evidence for this theory has come from a comparison of the sequences of the constant region sections (see Section 6.6.1) of the human $\gamma 1$ myeloma protein, Eu, which when aligned gave *ca.* 30% identity of sequence[37]. The constant region domains have been named C_L for the light chain and $C_H 1$, $C_H 2$, and $C_H 3$, numbering from the *N*-terminus of the heavy chain.

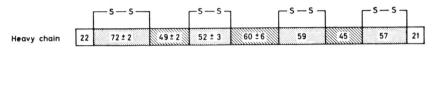

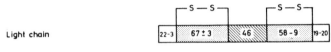

Figure 6.3 The pseudosubunit structure of human IgG chains. The hatched areas differentiate sections between S—S loops from sections within each loop (dotted areas). Numbers give the number of residues and the limits of variation in each section. (From Milstein and Svasti[35], by courtesy of Academic Press)

Evidence that, under carefully controlled conditions, proteolytic enzymes will split preferentially between the domains of both heavy and light chains has been obtained by a number of laboratories[38-42, 42a]. This implies that the domains are a feature of the physical structure being relatively-discrete folded units joined by more exposed stretches of peptide chain comparable to, but less clearly separated in the native molecule, than the Fab and Fc fragments.

Additional intrachain disulphide bonds have been found in the IgG of several species. In the rabbit γ-chain the position of inter- and intra-chain bonds are shown in Figure 6.4. In this case the interchain bonds were identified by isolation of the disulphide-bond-linked peptides after peptic digestion

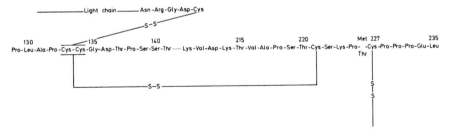

Figure 6.4 Position of the inter-chain disulphide bonds of rabbit IgG and of the additional intra-chain (positions 133/4 to 221) in the heavy chain which shows that the three inter-chains bonds, though sequentially distant must be closely grouped. (From O'Donnell, Frangione and Porter[43], by courtesy of The Biochemical Society)

at acid pH, conditions in which disulphide exchange is least likely to occur. Subsequent tryptic digestion and examination by the diagonal technique enabled the sequence arrangements of the cystine to be worked out[43]. The results were unequivocal except for the inter- and intra-chain bonds at positions 133 and 134, which could not be distinguished. A complete solution of the inter-chain bonds of a mouse IgG1 myeloma protein has been reported by Svasti and Milstein[44]. This is shown in Figure 6.5 and was achieved by

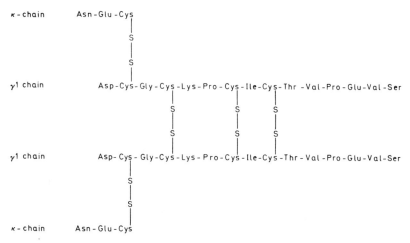

Figure 6.5 The inter-chain bonds of a mouse myeloma protein (IgG1,K) showing the parallel arrangement of the inter-heavy chain bonds. (From Svasti and Milstein[44], by courtesy of Springer Verlag)

splitting between the three inter-heavy chain bonds using either thermolysin or acid hydrolysis.

Rabbit IgG is unusual in having an extra intra-chain disulphide bond in all heavy chains and also in some κ-type light chains. Recent reports[45-47] suggest, surprisingly, that the additional disulphide bond of the κ-chains joins the C-terminal and N-terminal domains of the chain.

6.4.2 IgM

Treatment of IgM with reducing agents under appropriate conditions will give subunits consisting of two heavy and two light chains (IgMs) of sedimentation value 8S[48] rather than 19S or higher when isolated from serum. Unless very mild conditions of reduction are used, such as 10 mM cysteine or 0.125 mM dithiothreitol, substantial reduction of intra-subunit disulphide bonds, as well as inter-subunit bonds occurs[49]. Estimates of unit and subunit size have varied but exact figures are now available as the sequence of a μ-chain has been completed. The monomeric unit including the five polysaccharide units on the μ-chain has a mol. wt. of 191 200 and for the whole molecule of 956 000[36]. Disulphide bonds join the monomer units together and the cysteine residue concerned has been identified (Figure 6.6).

There are two inter-heavy chain disulphide bonds, one near the centre of the chain and a second between the penultimate residues at the carboxy terminal end of the μ-chains. The additional domain of the μ-chain means that this chain contains 580 amino acid residues compared to the 446 of the

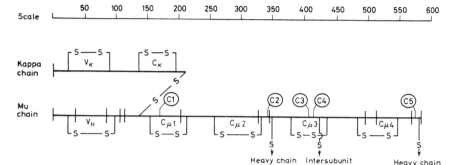

Figure 6.6 The inter-chain and intra-chain disulphide bonds of an IgM myeloma protein showing the position of the heavy–light and 2 heavy–heavy inter-chain bonds and the inter subunit bond. Ⓒ are polysaccharide substituents. The scale is in residue numbers. Vertical bars show position of methonine residue within the μ-chain. V_K, C_K, V_H, $C_{\mu 1}$, $C_{\mu 2}$, $C_{\mu 3}$, $C_{\mu 4}$ and $C_{\mu 5}$, are the domains of the IgM molecule and are about 115 residues in length. (From Putnam et al.[36], by courtesy of S. Karger)

$\gamma 1$-chain. The carbohydrate content is also substantially higher, 15% in the μ-chain as compared with 4% in the γ-chain, and is contained in five polysaccharide units in each μ-chain as shown in Figure 6.6.

6.4.3 IgA

IgA occurs in both blood and secretory fluids but in somewhat different forms˙ IgA of serum exists mainly as a monomer of mol. wt. 170 000 while the secretory (S) IgA exists mainly as a dimer of mol. wt. 385 000[50]. In both cases, higher aggregates are also found (See also Ref. 50a).

A comparison of the antigenic specificity of secretory and serum IgA showed that the former contained an additional component[51]. This has been shown to be due to an additional peptide chain now named secretory (S) piece.

The a-chain is intermediary in size and carbohydrate content between the μ-chain and the γ-chains. The molecular weight has been estimated as 54 000[52] and the carbohydrate content as 10%. Sequence data on a-chains is only just becoming available.[53].

6.4.3.1 Secretory piece

The additional antigenic material noted in S IgA compared to serum IgA was sought by examination of the reduced and alkylated human protein and was found to be eluted immediately after the heavy chain on Sephadex G100 in propionic acid. Re-running of the enriched fraction on Sephadex G200 in neutral salt solution separated aggregating heavy chains from S piece[22].

Cebra and Robbins[21] isolated S piece by dissociation of rabbit secretory IgA in 6 M guanidine without prior reduction and also from colostrum where it is found free in solution[52]. Free and bound S piece appear to be identical[54]. The S piece of rabbit IgA has been reported to be held only by non-covalent forces to the two IgA molecules[21], while that of human S IgA is held also by a disulphide bond[22].

In careful study of the component chains of rabbit S IgA O'Daly and Cebra[52] estimated the molecular weight of the S piece to be 60 000 and not 25 000 as reported earlier[50] and found that there was present in S IgA one mol S per four mol a-chain and four mol light chain. Although S piece and a-chain are similar in size and amino acid composition, tryptic peptides show a wide difference in pattern, implying considerable difference in sequence.

The observation that S piece is found free in colostrum in agammaglobuninemic patients suggests that it may have a function independent of its role in the structure of S IgA. It has been shown to be synthesised in epithelial not lymphocytic cells. The significance of S piece will remain open until some functional role has been attributed to it[22].

6.4.3.2 J Chain

The presence of a fast component when fully-reduced S IgA was electrophoresed in acrylamide gel in 8 M urea had been mentioned by Rejnek et al.[98] and by Cebra and Small[50], but in 1970 Halpern and Koshland examined it more carefully and suggested that it was an integral part of the molecule and named it J chain[56]. The presence of a similar component in human serum IgM and serum IgA has been reported by Mestecky et al.[57] and it has now been shown that J chain from human IgM and IgA myeloma proteins and S IgA are apparently identical as judged by chemical criteria and antigenic specificity[58]. It was also shown by the same criteria that J chain is a distinct component and not derived from a-chain or S piece. This component was named J as it is found only in polymeric immunoglobulins and it is believed that it may have a role in the joining of subunits through disulphide bond linkage. J chain has a high content of cystine.

There are at present discrepancies between the molecular weight reported by O'Daly and Cebra[52] for rabbit J chain (15 000) and for human J chain (24 000)[57, 58]. The former authors have suggested that this may be due to high values being given for glycoprotein when molecular weights are estimated by rate of movement in electrophoresis in acrylamide gels in solutions of sodium dodecylsulphate. There are also some differences in amino acid composition but these are probably due to species differences.

The content of J chain per mol S IgA was estimated from S IgA which had been totally reduced and reacted with ^{14}C iodoacetic acid[52]. Fractionation on acrylamide gel electrophoresis gave values from 0.7 to 0.95 mol J per mol S IgA, and it is probable that it is present at not more than 1 mol J chain per mol polymeric unit in both IgA and IgM. Estimation of the J chain in immunoglobulin polymers is difficult as it represents, on a weight basis only,

3–4% for S IgA and 1–2% for IgM. These estimates of one J chain molecule per mol S IgA and per mol IgM have been confirmed[59]. From the results of Putnam *et al.*[36] J chain would be expected to be joined through the half cystine at position Cys-424 in each of the ten μ chains of the IgM pentamer if it is an integral part of the structure. Recent evidence shows that J chain is synthesised by plasmacytoma cells which are synthesising IgM and suggests a close physiological relationship between J chain and the light and μ chains[60]. J chain has not been detected in any preparations of IgG.

6.4.4 IgD and IgE

These minor immunoglobulin classes are found as monomers in the blood but their molecular weights have been reported to be rather higher than IgG. For IgD, values range from 170 000 to 200 000[6], and for IgE 190 000[8] with values for the heavy chains of 60 000–70 000 for the δ-chain and for the ε-chain 70 000. In both cases the carbohydrate content is high, being *ca.* 15% of the heavy chain weight for both δ- and ε-chains.

6.5 CONFORMATION OF IMMUNOGLOBULIN MOLECULES

Estimates of the molecular weight of immunoglobulins, their subunits and peptide chains have become precise as their complete chemical structure has been determined. The relation of the subunits to each other, the interaction and the folding of the constituent chains is becoming more clear from studies by a variety of physical methods[61], but a full solution must await the completion of x-ray diffraction studies of crystals prepared from myeloma proteins.

6.5.1 IgG

The early observation that papain would split rabbit IgG into two Fab and one Fc piece[62] with little loss of peptide material suggested that this molecule consisted of three globular structures held together by short exposed sections of peptide chains. Hydrodynamic data supported this view[63] and it has been confirmed by electron-microscopic studies[64]. Satisfactory pictures were difficult to obtain by electron microscopy until Valentine and Green used rabbit anti-DNP antibodies after reaction with the bifunctional hapten DNPNH—$(CH_2)_8$—NHDNP. When equivalent mixtures of antibody and hapten were used, a series of ringed polymers were obtained which were stable and were easily visualised in the electron microscope. This showed (Figure 6.7) polymers ranging from dimers to large rings containing 10 or more molecules and presumably joined through their combining sites by the bifunctional hapten which was, of course, invisible. In the interpretative diagram (Figure 6.8), the position of the two Fab and one Fc section is shown. The Fc section was identified by treatment of the polymer with pepsin which removed it leaving the $(Fab)_2$ dimers still in a ring. The angle between

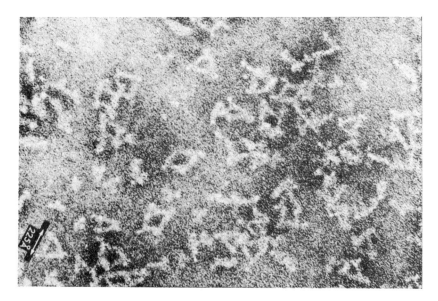

Figure 6.7 Electron-microscope picture of antibody complexes in the form of ring polymers of varying sizes formed between rabbit anti-DNP–lysine and the bifunctional haptene DNP–NH—[CH$_2$]$_8$—NH–DNP. Trimers and tetramers predominate but many other size polymers are visible. Magnification 275 000 diameters (reduced $\frac{1}{2}$ on reproduction) (From Valentine and Green[64] by courtesy of Academic Press

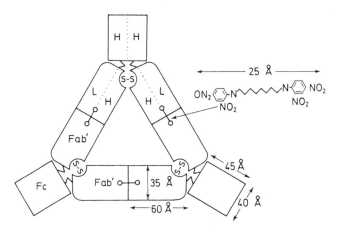

Figure 6.8 Diagram showing the arrangement of the antibody trimers in the electron microscope with the approximate sizes and arrangement of the enzymic fragments. (From Valentine and Green[64], by courtesy of Academic Press)

the two Fab sections varies from nearly 0 to 180°, i.e. the IgG molecule has a flexible Y shape with the angle between the Fab arms depending upon the reaction of the combining sites with the antigen. There is always uncertainty as to whether the picture of the dry material used in electron microscopy reflects the shape in solution but support for the Y conformation has come from birefringence studies[65] as well as the earlier evidence of the IgG being formed from three globular units.

Much difficulty has been met in obtaining crystals of immunoglobulins adequate for x-ray crystallographic studies. Preparations of immunoglobulins or of purified antibody from normal serum cannot be crystallised as they are complex mixtures of molecules. The Fc fragments from the IgG of most species, however, crystallise readily reflecting the much greater homogeneity in this section of the molecule. Crystals have also been obtained from myeloma proteins and their Fab fragments and from Bence–Jones proteins. In a recent symposium[66] the results from three laboratories using these pathological immunoglobulins were summarised. None had been taken beyond 6 Å resolution and hence detailed information had not been obtained but evidence was given for a three-armed structure for IgG comparable to the Y shape with the flexible arms at an angle of 180° [67, 67a].

6.5.2 IgM

Good electron-microscope pictures have been published of IgM[68-70] and agree that the molecule is spherical with five to ten projecting arms or with five arms each divided in two. The central portion appears to be hollow in some pictures[69]. Papain digestion of IgM gives Fab fragments and a polymeric Fc fragment[70a]. Together with electron-microscopic evidence this suggests that the five subunits are linked by disulphide bonds through the Fc sections, directly or via the J chain, with the ten Fab portions projecting from the ring, each with a combining site.

6.5.3 IgA

IgA myeloma proteins from both human and mouse serum[71, 72] give a less clear picture than those obtained with IgM, but it has been interpreted as due to mixtures of monomers, dimers and polymers. When the mouse myeloma protein MOPC 315, which has a high affinity for the DNP group, was examined in the presence of the bis-DNP hapten a dimer was obtained. Tetrads were also seen and it was suggested that two pairs of Fab units were joined by the divalent hapten and the two dimers held together by interaction between Fab or Fc fragments. Few cyclic structures such as those given by the bis-DNP hapten with IgG antibody could be seen. There was also evidence of a substructure in the Fab arms and it was suggested that this might be a reflection of the domains within the Fab fragments ($V_H V_L$ and $C_H 1 C_L$).

6.6 AMINO ACID SEQUENCE STUDIES

Amino acid sequence studies were necessary to establish the details of the polypeptide chain structure given above, and they have led to the discovery of a series of facts which are essential for the understanding of the mechanism of synthesis of immunoglobulins, their genetic origin and the structural basis of their biological activities. A summary will be attempted of this large mass of data and other references to it will be found in different chapters of this book.

6.6.1 Variable and constant regions

Perhaps the most surprising finding to come from sequence work came at the beginning when two human κ-type Bence–Jones proteins were examined[73, 74]. The sequences of the C-terminal 107 residues were identical for the two proteins, but there were a number of differences in the N-terminal 107 residues. This finding has been confirmed many times and has been extended to λ-chains and to heavy chains from several species. There is, therefore, a variable region in the N-terminal 105–115 residues of all immunoglobulin chains, i.e. two such variable regions in each Fab portion which contains the antibody combining site. The remainder of the molecule has a constant sequence in molecules of the same class, type and allotype. This phenomenon of a variable region is very remarkable and offers a structural basis for the very wide range of combining sites, as will be discussed later. It also raises profound problems as to the genetic origin of these multiple-form proteins in what appears to be, at present, a unique phenomenon in biology.

6.6.2 Variable region sequences

Extensive collection of sequence data has brought out the following features of the variable regions:

6.6.2.1 Subgroups

As more information was obtained more positions were found to vary in the N-terminal section of human κ-chains Deletions and insertions were also found so that the length of the variable region ranged over *ca.* 105–110 residues of which 70 or more differed between individual proteins. However, some order was found when it was recognised that the sequences could be broken down into three families or subgroups, the criteria being that members of a subgroup resembled each other more closely than they do any member of another subgroup. It became possible to recognise subgroup characteristic residues including insertions and deletions in different positions in the variable region. This is illustrated for human κ-chain[75] in Figure 6.9. Milstein and Deverson[76] have suggested that the $\kappa1$ subgroup should be

Amino terminal position

```
                    10                    20                    30              40
Vκ₁ Subgroup
ROY    D I Q M T Q S P S S L S A S V G D R Y T I T C Q A S Q D I S - - - - - - - - I F L N W Y Q Q K P
AG     D I Q M T Q S P S S L S A S V G D R Y T I T C Q A S Q D I N - - - - - - - - H Y L N W Y Q Q G P
EU     B I Z M T Z S P S T L S A S V G B R Y T I T C R A S Z S I B - - - - - - - - T W L A W Y Z Z K P
BJ     D V Q M T Z S P S S L S A S V G D R Y T I T C Q A S Q D I N - - - - - - - - K Y
OU     D I Q M T Z S P S S L S A S V G D R Y T I T C R A S Z T I S - - - - - - - - S W L B W Y Z(Z K P)
HBJ4   D I Q M T Q S P S T L(S A S V G B R Y T I T)D C R A S Q B I B - - - - - - - - B W L A W Y Q E L P
DAV    D I Q M T Q S P S T L S T V Y G D R Y T I T C D A S Q B I B - - - - - - - - S W L I W Y Q Q Y P
FIN    D I Q M T Q S P S S L S A S V G D R I T I T C D A S Q B I B - - - - - - - - S W L I W Y Q Q Y P
KER    D I Q M T Q S P S S L S A S V G D R Y T I T C Q A S Q B I K - - - - - - - - D F
TRA    D I Q M T Q S P S S L S A S V G D R Y T I T C
CON    D I Q M T Q S P S S L S A S V G D R Y T I T
LUX    D I Q L T Q S P S F S S L S A S V G D R Y T I T
BEL    B I Z L T Z S P S S L S A S V G D R Y T I T C Z A S Z B I S - - - - - K - - S S L A W Y Z Z K P
PAUL   D I Q M T Q S P Z T L S A S V G D R Y T I T C R A S Q S I S - - - - - S S L A W Y Q Q K P

Vκ₁₁ Subgroup
Ti     E I V L T Q S P G T L S L S P G E R A T L S C R A S Q S V S - - - - - N S F L A W Y Q Q K P
FR4    E(I V L)T Q S P G T L S L S P G E R A T L S C R A S Q S V R - - - - - N N Y L A W Y Q Q R P
B6     Z I V L T Z S P G T L S L S P G Z R A A L S C R A S Q S V S - - - - - G N Y L A W Y Q Q K P
RAD    E I V L T Q S P G T L S L S P G D R A T L S C R A S Q - V S - - - - - S N S Y L A W Y Q Q K P
CAS    E I V L T Q S P A T L S L S P G E R A T L S
SMI    E I V L T Q S P A T L S L S P G E R A T L S
DIL    E I V L T Q S P G T L S L S P G D R A T L S C R A S Q S L S - - - - - - - S K S L S W Y Z Z K P
NIG    K I V L T Q S P A T L S L S P G E R A T L S
GRA    E M V M T Q S P A T L S M S P G E R A T L S

Vκ₁₁₁ Subgroup
CUM    E D I V M T Q T P L S L P V T P G E P A S I S C R S S Q S L L A S G D G N T Y L N W Y L Q K A
TEW    D I V M T Q S P L S L P V T P G E P A S I S C R S S Q - - - H(G B)S - - - F L N W Y L Q K P
MIL    D I V L T Q S P L S L P V T P G E P A S I S C R S S Q N L L Z S - B G B - Y L D W Y L Z K P
MAN    D I V M T Q S P L S L P V T P G E P A S I S C R
BATES  D I V M T Q S P L S L P V T P G E P A S I S G R S S Q(S)L L H(S)B G B B - Y L B - Y L Z K P
```

Figure 6.9 Sequence data on the *N*-terminal residue of human *κ*-chains showing how they can be classified into three subgroups on the basis of sequence homology. Subgroup specific residue are underlined and deletions are shown by dashes.

Key to one letter amino acid code:

A Ala	G Gly	N Asn	V Val
B Asx	H His	P Pro	W Trp
C Cys	I Ile	Q Gln	Y Tyr
D Asp	K Lys	R Arg	Z Glx
E Glu	L Leu	S Ser	
F Phe	M Met	T Thr	

(From Hood and Prahl[75], by courtesy of Academic Press)

subdivided so that there are a total of four subgroups in the human κ-chains.

A similar phenomenon occurs in the human λ-chain where four or five subgroups have been found, and also in human heavy chains. In the latter there are three subgroups, V_HI and V_HII have N-terminal pyrollidone carboxylic acid (P.C.A) and V_HIII N-terminal glutamic acid, aspartic acid or alanine[77, 78]. A fourth subgroup also with N-terminal P.C.A. has been reported in μ-chains[79].

There is a striking contrast between the heavy and light chains in that the subgroup sequences of the κ- and λ-chains are distinct while those of the μ- and γ-chains are common. Incomplete data suggests that the subgroups of the a-chain will also be common with those of the γ-chain and μ-chains. That is, heavy chains differing markedly in the sequence of the constant region (35% homology has been found between μ- and γ-chains) may have as much as 80% homology in the variable region when sharing a common subgroup.

No evidence of subgroups in the variable region of the heavy chains from rabbit immunoglobulin has been recognised with the possible exception of the allotype blank molecules, i.e. molecules carrying no allotypic markers which are discussed later, but as myeloma proteins have not been obtained from this species, the presence of subgroups would not be easy to detect. Kehoe and Capra[78] have partially sequenced a number of myeloma protein heavy chains from cats and dogs. They found a surprising similarity of sequence in the variable regions with no evidence of subgroups in the proteins from either species. There is a rather close similarity of the N-terminal 30 residues of these cat and dog proteins to the sequences of the V_HIII subgroups of the human protein. Thus only in the human immunoglobulins is there clear evidence so far of subgroups in the heavy-chain variable region.

Milstein[80] found that subgroup characteristic sequences of two subgroups of the human κ-chains were always present in the immunoglobulins from the serum of individual normal human subjects showing that these subgroups were not allelic. This has been confirmed for the heavy-chain subgroups[81] and is no doubt also true of the λ-subgroups.

The generality of the subgroup phenomena, the significance of sequences which do not fit exactly and may not fall unequivocally in a given subgroup, and the implication for theories of the genetic origin of immunoglobulins are topics of continued debate and are discussed in Chapter 7.

6.6.2.2   Constant residues

It follows from the above that there will also be found in the variable region, positions which are constant within subgroups and also constant to all subgroups of, say, human κ-chains.

The most striking constant feature is the disulphide bond loop between half-cystine residues at positions 22 and 88. The numbering may differ slightly between individuals proteins but this feature is constant in the sense that it is always present and the half-cystine residues are in very similar sequences such as Thr-Cys in the human κ-subgroup V_{KI} and Ser-Cys-Arg in V_{KII} and V_{KIII} at position 22 (Figure 6.9) and Tyr-Tyr-Cys-Gln in all three subgroups at position 88.

Other very conservative sequences may be seen. Kabat[82] has drawn particular attention to glycine residues, and such sequences may be essential in maintaining structural features necessary for the stability of the whole section of the molecule.

6.6.2.3 Hypervariable regions

Conversely short sections of the variable regions show very marked differences in sequence between individual proteins. This is illustrated most clearly perhaps by the plot of variability against residue position made by Wu and Kabat[83]. Data from κ- and λ-light chains of both human and mouse immunoglobulins have been used. It is apparent that there are three peaks of hypervariability around positions 28, 50 and 96 and the latter is much greater than the other two. Heavy-chain variable sections show the same phenomenon although the variability about position 50 is not so obvious from the limited data available to date[84].

The region of greatest hypervariability in the heavy chain, in approximately position 95–110, seems to be larger than the equivalent section in the light chains[85]. In sequence studies of normal rabbit heavy chains, Mole et al.[86] drew attention to the multiple sequences in positions 32–35, 50–52 and to the apparently most variable region 95–110 where no coherent sequence could be obtained. Kehoe and Capra[87] have suggested that there is a further hypervariable region in position 86–91. Mole et al. found alternative residues in positions 79 and 80 (equivalent to 85–86 on the numbering of Kehoe and Capra[87], but the next five residues appeared to correlate with allotype and were apparently present in near 100% yield. This is not in agreement with the suggestion of hypervariable sections in that position. However, in preliminary data on homogeneous rabbit anti-pneumococcal polysaccharide antibodies Strosberg et al.[88] failed to find these allotype related sequences in this section. More evidence will be needed to resolve these discrepancies.

Not surprisingly the conclusion has been drawn that these hypervariable positions are likely to be in the combining site and directly concerned in determining specificity.

6.6.2.4 Rabbit allotypes

As mentioned, there is no evidence of subgroups except possibly the allotype blank molecules in the heavy-chain variable region of rabbit immunoglobulins. However, there appear to be three variable-region sequences which in contrast to the human κ-chain subgroups are allelic. As discussed in Chapter 7, allotypic variants in the rabbit heavy chain were detected serologically and particular interest has centred on them as evidence has built up to suggest that they may be genetic markers of the heavy chain variable region. If correct, this makes them valuable characteristics in determining the genetic origin of the variable region. There are three alleles at one locus, the a locus Aa1, Aa2, Aa3. There are also in all individuals, blank molecules which do not carry any of the three allelic antigenic specificities. Blank molecules form

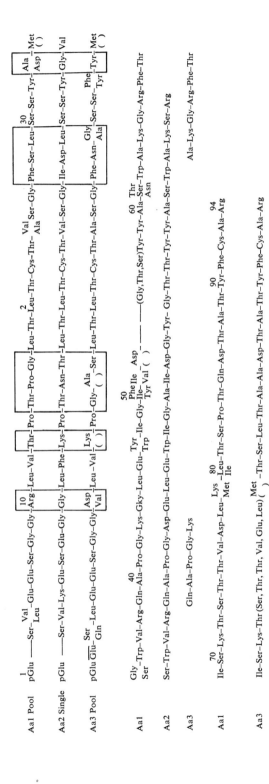

Figure 6.10 Sequence of the heavy chain variable regions of the three allotypic forms of rabbit IgG. Changes in the residues in boxes appear to correlate with the A1, A2 and A3 allotypic specificities. Another apparent correlation in residues 80–85 between A1 and A3 specificities has subsequently been shown not to be common to homogeneous antibodies showing these specificities. It is probable that they represent a distinct inherited variation.

10–20% of the total IgG in normal serum but the concentration can be raised, by suppression of the other alleles, to near 100%. It seems likely that the blank molecules are the products of a distinct locus and may therefore be equivalent to a subgroup.

Sequence data is now available on most of the variable regions of each of the three alleles and is shown in Figure 6.10. Much of the work has been carried out by using IgG from the normal sera of rabbits of given allotype and hence has met the difficulties of sequencing proteins of mixed sequence. A coherent sequence has in fact been obtained for most of the first 94 residues of both the Aa1 and Aa3 allotypes. Alternative residues have been recognised in a variety of positions but there appears to be much less complexity than would have been expected. Where the complexity has been obvious, it coincides with the most variable section recognised from work with human myeloma proteins as discussed above. In particular, no coherent sequence could be established between positions 95–110.

If the antigenic specificities of the three allotypes are determined by certain sequences in the variable region, these sections should be absolutely stable in a given allotype and be common to all molecules, with the exception of the small percentage of blank molecules which are always present. It is important, therefore, to establish the yield of peptides obtained to check if alternative sequences over the same section may have been missed. This is difficult as the N-terminal residue is pyrollidone carboxylic acid and sequential degradation is not possible. An estimate of the yield could be made of the section 85–94 however, by reason of the half-cystine at 92. This residue, after reduction was reacted with [^{14}C]iodoacetate and then the S-carboxymethyl cystine containing peptides could be estimated by the radioactivity. With this method only the sequences shown in Figure 6.10 were detected and hence are believed to account for 80% or more of this section.

From Figure 6.10, it can been seen that there are some 16 allotype related positions scattered throughout the variable region but absent from the middle section. In six of these, however, alternative residues have been found and hence they are unlikely to be determinants of the allotypic antigenic specificities. Only a single sequence was obtained from the Aa2 allotypic heavy chain as it was obtained from an antistreptococcal carbohydrate antibody which appeared from various criteria to be homegeneous[89]. Differences in sequence between allotype A2 and A1 (or A3) were found in the same regions as those between A1 and A3.

A sequence of the N-terminal 59 residues of the heavy chains of a homogeneous rabbit antipneumococcal polysaccharide[90] agrees closely with the sequence for pooled immunoglobulins of allotype A1, the differences being near position 50 which has been identified as a hypervariable region. These results would be in agreement with the presence of allotype related residues in the N-terminal 34. However, preliminary data[88] on the sequences of another homogeneous antipolysaccharide antibody do not confirm the presence of sequences related to the A1 and A3 specificities in positions 80–85. It is possible that the differences found by Mole et al.[86] are genetic variants of another locus closely linked to that of the 'a' locus.

Proof that these sequence differences are indeed the structural basis of the different allotypic specificities has not been obtained and could have only been shown if the isolated peptides retained affinity for anti-allotypic sera. This cannot be demonstrated presumably because their steric structure depends on the integrity of larger sections of the molecule. An attempt is therefore being made to follow chemically the inheritance of the ^{14}C-labelled peptides from position 80–94[91] and if successful will eliminate the ambiguity of the correlation of sequence with allotype. It is of considerable interest to decide if these variable regions do indeed carry genetic markers and investigations are now being extended to mouse κ-chain[92] where evidence has been found of an inherited sequence variation near the half-cystine residue at position 23.

6.6.3 Constant-region sequence studies

The differences in sequence between constant regions reflects as expected the antigenic differences which have been used to classify the different forms of immunoglobulins.

6.6.3.1 Type and subtype

Comparisons of complete sequences are available for human κ- and λ-chains and only 40 % homology was found between the constant regions (see Ref. 31). This considerable difference is remarkable as the κ- and λ-chains fulfil an apparently identical function associating with heavy chains of any class or subclass. With rare exceptions, there is no suggestion of any difference in antibody specificity or other biological activities between immunoglobulins with either κ- or λ-chains, nor is there any evidence of differences in stability or other physical properties of the molecules. In contrast to the differences in the heavy-chain classes, which have been found to be reflected in their biological properties there is no apparent advantage in the evolutionary development of the two forms of light chains. In horses nearly 100 % of the light chains in the immunoglobulins have λ-chains while in mice the reverse is true with almost 100 % κ-chains but there is no evidence of any difference in the effectiveness of the immune reaction of these two species.

No sequence differences within the constant regions of human κ-chains have been established except the allelic Inv variations referred to later. In the human λ-chain there are, however, several examples of subtypes present in all individuals and with differences in sequence. In the human λ-chains, antigenically distinct $0z^+$ and $0z^-$ forms were found to correlate with a lysine and arginine residue respectively in position 191 and both were present in the immunoglobulin of all normal individuals investigated[93]. More recently there have been two reports of a glycine to serine change at position 153 and again both variants were present in all individuals studied[94]. There was no linkage between the serine–glycine and the lysine–arginine changes, three of the four possible variants were identified[95].

Much more extensive sequence differences have been found between two mouse λ-proteins[96]. The two chains MOPC 104[97] and MOPC 315[96] were identified as λ on the grounds that they showed much stronger homology to human λ-chains than to mouse κ-chains, yet they differed from each other in 27% of residue positions in the constant region.

It appears probable that both forms of λ-chain, designated λ1 for the most common 104 subtype and λ2 for the rare 315 subtype, are present in normal serum. However, less than 0.1% of the immunoglobulin of the λ2 subtype was detected serologically in serum from normal BALB/C and C57BL/6 mice and more evidence on this point will be needed to prove that this substantially different form is certainly a λ-subtype.

Although subtypes have not been found in human κ-chains, they do appear to exist in rabbit κ-chains[55]. If after oxidative sulphitolysis, rabbit IgG is fractionated on Sephadex columns in urea formate solution, two light-chain fractions can be distinguished. The first contains the λ-chain and a fraction of κ-chains K_A with five half-cystine residues per mol and the second K_B, κ-chains with seven half-cystine residues. Other significant differences in amino acid content between K_A and K_B fractions were also noted but both fractions carried the four allotypic specificities b4, b5, b6 and b9. The available evidence suggests that the allelic markers are due to sequence changes in the constant region of the κ-chain and there is evidence that the additional disulphide bond of the K_B fraction may link the constant and variable regions[46, 46a, 47]. It is not therefore clear whether K_A and K_B are subtypes of the constant region which, remarkably, share genetic markers or subgroups of the variable regions or a composite of both.

6.6.3.2 Class and subclass

The division into classes is common to the immunoglobulins of all species examined but substantial sequence data is available only for the γ-chains and one human μ-chain. The work on the latter is only just reaching completion and emphasises the surprisingly large differences between the two chains. The constant region of the γ1-chain contains 328 residues[32] and that of the μ-chain 460 residues[36]. The γ1-chain has only one oligosaccharide group and the μ-chain five. The μ-chain has an additional domain and an inter-unit disulphide bond in addition to the interchain bonds (Figure 6.6). Only 24–40% sequence homology can be recognised between equivalent sections of the γ- and μ-chain constant regions and a pentapeptide is the longest identical sequence. These differences offer a striking contrast to the variable region where nearly 80% homology of sequence with a γ1-variable region is found. Presumably this reflects the identity of function of the variable region in forming a combining site in both immunoglobulins and the different biological activities of the constant regions of IgM and IgG.

Subclasses have been recognised in IgG of most species examined, the exception being rabbit where neither serological nor chemical studies have picked out subclasses so far. Subclasses have been distinguished in IgA of several species and also possibly in human IgM. Sequence data is available only for the human IgG subclasses γ1, γ2, γ3 and γ4. The most obvious structural difference between them is in the distribution of the interchain disulphide bonds, (Figure 6.2) and contrasts with the close similarity in position and in adjacent sequences of the three intrachain disulphide bonds

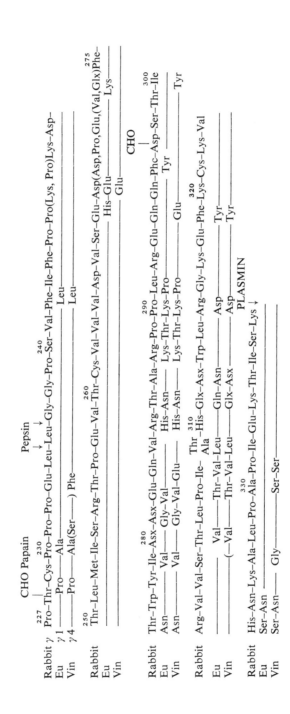

Figure 6.11 *N*-terminal sequence of the Fc fraction of rabbit γ-chain, the human γ1 myeloma Eu[32] and the human γ4 myeloma. (Vin)[101]

of the constant region. Only the $\gamma1$ constant region has been sequenced completely but a large part of the $\gamma4$ sequence has been published and shows differences from the $\gamma1$-sequence in only 13 positions of the 216 residues identified in the Fc region. Differences in the biological properties of the subclasses have been observed such as the inability of IgG4 to fix complement and of IgG2 to effect passive cutaneous anaphylaxis. No obvious correlation has been found between sequence of IgG4 and IgG1 and the capacity to bind complement. This property is carried by the Fc region and probably by the N-terminal half of the Fc the C_H2 domain[41, 42a, 99, 100]. However, a comparison of the sequence of this section from $\gamma1$, $\gamma4$, and rabbit heavy chain fails to reveal any major difference between $\gamma4$ which will not bind complement and the other two which will[101, 102] (Figure 6.11). The binding of Clq^-, the first subcomponent of complement which is believed to interact with aggregated IgG or Fc and initiate the sequential activation of C1r and $C1s^-$ would be expected to depend upon the conformation of a substantial section of peptide chain. The only sequence differences which are unique to $\gamma4$ are: in positions 232–234, $\gamma4$ Ser-Glu-Phe, others Pro-Glu-Leu; position 283 $\gamma4$ Glu, others Gln; position 327 $\gamma4$ Gly others Ala; positions 331–332 $\gamma4$ Ser-Ser other Ala-Pro.

Positions 232–234 are the C-terminal end of the pepsin product (Fab$_2'$) which will not bind Clq[103], and hence are unlikely to be involved. Utsumi[99] showed by progressive degradation of rabbit Fc fragment with papain that complement fixing ability was lost when residues N-terminal to position 280 were removed thus apparently excluding the other position where differences occur, from direct involvement. Secondary configurational changes could follow these enzymic splits and cause functional residues still present to lose their binding activity. It seems likely that very small structural changes may be responsible for the differences between ability to bind or not to bind Clq by the aggregated proteins. The same comment is likely to apply to other differences in the biological properties of all the subclasses as structural differences between them seem to be small.

Partial sequences around the interchain disulphide bonds have been obtained for the human IgA subclasses Al and A2. Differences were noted between the hinge region peptides but these are due to an allelic difference in A2 subclass (Am$^+$ with no heavy-light disulphide bond, Am$^-$ with the bond) as well as to subclass differences[104, 105].

6.6.3.3 Allotypic variants in the constant regions

The considerable sequence differences which appear to correlate with allelic difference in the variable region of rabbit IgG have been discussed above. Much clearer information is available for the allelic changes found in the constant regions of human and rabbit heavy and light chains. This is due to the presence of single unequivocal sequences for the constant region and also due to the much more limited changes observed. With the exception of the 'b' locus allotypes of the rabbit light chain, all other allotypes in the constant region have been detected by the technique of inhibition of agglutination rather than by the precipitation methods used for the rabbit 'a' and 'b'

Table 6.2 Allotype related sequence changes in the constant region of human γ-chains

	Residue position	Residue	Gm group	References
$\gamma 1$ Chain				
	214	Arg	4^+	130
		Lys	4^-	32
	356, 357, 358	-Asn-Glu-Leu	1^+	131
		-Glu-Glu-Met-	1^-	138
$\gamma 3$ Chain				
	11 from C-terminus	Phe	5	132
		Tyr	21	

Table 6.3 Allotype related sequence changes in the constant region of rabbit γ-chains

Residue position	Residue	Allotype	Ref.
214	Met	A11	133
	Thr	A12	
309	Thr	A14	97
	Ala	A15	

Table 6.4 Alloytpe related sequence changes in the constant region of rabbit κ-chains

Residue position	Residue	Allotype	Ref.
C-terminus	Phe-Asn-Arg-Gly-Asp-Cys	A b4	134
	Phe-Ser-Arg-Lys-Asn-Cys	A b5	135
	Ser-Arg-Lys-Ser-Cys	A b6	

Table 6.5 Allotype related sequence change in the constant region of human κ-chains

Residue position	Residue	Allotype	Ref.
191	Leu	Inv 1,2	136
	Val	Inv 3	137

locus allotypes. In the latter case, it is probable that only specificities depending on multiple differences would be found by using precipitating sera. With inhibition techniques, single residue changes (double in the whole molecule) should be detected and the results confirm this expectation. Tables 6.2., 6.3, 6.4 and 6.5 summarise the allotype related sequence changes reported for human γ- and κ-chains and rabbit γ- and κ-chains.

It will be seen that no distinction is made between specificities Inv 1 and Inv 2. These specificities are closely related and the significance of the distinction between them is uncertain[15]. The antigenic distinction recognised by the anti-Inv serum illustrates the extreme sensitivity of the serological methods in detecting very small structural differences in proteins.

Only fragmentary sequences are available on rabbit light chains; κ-chains carry the 'b' locus specificities and differences are apparent near the C-terminus as shown in Table 6.4. Another allotype related sequence change has been found adjacent to the additional cystine linking position 171 in the constant region with the variable region[45-47]. In b4 and b5 κ-chains, position 169 is alanine and aspartic acid respectively. However, in homogeneous antibenzoate antibody of b4 allotype, the equivalent cysteic acid containing peptide did not contain alanine suggesting that this sequence change could not be characteristic of the allotype. More information will be needed to clarify this point which is similar to the findings with the 'a' locus specificities referred to above where an apparent allotype related sequence was not found in homogeneous antibodies of the same allotypic specificity.

Examples of allotype related change in the constant region of human and rabbit γ-chains are shown in Tables 6.2. and 6.3. It should again be emphasised that in no case have small peptides which include these residue changes been obtained and found to inhibit antiallotypic serum, presumably because larger segments of peptide chain are necessary to maintain the conformation of the allotypic antigenic sites. This leaves the interpretation of the sequence studies somewhat uncertain.

6.7 THE POLYSACCHARIDE CONTENT OF IMMUNOGLOBULINS

All immunoglobulins are glycoproteins, the content of carbohydrate varying considerably between the different classes. There are, however, obvious differences in the percentage of carbohydrate between myeloma proteins of the same class and it is most probable that there are also marked variations between individual molecules in preparations of normal immunoglobulins. No convincing explanation has yet been offered of the biological role of these polysaccharide substituents.

6.7.1 Carbohydrate content

Table 6.6 lists the analysis of the carbohydrate content of the different classes of human immunoglobulin expressed as mol sugar residue per mol monomer.

Table 6.6 Carbohydrate content of human immunoglobulins (mol sugar residue/mol monomer)

Protein	Fucose	Mannose	Galactose	N-acetyl-glucosamine	N-acetyl-galactosamine	N-acetyl neuraminic acid	TOTAL
Normal IgG	2	9	3	7	0	1	22
Range of IgG1 myelomas	1.3–3.5	5.0–12.0	1.5–7.1	4.0–9.5	0	0–3.5	11.8–35.6
Normal IgM	Present	36	12	38	0	6	102
Range of IgM myelomas	3–6	27–41	9–15	24–32	0	8–17	71–111
Range of serum IgA myelomas	1–2	12–16	12	12–15	6–9	5–9	48–63
Range of secretory IgA myelomas	8–9	15–16	16–19	17–18	3–4	4–7	63–73
IgD myeloma	1	19	13	14	9	18	74
IgE myeloma	4	36	17	36	0	18	111

Abstracted from tables published by Clamp and Johnson[104]

There is a four to fivefold difference between the total content of IgG compared to IgM and IgE, with IgA and IgD having intermediary values. The variation between individual proteins is threefold within one subclass IgG 1. No significant difference in average carbohydrate content has been found between the IgG subclasses.

Sequence studies, particularly of human IgG myeloma proteins have shown that varying numbers of polysaccharide units may be present. In the majority of cases no carbohydrate has been detected in Bence–Jones proteins or on light chains of myeloma proteins, but in some cases it is present and has been shown to be attached to an aspartic acid or asparagine residue at position 28 in a mouse Bence–Jones protein[107] and at position 84 in human Bence–Jones protein[108]. In two other Bence–Jones proteins carbohydrate was found attached in positions 30 and 71[108a], i.e. in all cases in the variable region of the chains.

Carbohydrate is always covalently attached to heavy chains and in the γ-chain of the IgG1 myeloma protein Eu it was attached only to an aspartic acid or asparagine residue at position 297. None was present on the light chain of Eu[32]. In rabbit IgG, the major polysaccharide unit is in an equivalent position in the N-terminal domain of the Fc[34], and indeed the sequence around the aspartic acid residue to which the carbohydrate is attached is very similar in the γ-chains of both species.

Additional polysaccharide units have been reported in γ chains, one in the variable region of IgG1 myeloma protein Cor attached to an aspartic acid residue at position 62[109]. Another on a threonine residue adjacent to the half-cystine residue of the heavy-heavy interchain bond in the hinge region of the γ-chain from pooled rabbit IgG[110] and a further unit also in the rabbit γ-chain but attached to an asparagine residue in the Fd section[111]. These authors also gave evidence showing that the polysaccharide of the hinge region may be asymmetrically attached to only one heavy chain in an IgG molecule.

The solution of the sequence of a μ-chain from an IgM myeloma protein has led to the placing of five polysaccharide units in this chain at position 170, 342, 405, 412 and 574[36] all in the constant region.

Few sequence studies are available in IgA, but evidence has been given of a polysaccharide unit attached to a serine residue in a proline-rich peptide, presumably from the hinge region[104]. The secretary piece contains 11.6% carbohydrate but this does not account fully for the difference in carbohydrate content between serum and secretory IgA[112]. J piece is also a glycoprotein but the content is so small that it is unlikely to explain the deficiency suggesting that the α chains of the two forms of IgA may differ in carbohydrate content.

6.7.2 Linkage of polysaccharide to protein

In most cases the polysaccharide has been found attached via N-acetyl glucosamine to an aspartic acid or asparagine residue and it is likely that there is a glycosylamine bond present as shown in ovalbumin[113] but no direct evidence has been reported. Press and Hogg[109] drew attention to the similarity of sequence to which the carbohydrate was attached.

Cor Fd section	Tyr-Asx-Thr-Ser
Eu Fc section	Tyr-Asx-Ser-Thr
Rabbit Fc section	Phe-Asx-Ser-Thr
Mouse light chain	Glu-Asx-Ile-Ser

They suggested that this sequence may be a necessary but not sufficient feature for the enzyme-catalysed reaction of the N-acetylglucosamine residue with asparagine. If this is correct, additional carbohydrate units attached to asparagine would be expected to occur only in the variable region where such tetrapeptides might appear. From the limited data available this is correct.

Attachment of polysaccharide occurs also though an O-glycosidic linkage involving N-acetylgalactosamine and a serine or threonine residue. This appears to be the linkage of the polysaccharide in the hinge region of rabbit IgG[110] and also in a glycopeptide, from the heavy-chain disease protein Zuc, which contains no asparagine but two serine residues[113a]. As the sequence requirements for the enzymic condensation of a galactosamine residue on to a hydroxyamino acid do not seem to be exacting additional polysaccharide units bound through this linkage may well appear in either the variable or constant regions.

6.7.3 The polysaccharide units

Clamp and Johnson[106] have postulated three types of polysaccharide units in immunoglobulins.

(a) CA which has a complex heavily-branching structure containing 1 fucose, 3 mannose, 2 galactose, 3–4 N-acetylglucosamine and 0–2 sialic acid. This CA unit appears to be present in all immunoglobulins.

(b) CB is a much simpler structure containing only mannose and N-acetylglucosamine. It is found in IgM and IgE and may be present in other classes.

(c) CC is less well defined but appears to be similar to CB. However, it also contains some galactose, N-acetylgalactosamine and perhaps also sialic acid and mannose. It is found in the hinge region of IgA and possibly also of rabbit IgG.

A full discussion of immunoglobulins as glycoproteins will be found in the article of Clamp and Johnson[106].

6.8 STRUCTURE OF THE COMBINING SITE

The combining site is the essential unique feature of antibody structure. As information accumulated it became less easy to envisage how molecules with the same peptide chain structure and very similar amino acid composition could show such a wide range of combining specificity. The discovery of the phenomenon of the variable region at the N-terminal ends of the light and heavy chains immediately offered an explanation. From studies of the catalytic sites of enzymes, it was apparent that the specific affinity of the combining site would depend upon the shape of the site and distribution of the different amino acid site chains in it[85, 114, 115]. Clearly the range of possibilities provided by the variable regions of the two chains was very large indeed. Direct proof that the combining sites are entirely formed from the variable region has been obtained by Inbar et al.[116]. The mouse myeloma protein MOPC 315 with high affinity for DNP-lysine was used. The Fab' fragment was digested with pepsin for 4 h at pH 3.6 and fractionated on a DNP–lysine–Sepharose column. Material bound to the column was eluted with DNP–glycine and ran on a Sephadex G75 column. The major peak had a mol. wt. of 29 000 and was dissociated by sodium dodecyl sulphate into half this size. The fragment was named Fv as one chain had the same N-terminal residues as the whole heavy chain. The other was blocked as in the whole light chain and hence it was concluded that Fv was formed from the variable region of both chains. A short section of constant region may be included as the molecular weight suggests that the Fv contains 260 residues and the variable regions together contain about 225 residues. The binding capacity was similar to that of Fab showing that the whole of the combining site was contained in the Fv fragment. That an enzyme split can be obtained in this position is in agreement with the domain hypothesis discussed earlier. These observations exclude all but a very small number of residues in the constant region from taking any part in the structure of the combining site.

6.8.1 Size of antibody-combining site

The size of the combining site has been estimated by investigation of the size of haptenes, polysaccharides or peptides which would inhibit most effectively the combination of antigen with its specific antibody. This has led to the view that hexasaccharides, hexapeptides and haptenes of equivalent size approximately fill the antibody combining site. Larger molecules which include the antigenic sites are not more effective inhibitors.

There is evidence that there is a hydrophobic region in or close to the combining site. Benjamini et al.[117] showed that a decapeptide from positions 103–112 in the peptide chain of tobacco mosaic virus (T.M.V.) would inhibit the combination of T.M.V. with its antisera. The C-terminal tripeptide from this sequence Ala-Thr-Arg showed no affinity for the antibody but if the amino group was substituted with an octanyl group, binding could be demonstrated. The specificity depended on the tripeptide sequence and was lost if alanine was removed. The considerable rise in binding affinity on attaching the octanyl group is assumed to be due to an interaction with adjacent hydrophobic residues. Parker and Osterland[118] also suggested that there were hydrophobic regions on the surface of the IgG molecules from studying the binding of 8-aminonaphthalene 1-sulphonate (ANS). One mol was bound per Fab' fragment and the affinity was rather higher with anti-DNP antibody than with inert IgG. This suggests that there might be some cross reaction between the antibody site and the ANS group and that therefore the hydrophobic binding site might be part of the combining site. It was not, however, possible to prove this last point.

The maximum size of the antigenic site, which the antibody-combining site can accommodate is very similar to the maximum size of substrates which are being found to fit the catalytic sites of hydrolytic enzymes. In the case of lysozyme, for example, the enzyme for which the most detailed information is available[119], the catalytic site is a cleft in the molecule and it will accommodate a hexasaccharide. Study of the molecular model derived from x-ray diffraction of lysozyme crystals shows that 15–20 amino acid residues line the catalytic cleft. It is likely that a similar number of residues are directly concerned in the structure of the antibody combining site. The residues in lysozome are not adjacent in the peptide chain but are brought together by the complex folding of the chain. Similarly in the antibody site both the heavy and light chain contribute residues to the site as the presence of the variable regions in both chains suggest and several lines of evidence show that sequentially unrelated segments are concerned. Indirect evidence is given by the marked stabilising effects of a hapten when in combination in the antibody. Cathou and Werner[120], observed that solutions of 4 M guanidine HCl would disrupt the native structure of rabbit anti-DNP antibodies, as judged by circular dichroism measurements, but if hapten was present little change occurred. This implies that the hapten by its binding to different segments forming part of the combining site stabilises the whole structure.

The sections of the variable region which are in the combining site are assumed to be the hypervariable portions discussed earlier. Three were identified in the light chain by the plot of Wu and Kabat[83] and it is probable that there is a similar number in the variable region of the heavy chains[84]. Together these six hypervariable sections could well contribute some 20 residues to the number likely to be directly involved in the combining site. If hypervariability is accepted as evidence for the direct involvement of a position, then the positions 95–110 in the heavy chain appear to have the highest linear concentration with perhaps five or six hypervariable positions in this segment and one or two contributed by the other five sections from the light and heavy chains.

6.8.2 Affinity labelling of antibodies and myeloma proteins

Visualisation of the combining site must await the successful completion of the x-ray crystallographic studies from which a molecular model of the Fab fragment can be deduced. Identification of the combining site ought to be possible by study of the crystals with and without bound hapten in a manner analogous to the study of lysozyme in the presence of competitive inhibitors[119] Such crystals have in fact been obtained using the Fab fragment from the mouse myeloma protein MOPC 315 which has been crystallised in the absence and in the presence of DNP–lysine. In the latter case crystals containing 1 mol of hapten were obtained[121] but it is uncertain whether they are suitable for crystallographic study.

In the meantime, valuable information on the structure of the site can be obtained by the use of affinity-labelling methods. In this technique, a hapten into which a reactive group has been introduced combines with its specific antibody. Subsequent covalent reaction between the reactive grouping and an amino acid residue in or near the combining site should occur. Subsequent enzymic hydrolysis and characterisation of the labelled peptides should enable the reacted amino acid residues to be identified in the sequence of the variable region.

The method has been used both with mouse myeloma proteins showing high affinity for haptenic groups and with antibodies synthesised in rabbits and pigs. The most popular reagents chosen have been a haptene with a substituted diazo group[122] or with a bromacetyl derivative[123] (Figure 6.12). Also

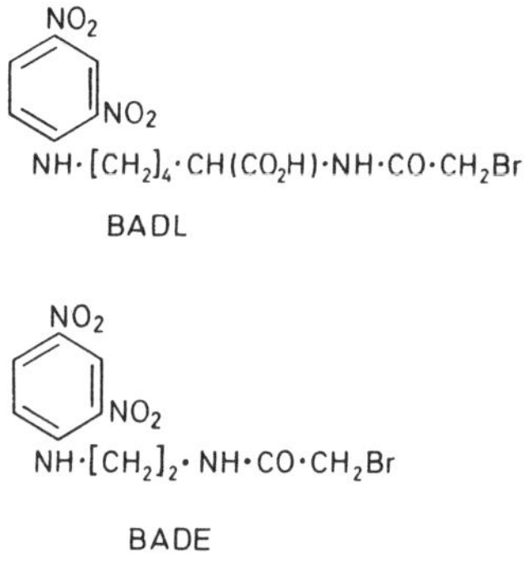

Figure 6.12 Bromacetyl derivatives of the dinitrophenyl haptene have been used as affinity-labelling reagents. The varying distance between the haptenic group and the reactive group facilitate the mapping of the position of the combining site.
Bromacetyl–DNP–lysine   BADL
Bromacetyl–DNP–ethylene diamine BADE

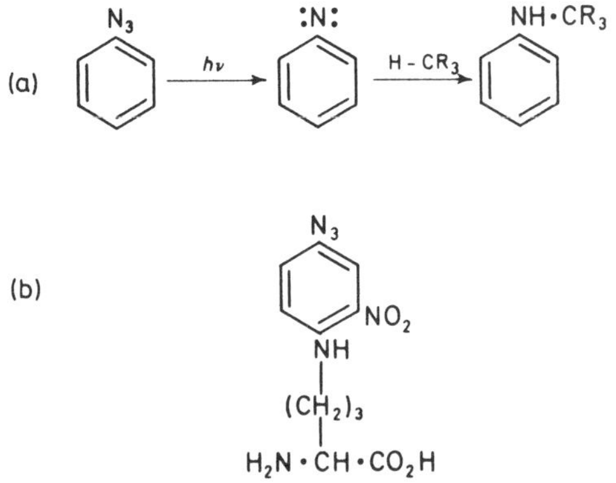

Figure 6.13 An aromatic azide has been used as an affinity labelling reagent. (a) activation of the azide by light to give a nitrene able to insert into any C—H bond. (b) the haptene used was nitroazidophenyl-lysine

used have been two photoactivated reagents one of them an aromatic azide[124,125] (Figure 6.13).

The diazo and bromacetyl derivatives are limited in that they react only with lysine, tyrosine and histidine residues. The bromacetyl derivatives have the advantage that the length of side chain between the haptene and the reactive group can be varied (Figure 6.13) and hence the distance between the combining site and the nearest tyrosine or lysine residue judged[115]. Reaction with histidine has been reported only for one horse antibody[126] and indeed from the sequence information available few histidine residues if any are present in the variable region.

A difficulty in such mapping experiments is that the combining site binds the haptene reversibly and hence it may function in part to concentrate rather than hold rigidly the labelling reagent. Such a mechanism was suggested by the specific reaction of the mouse myeloma protein 315 with m-nitrobenzene-diazonium fluoroborate. The reacted protein showed a 50-fold drop in affinity for the hapten but the number of combining sites was unchanged[127]. Apparently the hapten part of the covalently bound reagent was obstructing or altering the combining site but was not filling the site.

In spite of this limitation, interesting results were obtained using the bromacetyl reagents of varying length. Most notably BADL labelled only the heavy chain of myeloma protein 315 reacting with a lysine residue while BADE labelled only the light chain on tyrosine in position 35[123]. This suggested that the distance between lysine and tyrosine residues should be the difference in length of the two reagents, i.e. 5 Å. Givol et al.[128] synthesised the bifunctional reagent, $DNPNH—[CH_2]_2CH(NH \cdot CO \cdot CH_2Br) \cdot CO \cdot [NH]_2Br(DIBAB)$ which should react with and cross-link the lysine and tyrosine residues of the heavy and light chain, respectively. They found that more than half of the 315 molecules were in fact cross-linked and were able to show that reaction had occurred through the residues predicted. Caution is necessary in drawing too precise conclusions on the structure of the combining site because as Givol[114] has pointed out two reagents of different length, m-nitrobenzenediazonium fluoroborate and BADE, both react with the light-chain tyrosine residue in position 35. It is assumed that BADE must be in a coiled configuration so that its length is in fact the same as that of the diazonium reagent but this is not easily verified and arguments become circular.

Perhaps of greatest interest would be to label the contact amino acids in the combining site if this were possible and to get direct information as to how many residues are concerned, how much they differ from specificity to specificity and what type of bonding is likely between the contact residues and a haptenic group. Labelling with the reagents discussed above where the reactive group is attached to the haptenic group but is not part of it, is unlikely to give this information. The amino acid residues which have been labelled have all been in rather constant positions and presumably are close to, but not part of, the contact residues. More promising in this respect would be a labelling reagent which would be used as the specificity determinant of the hapten in an inert form so that it could be attached to a protein and used to raise specific antibodies. If after binding to the isolated antibody, the specificity determinant could be activated there would be a possibility of reaction with the contact residues in the combining site. It would be necessary that the activated groups should be highly reactive. Also the rate of reaction would have to be high relative to the rate of dissociation of hapten and antibody. The aryl azide (Figure 6.13) is a possible candidate. Antibodies can be raised in rabbits against the haptenic group 2-nitro-azidophenyl (NAP) when coupled to lysine residues in a protein and subsequently the antibodies may be purified by affinity chromatography. The antibodies show an affinity of ca. 10^7 1 mol^{-1} but the half-life of the aryl nitrene formed by photolysis at 400 mm may be as long as 10^{-4} s.

Doubts have been raised as to whether reaction will occur primarily in the site or will be with adjacent residues near the site as the reagent dissociates from the combining site. In the early experiments, a substantial part of the label (ca. 20%) was found to be attached to the half-cystine and alanine residue in the stable sequence Phe-Cys-Ala-Arg immediately prior to the most hypervariable part of the heavy chain starting at position 95. It is unlikely, although not impossible, that this sequence can contribute directly to the contact residues as it appears to be common to antibodies of all specificities. In later experiments, however, little labelling ($< 5\%$) has been identified on stable residues and it seems probable that it is almost entirely on the variable residues as would be expected. Singer and colleagues[134] have used an aryl azide attached to a trimethyl or triethyl ammonium group as an affinity label for acetylcholine esterase and acetylcholine receptor in frog sartorius muscle. The reagent gave an apparently specific reaction and inhibition of activity but the degree of labelling was very high and clearly in large part non-specific. The labelling was substantially reduced by addition of a large excess of p-aminobenzoate but so also was the inhibition of activity. These results were interpreted as evidence that the reagent came out of the binding site after activation and reacted with adjacent residues or with whatever substances were in excess such as p-aminobenzoate. This work is in contrast with that with antibodies where labelling is less than expected and there is little evidence of non-specific reaction. In the choline ester receptor site in muscle, the aryl azide is not bound in the site in contrast to the antibody site where the specific affinity is for the reactive group.

No myeloma protein able to bind the NAP–haptene has been found to date and hence work has been confined to natural antibodies which contain molecules with a wide range of specificities and binding affinities. Though all bind two molecules of NAP–lysine per molecule of antibody on irradiation only *ca.* 35% of the antibodies form a covalent bond with the haptene. The reacted molecules can be separated as they no longer bind to an anti-DNP immuno-absorbent column and have 1.6–2 molecules of haptene bound per molecule of antibody. The 60% of the molecules which are retained on the column have about 0.2 molecules of haptene bound per molecule of antibody and will bind non-covalently an additional 1.8 molecules of haptene but on irradiation no further covalent reaction takes place. Apparently two classes of antibody molecules exist which differ presumably in the orientation of the haptene in the site. In one case the nitrene can react with an amino acid residue to give a covalent bond and in the second the orientation appears to be such that reaction occurs preferentially with a solvent molecule.

The conclusions from the different affinity labelling studies are all in agreement with each other and with the data discussed earlier concerning the evidence on the nature of the binding site.

Using substituted haptenes, the reactive residues are the tyrosine at position 35 in the light chain of both a mouse myeloma protein and of pig anti-DNP antibodies. A tyrosine in the heavy chain adjacent to the most variable region has been labelled in pig antibodies and other neighbouring residues in rabbit anti-NAP antibodies. With natural antibodies the labelling is usually several times higher on the heavy chain than on the light chain. With mouse myeloma proteins either heavy or light chains may be labelled depending on the reagent used and in the heavy chain a lysine residue near the hypervariable region of the position 50–52 is reactive.

There is little doubt that the hypervariable regions do form the combining site but whether it will be feasible to work out the individual contributions of these six or more hypervariable segments and then of each of the residues in these segments to the specificity of the site using photo affinity techniques is not yet clear. It is, however, likely that a combination of all the available methods, particularly x-ray studies of crystalline myeloma proteins will soon make possible a clear description of a combining site and of the structural variation within it which makes possible the wide range of combining specificity.

6.9 CONCLUSION

The structure of immunoglobulins is now largely known and provides an explanation in chemical terms of most of their complexities. It is likely that the structural basis of the principal biological activity of immunoglobulins, their specific combining power, will soon be available.

Very much less is known of the mechanism of their other important physiological properties, such as (a) the fixation of complement by antibody-antigen aggregates; (b) the capacity of immunoglobulins to pass through membranes, e.g. from mother to foetus or through the gut of new born mammals; (c) the binding of immunoglobulins to cell surfaces to give rise, after combination with antigen, to allergic reactions; and (d) the role of immunoglobulins as receptors on B lymphocytes.

Most of these reactions are likely to be due to structural features in the Fc section of the molecule and much of the future interest in structural studies may be concerned with the conformation of the Fc and the mechanism of its interaction with macromolecules and with membranes of different types.

Of equal interest will be a clear identification of the structural basis of the allelic variants of immunoglobulins, particularly those of the variable regions. It is not yet certain that such sequence variations as have been found in the variable regions of the immunoglobulins of some species are markers for structural genes. There are inconsistencies and apparently incomprehensible features, the understanding of which in structural terms is likely to make an essential contribution to a solution of the genetic origin of immunoglobulins, one of the most interesting features of immunology.

References

1. Colloque sur les réactions immunitaires chez les invertébrés. (1971). *Arch. Zool. Exp. Gen.* **112**, 55
2. Krause, R. M. (1970). *Advan. Immunol.,* **12**, 1
3. Heidelberger, M. and Pederson, K. O. (1937). *J. Exp. Med.,* **65**, 393
4. Grabar, P. and Williams, C. A. (1953). *Biochim. Biophys. Acta,* **10**, 193
5. Rowe, D. S. and Fahey, J. D. (1965). *J. Exp. Med.,* **121**, 171
6. Spiegelberg, H. L. (1972). *Contemporary Topics in Immunochemistry,* **1**, 165
7. Ishizaka, K. and Ishizaka, T. (1971). *Progress in Immunology* (B. Amos, editor) (New York: Academic Press)
8. Bennich, H. and Johansson, S. G. O. (1971). *Advan. Immunol.,* **13**, 1
9. Johansson, S. G. O. and Bennich, H. (1967). *Immunology,* **13**, 381
10. Bennich, H., Ishizaka, K., Ishizaka, T. and Johansson, S. G. O. (1969). *J. Immunol.,* **102**, 826
11. Ishizaka, T., Ishizaka, K., Salmon, S. and Fudenberg, H. (1967). *J. Immunol.,* **99**, 82
12. Oudin, J. (1960). *J. Exp. Med.,* **112**, 107, 125
13. Oudin, J. (1960). *C.R. Acad. Sci. Paris,* **250**, 770
14. Grubb, R. (1956). *Acta Path.,* **39**, 195

15. Grubb, R. (1970). The Genetic Markers of Human Immunoglobulins. Molecular Biology Biochemistry and Biophysics, Vol. 9 (Berlin: Springer-Verlag)
16. Kunkel, H. G., Mannick, M. and Williams, R. C. (1963). *Science*, **140**, 1218
17. Oudin, J. and Michel, M. (1963). *C.R. Acad. Sci. Paris*, **257**, 805
18. Weigert, M. G., Cesari, I. M., Yonkovich, S. J. and Cohn, M. (1971). *Nature (London)* **228**, 1045
19. Appella, E. (1971). *Proc. Nat. Acad. Sci. (USA)*, **68**, 590
20. Gell, P. G. H. and Kelus, A. S. (1964). *Nature (London)* **201**, 687
21. Cebra, J. J. and Robbins, J. B. (1966). *J. Immunol.*, **97**, 12
22. Tomasi, T. B. and Bienenstock, J. (1968). *Advan. Immunol.*, **9**, 1
23. Sober, H. A., Gutter, F. J., Wyckoff, M. M. and Peterson, E. A. (1956). *J. Amer. Chem. Soc.*, **78**, 756
24. Chaplin, H., Cohen, S. and Press, E. M. (1965). *Biochem. J.*, **95**, 256
25. Vreisman, P. C. C. V. B. and Feldman, J. D. (1972). *Immunochem.*, **9**, 525
26. Ishizaka, K. and Ishizaka, T. (1967). *J. Immunol.*, **99**, 1187
27. Jones, V. E. and Edwards, A. J. (1971). *Immunology*, **21**, 383
28. Ito, K., Wicher, K. and Arbesman, C. E. (1969). *J. Immunol.*, **103**, 622
29. Cohen, S. and Porter, R. R. (1964). *Advan. Immunol.*, **4**, 287
30. Cohen, S. and Milstein, C. (1967). *Advan. Immunol.*, **7**, 1
31. Milstein, C. and Pink, J. R. L. (1970). *Prog. Biophys. Molec. Biol.*, **21**, 211
32. Edelman, G. M., Cunningham, B. A., Gall, W. E., Gottlieb, P. D., Rutihauser, U. and Waxdal, M. J. (1969). *Proc. Nat. Acad. Sci. (USA)*, **63**, 78
33. Brown, J. R. and Hartley, B. S. (1966). *Biochem. J.*, **101**, 214
34. Hill, R. L., Delaney, R., Fellows, R. E. and Lebowitz, H. E. (1966). *Proc. Nat. Acad. Sci. (USA)* **56**, 1762
35. Milstein, C. and Svasti, J. (1971). *Progress in Immunology*, 33 (B. Amos, editor) (New York: Academic Press)
36. Putnam, F. W., Shinoda, T., Shimizu, A., Paul, C., Florent, G. and Roff, E. (1973). in *Specific Receptors of Antibodies. Antigens and Cells*, (D. Pressman, editor) (Basel: S. Karger)
37. Rutishauser, U., Cunningham, B. A., Bennett, J. C., Konisberg, W. H. and Edelman, G. M. (1970). *Biochemistry*, **9**, 3171
38. Solomon, A. and McLaughlin, C. L. (1969). *J. Biol. Chem.*, **244**, 3393
39. Björk, I. (1970). *Fed. Proc. (Fed. Amer. Soc. Exp. Biol.)*, **29**, 773
40. Turner, M. W. and Bennich, H. (1968). *Biochem. J.*, **107**, 171
41. Connell, G. E. and Porter, R. R. (1971). *Biochem. J.*, **124**, 53 P
42. Gall, W. E. and D'Eustachio, P. (1972). *Biochemistry*, **11**, 4621
42a. Ellerson, J. R., Yasmeen, D., Painter, R. H. and Dorrington, K. J. (1972). *FEBS Lett.*, **24**, 318
43. O'Donnell, I. J., Frangione, B. and Porter, R. R. (1970). *Biochem. J.*, **116**, 261
44. Svasti, J. and Milstein, C. (1972). *Europ. J. Biochem.*, **31**, 405
45. Fraser, K., Strosberg, A. D., Margolies, M. N., Perry, D. and Haber, E. (1972). *Fed. Proc. (Fed. Amer. Soc. Exp. Biol.)* **31**, 742
46. Poulsen, K. and Haber, E. (1972). *Fed Proc. (Fed. Amer. Soc. Exp. Biol.)* **31**, 772
46a. Strosberg, A. D., Fraser, K. J., Margolies, M. N. and Haber, E. (1972). *Biochemistry*, **11**, 4978
47. Lamm, M. E. and Frangione, B. (1972). *Biochem. J.*, **128**, 1357
48. Deutsch, H. F. and Morton, J. I. (1957). *Science*, **125**, 600
49. Metzger, H. (1970). *Advan. Immunol.*, **12**, 57
50. Cebra, J. J. and Small, P. A. (1967). *Biochemistry*, **6**, 503
50a. Tomasi, T. B. and Grey, H. M. (1972). *Progress in Allergy*, **16**, 81
51. Tomasi, T. B., Tan, E. M., Solomon, A. and Prendergast, R. A. (1965). *J. Exp. Med.*, **121**, 101
52. O'Daly, J. A. and Cebra, J. J. (1971). *Biochemistry*, **10**, 3843
53. Chuang, C-Y., Capra, J. D. and Kehoe, J. M. (1973). *Science*
54. Lamm, M. E. and Greenberg, J. (1972). *Biochemistry*, **11**, 2744
55. Rejnek, J., Appella, E., Mage, R. G. and Reisfeld, R. A. (1969). *Biochemistry*, **8**, 2712.
56. Halpern, M. S. and Koshland, M. E. (1970). *Nature (London)*, **228**, 1276
57. Mestecky, J., Zikan, J. and Butler, W. T. (1971). *Science*, **171**, 1163
58. Morrison, S. L. and Koshland, M. E. (1972). *Proc. Nat. Acad. Sci. (USA)*, **69**, 124

59. Mestecky, J., Zikan, J., Butler, W. T. and Kulhavy, R. (1972). *Immunochemistry*, **9**, 883
60. Parkhouse, R. M. E. (1972). *Nature New Biol.*, **236**, 9
61. Dorrington, K. J. and Tanford, C. (1970). *Advan. Immunol.*, **12**, 333
62. Porter, R. R. (1959). *Biochem. J.*, **73**, 119
63. Noelken, M. E., Nelson, C. A., Buckley, C. E. and Tanford, C. (1965). *J. Biol. Chem.*, **240**, 218
64. Valentine, R. C. and Green, M. N. (1967). *J. Molec. Biol.*, **27**, 615
65. Cathou, R. E. and O'Konski, C. T. (1970). *J. Molec. Biol.*, **48**, 125
66. *Cold Spring Harbor Symp. Quant. Biol.*, **36**, (1971). *Structure and function of proteins at the three-dimensional level*
67. Sarma, V. R., Davies, D. R., Labaw, L. W., Silverton, E. W. and Terry, W. D. (1971). *Cold Spring Harbor Symp. Quant. Biol.*, **36**, 413
67a. Poljack, R. T., Amzel, L. M., Avey, H. P., Becka, L. N. and Nisonoff, A. (1972). *Nature New Biol.*, **235**, 137
68. Feinstein, A. and Munn, E. A. (1969). *Nature (London)*, **224**, 1307
69. Chesebro, B. and Svehag, S-E. (1969). *J. Immunol.*, **102**, 1064
70. Green, N. M. (1969) *Advan. Immunol.*, **11**, 1
70a. Mihaesco, C. and Seligman, M. (1966). *C.R. Acad. Sci. Paris*, **162**, 2661
71. Dourmashkin, R. R., Virella, G. and Parkhouse, R. M. E. (1971). *J. Molec. Biol.*, **56**, 207
72. Green, N. M., Dourmashkin, R. R. and Parkhouse, R. M. E. (1971). *J. Molec. Biol.*, **56**, 203
73. Hilschmann, N. and Craig, L. C. (1965). *Proc. Nat Acad. Sci. (USA)*, **53**, 1403
74. Titani, K., Whitley, E., Avogardo, L. and Putnam, F. W. (1965). *Science*, **149**, 1090
75. Hood, L. and Prahl, J. (1971). *Advan. Immunol.*, **14**, 291
76. Milstein, C. P. and Deverson, E. V. (1971). *Biochem. J.*, **123**, 945
77. Wang, A. C., Pink, J. R. L., Fudenberg, H. H. and Ohms, J. (1970). *Proc. Nat. Acad. Sci. (USA)*, **66**, 657
78. Kehoe, J. M. and Capra, J. D. (1972). *Proc. Nat. Acad. Sci. (USA)*, **69**, 2052
79. Bennett, J. C. (1968). *Biochemistry*, **7**, 3340
80. Milstein, C., Milstein, C. P. and Feinstein, A. (1969). *Nature (London)*, **221**, 153
81. Wang, A. C., Fudenberg, H. H. and Pink, J. R. L. (1971). *Proc. Nat. Acad. Sci. (USA)* **68**, 1143
82. Kabat, E. A. (1967). *Proc. Nat. Acad. Sci. (USA)*, **58**, 229
83. Wu, T. T. and Kabat, E. A. (1970). *J. Exp. Med.*, **132**, 211
84. Kabat, E. A. and Wu, T. T. (1971). *Annal. N.Y. Acad. Sci.*, **190**, 382
85. Porter, R. R. (1969–70). *Harvey Lectures, Series*, **65**, 157
86. Mole, L. E., Jackson, S. A., Porter, R. R. and Wilkinson J. M. (1971). *Biochem. J.*, **124**, 301
87. Kehoe, J. M. and Capra, J. D. (1971). *Proc. Nat. Acad. Sci. (USA)*, **68**, 2019
88. Strosberg, A. D., Jaton, J-C., Capra, J. D. and Haber, E. (1972). *Fed. Proc. (Fed. Amer. Soc. Exp. Biol.)*, **31**, 771 abs.
89. Fleischman, J. B. (1971). *Biochemistry*, **10**, 2753
90. Jaton, J-C. and Braun, D. G. (1972). *Biochem. J.*, **130**, 539
91. Mole, L. E. (1973). *Unpublished work*.
92. Edelman, G. M. and Gottleib, P. D. (1970). *Proc. Nat. Acad. Sci. (USA)*, **67**, 1192
93. Ein, D. (1968). *Proc. Nat. Acad. Sci. (USA)*, **60**, 982
94. Gibson, D., Levanon, M. and Smithies, O. (1971). *Biochemistry*, **10**, 3114
95. Hess, M., Hilschmann, N., Rivat, L., Rivat, C. and Ropartz, C. (1971). *Nature New Biol.*, **234**, 58
96. Schulenburg, E. P., Simms, E. S., Lynch, R. G., Bradshaw, R. A. and Eisen, H. N. (1971). *Proc. Nat. Acad. Sci. (USA)*, **68**, 2623
97. Appella, E., Chersi, A., Mage, R. G. and Dubiski, S. (1971). *Proc. Nat. Acad. Sci. (USA)*, **68**, 1341
98. Rejnek, J., Kostka, J. and Kotýnek, O. (1966). *Nature (London)*, **209**, 926
99. Utsumi, S. (1969). *Biochem. J.*, **112**, 343
100. Kehoe, J. M. and Fougereau, M. (1969). *Nature (London)*, **224**, 1212
101. Pink, J. R. L., Buttery, S. H., De Vries, G. M. and Milstein, C. (1970). *Biochem. J.*, **117**, 33

102. Mole, L. E. (1971). *D. Phil. Thesis Oxford University*
103. Reid, K. B. M. (1971). *Immunology*, **20**, 649
104. Wolfenstein, C., Frangione, B., Mihaesco, E. and Franklin, E. C. (1971). *Biochemistry*, **10**, 4140
105. Wolfenstein-Todel, C., Frangione, B. and Franklin, E. C. (1972). *Biochemistry*,
106. Clamp, J. R. and Johnson, I. (1972). *Glycoproteins*, 2nd edn, (Gotschalk, A., editor) (Amsterdam: Elsevier Publishing Company)
107. Melchers, F. (1969). *Biochemistry*, **8**, 938
108. Edmundson, A. B., Sheber, F. A., Ely, K. R., Simonds, N. B., Hutson, N. K. and Rossiter, J. L. (1968). *Arch. Biochem. Biophys.*, **127**, 725
108a. Milstein, C. P. and Milstein, C. (1971). *Biochem. J.*, **121**, 211
109. Press, E. M. and Hogg, N. M. (1970). *Biochem. J.*, **117**, 641
110. Smyth, D. S. and Utsumi, S. (1967). *Nature (London)*, **216**, 332
111. Fanger, M. W. and Smyth, D. G. (1972). *Biochem. J.*, **127**, 757
112. Munster, P. J. J. van, Stoelinga, G. B. A., Clamp, J. R., Gerding, J. J. Th., Reijnen, J. C. M. and Voss, M. (1972). *Immunology*, **23**, 249
113. Neuberger, A., Gottschalk, A. and Marshall, R. D. (1966). *Glycoproteins*, 273, (A. Gottschalk, editor) (Amsterdam: Elsevier Publishing Company)
113a. Frangione, B. and Milstein, C. (1969). *Nature* **224**, 597
114. Givol, D. (1973). *Contemporary Topics in Immunochemistry*, **2**
115. Porter, R. R. (1972). *Contemporary Topics in Immunochemistry*, **1**, 145
116. Inbar, D., Hochman, J. and Givol, D. (1972). *Proc. Nat. Acad. Sci. (USA)* **69**, 2659
116a. Hochman, J., Inbar, D. and Givol, D. (1973). *Biochemistry* **12**, 1130
117. Benjamini, E., Shimizu, M., Young, J. D. and Leung, C. Y. (1969). *Biochemistry*, **8**, 2242
118. Parker, C. W. and Osterland, C. K. (1970). *Biochemistry*, **9**, 1704
119. North, A. C. T. and Phillips, D. C. (1969). *Prog. Biophys. Molec. Biol.*, **19**, 1
120. Cathou, R. E. and Werner, T. C. (1970). *Biochemistry*, **9**, 3149
121. Inbar, D., Rotman, M. and Givol, D. (1971). *J. Biol. Chem.*, **246**, 6272
122. Wofsy, L., Metzger, H. and Singer, S. J. (1962). *Biochemistry*, **1**, 1031
123. Haimovich, J., Givol, D. and Eisen, H. N. (1970). *Proc. Nat. Acad. Sci. (USA)*, **67**, 1656
124. Fleet, G. W. J., Knowles, J. R. and Porter, R. R. (1969). *Nature (London)*, **224**, 511
124a. Fleet, G. W. T., Knowles, J. R. and Porter, R. R. (1972). *Biochem. J.*, **128**, 499
125. Converse, C. A. and Richards, F. F. (1969). *Biochemistry*, **8**, 4431
126. Wofsy, L. and Parker, D. C. (1967). *Cold Spring Harbor Symp. Quant. Biol.*, **32**, 111
127. Goetzl, E. J. and Metzger, H. (1970). *Biochemistry*, **9**, 1267, 3862
128. Givol, D., Strausbauch, P. H., Hurwitz, E., Wilchek, M., Haimovich, J. and Eisen, H. N. (1971). *Biochemistry*, **10**, 3461
129. Press, E. M., Fleet, G. W. J. and Fisher, C. E. (1971). *Progress in Immunology*, 233 (B. D. Amos, editor) (New York: Academic Press)
130. Press, E. M. and Hogg, N. M. (1969). *Nature (London)*, **223**, 807
131. Thorpe, N. O. and Deutsch, H. F. (1966). *Immunochemistry*, **3**, 329
132. Prahl, J. W. (1967). *Biochem. J.*, **105**, 1019
133. Prahl, J. W., Mandy, M. J. and Todd, C. W. (1969). *Biochemistry*, **8**, 4935
134. Frangione, B. (1969). *FEBS Lett.*, **3**, 341
135. Appella, E., Rejnek, J. and Reisfeld, R. A. (1969). *J. Molec. Biol.*, **41**, 473
136. Milstein, C. (1966). *Nature (London)*, **209**, 370
137. Baglioni, C., Alescio Zonta, L., Cioli, D. and Carbonara, A. (1966). *Science*, **152**, 1517
138. Frangione, B., Franklin, E. C., Findenberg, H. H. and Koshland, M. E. (1966). *J. Exp. Med.*, **124**, 715
139. Kiefer, H., Lindstrom, J., Lennox, E. S. and Singer, S. J. (1970). *PNAS* **67**, 1688. Also Singer S. J. (1972). Personal communication

7
Genetics of Immunoglobulins and of the Immune Response

C. MILSTEIN
Medical Research Council, Cambridge

and

A. J. MUNRO
Department of Pathology, Cambridge

7.1   INTRODUCTION

The induction of an immune response is a complex process. To induce cell proliferation and the secretion of circulating antibody most antigens have to react with receptors on two classes of lymphocytes (T and B cells). Each step of this process is likely to be under the control of a number of genes. The most obvious are the genes coding for circulating antibodies, which involve genes for the variable and constant sections of the immunoglobulin (Ig) chains. Models for the arrangement of these genes have been produced and are now generally accepted. However, the number of genes coding for the variable section is still controversial, and is closely connected with the problem of the origin of antibody diversity. The antigen receptors on a B lymphocyte, the line of cells responsible for secreting circulating antibody, are thought to be identical to the antibody molecules it secretes. Consequently, the same genes code for the receptors on B cells and circulating antibodies. However, the expression of functional receptors on the surface of cells and the process of secretion of antibodies are likely to be controlled by separate genes.

The genes involved in other steps of the response are much less well defined, and so far the products of these genes have not been identified. The evidence for the existence of such genes comes from the genetic analysis of the immune response. The ability to respond to a specific antigen has been the subject of recent extensive research in mice and guinea-pigs, and in many cases has been shown to be controlled by a single (complex) genetic locus. The characteristic property of this locus is that it is closely linked to the genes which code for the major histocompatibility antigens. It has been suggested that the genes in this locus code for antigen receptors on T cells, but this is not generally accepted.

7.2   THE Ig GENES

For a sequence of amino acids in a polypeptide chain, there is a corresponding sequence of nucleotides in the DNA of the cell which makes that polypeptide chain. Somatic cells of higher organisms are diploid and each cell contains two copies of each gene, one paternal and the other maternal. If for a particular gene these two copies differ, the individual may make two forms of the corresponding polypeptide chain differing perhaps by a single amino acid. If they represent allelic forms of the same gene they will occur on different chromosomes and will segregate in a Mendelian fashion. Segregation analysis (either by family or population studies) is used to distinguish between allelic forms of one gene and two closely-related genes present on each of the parental chromosomes (Figure 7.1).

As first observed with kappa chains[1] all Ig chains contain a variable section and a constant section (see Chapter 6). Analysis of amino acid sequences and of the segregation of markers shows that a different number of genes code for V- and C-sections. This paradoxical situation will be discussed extensively below and has led to the conclusion that both sections are coded for by different genes, the C-genes and the V-genes. So far this is the only case where the genetic information for a single polypeptide chain is held as two separate germ-line genes.

7.2.1 C-genes

7.2.1.1 κ-light chains

The analysis of the amino acid sequence of the constant section of human κ-chains shows an amino acid substitution (Val/Leu) at position 191 which correlates with the Inv allotypes[2, 3]. Family studies show that this marker segregates in a true allelic fashion (see Figure 7.1)[4-6]. This suggests that there is only one C-gene for κ-chains in the haploid set of chromosomes. Rabbits and rats are the other species with known allotypes on their κ-chains (see Tables 7.1 and 7.2). Although the correlation between chemical and serological evidence may not be so simple and clear cut as in human κ-chains, the

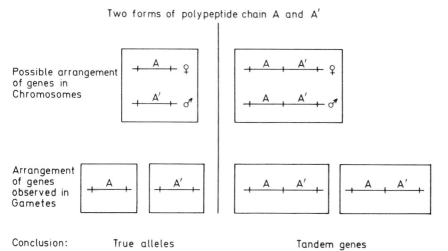

Figure 7.1 A test for alleles or tandem genes. The diagram illustrates the possible arrangement of the genes on the chromosomes of an individual carrying two similar but not identical forms of a polypeptide chain: A and A'. The distribution of the genes in the gametes can be measured by either family studies or population studies. True alleles generally give rise to homozygous individuals accounting for at least 50% of the offspring or of the total population. It should be noted that in the case of tandem genes, A on the paternal chromosome is a 'pseudo-allele' of A' on the maternal chromosome and vice versa

Table 7.1   The class or type of immunoglobulin chain carrying allotypic markers in different species. No allotypes yet found indicated by a dash

| Species | Immunoglobulin chain | | | | |
| | Light chains | | Heavy chains | | |
	κ	λ	μ	a	γ
Man	+	—	—	+	+
Mouse	—	—	—	+	+
Rabbit	+	+	+	+	+
Rat	+	—	—	—	—

Table 7.2   The more common allotypic determinants found on rabbit Ig chains

Genetic locus	Chain involved	Allotypes
'a' locus	Heavy chain V-section	a1, a2, a3
'b' locus	κ-light chains	b4, b5, b6, b9
'c' locus	λ-light chains	c7, c21
'd' locus	γ-chain C-section	d8, d10, d11, d12
'e' locus	γ-chain C-section	e14, e15
'f' locus	a-chain C-section	f71, f72, f73, f74, f75
'Ms' locus	μ-chain C-section	Ms1, Ms2, Ms4, Ms5, Ms6

Ms3 is only expressed when particular light chains carrying the b4 determinants are combined with μ-chains

segregation of these markers also suggests a single C-gene for the κ-chain of these species[7-9]. So far no evidence is available on the number of C_κ-genes in other species because no allotypic markers have been detected.

7.2.1.2   λ-light chains

Human λ-chains are thought to be coded for by at least three C-genes. The evidence for this comes from the presence of serological markers correlated with well defined amino acid substitutions which occur in all individuals (Figure 7.1)[10-12]. The fact that these sequences differ in only one or two residues suggests that the genes which code for these sequences result from a recent expansion of a single gene. In rabbits it is not yet clear if there is only one C_λ-gene characterised by the segregation of the λ-chain allotype markers C7 and C21[9]. Sequence studies of mouse myeloma proteins show the presence of two C_λ-sections[13, 14]. Both are λ-like when compared with human λ and have been designated C_λI and C_λII. Comparison of the two sequences indicates that the two corresponding genes differ by at least 34 nucleotides. The difference between human C_λ and mouse C_λI or C_λII is at least 42 nucleotides, suggesting that a gene duplication of the C_λ-gene occurred in the mouse evolutionary line shortly after the divergence of human and mouse lines. However, no segregation studies have been performed and the possibility that C_λI and C_λII are alleles is not completely excluded.

7.2.1.3 *Heavy chains*

The class and subclass of heavy chains are defined by amino acid sequence. In humans there are a large number of allotypes associated with most subclasses of γ- and α-chains (Gm and Am systems respectively), but none so far have been found in the μ-class (Tables 7.1 and 7.3). In some cases the markers have been correlated with specific amino acid changes (see Chapter 6). These markers segregate in a normal Mendelian manner, suggesting that

Table 7.3 **Most commonly used human allotypes. Original and new recommended nomenclature[146] are included. The so-called 'non markers' are not included. These are usually the allelic form of one of the markers which contains an antigenic structure also present in other subclasses. For instance, the 'non a' antiserum recognises the allele of Gm(a) on γ1 but also recognises all γ2 and γ3 chains irrespective of genetic origin. The subject is extensively reviewed in Ref. 15**

Markers	Original	New	Chain
	a	1	
	x	2	
	b² or bʷ	3	γ1
	f	4	
	z	17	
Gm	n	23	γ2
	b, b′	5	
	c	6	γ3
	g	21	
	b°		
Am	1 or +	1	α2
	1	1	
InV	a	2	κ
	b	3	

there is only one C-gene in each case (Figure 7.1) (For reviews see Refs. 15 and 16). There are interesting exceptions which occur in rare families. At two places in the C-section of γ_1-chains, certain amino acid differences are recognised as genetically inherited Gm markers. At each site there are two alternative forms, Gm(a) or Gm(non-a) at one site, and Gm(f) or Gm(z) at the other. In Caucasians, the γ_1-chains carry either Gm(z) and Gm(a) or Gm(f) and Gm(non-a), but a rare complex which contains the four markers has been shown to be inherited as a stable unit. This has been interpreted as a recent duplication arising from an unequal cross-over between the two allelic forms (see Figure 7.2)[17]. An event of this type will give rise to one chromosome with an additional segment, and the other chromosome with a deletion in the homologous site. There is evidence in other rare families for inheritable deletions in the heavy chain C-genes[15]. In one case the γ_3 C-gene, and in other cases the γ_1 C-gene, appear to be absent.

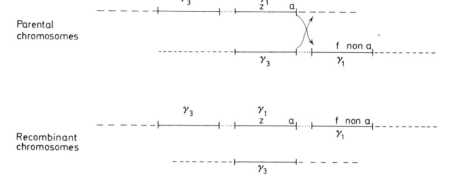

Figure 7.2 Unequal cross-over between allelic genes. The diagram illustrates the possible mispairing of tandem genes to give rise to the duplication which accounts for the stable inheritance of all four $\gamma1$ genetic markers (z, a, f and 'non-a'). On the other hand, the chromosome carrying the deletion of the $\gamma1$ gene could account for the observed absence of IgG1 in other families

In rabbits there are allotypic markers associated with the C-section of γ-[18, 19], a-[20] and μ-[21] chains (Table 7.2), some of which have been correlated with amino acid changes (see Chapter 6). All these markers segregate in the manner expected for single genes (Figure 7.1). In the mouse there are markers in most of the γ-subclasses and on a-chains, but none have been found on μ-chains (Table 7.4). Again, the segregation of these markers suggests single C-genes[22-24].

Table 7.4 The allotypic determinants found on the immunoglobulin heavy chains of prototype inbred mouse strains. The numbers define different specific antigenic determinants (sp. det.) The Ig-4 markers are defined by the electrophoretic mobility of the $\gamma1$ chain: f, fast; s, slow[24]. An alternative nomenclature is also in use[23,147] where γF, γG and γH refer to $\gamma1$, $\gamma2a$ and $\gamma2b$ respectively. A detailed comparison of these two nomenclatures is given in Ref. 24.

Genetic locus	Ig-1		Ig-2		Ig-3		Ig-4
Chains involved	$\gamma2a$		a		$\gamma2b$		$\gamma1$
	Sp. det.	Allele	Sp. det.	Allele	Sp. det.	Allele	Allele
BALB/C	1, 6, 7, 8, 10, 12	Ig1ᵃ	2, 3, 4	Ig2ᵃʰ	1, 2, 4, 7, 8	Ig3ᵃᶜʰ	f
C57BL/10J	4, 7	Ig1ᵇ	—	Ig2ᵇ	4, 7, 8, 9	Ig3ᵇ	s
DBA/2J	2, 3, 7	Ig1ᶜ	1	Ig2ᶜᵍ	1, 2, 4, 7, 8	Ig3ᵃᶜʰ	f
AKR/J	1, 2, 5, 7, 12	Ig1ᵈ	3	Ig2ᵈᵉ	1, 3, 7, 8	Ig3ᵈ	f
A/J	1, 2, 5, 6, 7, 8, 12	Ig1ᵉ	3	Ig2ᵈᵉ	1, 3, 7	Ig3ᵉ	f
CE/J	1, 2, 8, 11	Ig1ᶠ	4	Ig2ᶠ	1, 2, 3, 4	Ig3ᶠ	f
R111/J	2, 3	Ig1ᵍ	1	Ig2ᶜᵍ	1, 2, 4?	Ig3ᵍ	f
SEA/Gn	1, 2, 6, 7, 10, 12	Ig1ʰ	2, 3, 4	Ig2ᵃʰ	1, 2, 4, 7, 8	Ig3ᵃᶜʰ	f

7.2.1.4 C-gene linkage groups

The allotypic markers can be used in family studies to establish the arrange-ment of the different C-genes and their location relative to other genes. In rabbits, it has been shown that the C-genes for κ, λ and heavy chains all segregate independently from each other, showing that these genes are un-linked[9]. For example, a rabbit heterozygous for allelic markers in κ- and λ-chains will produce in its haploid cells (sperm or ovum) all four possible combinations of markers. Figure 7.3 illustrates the principles behind these

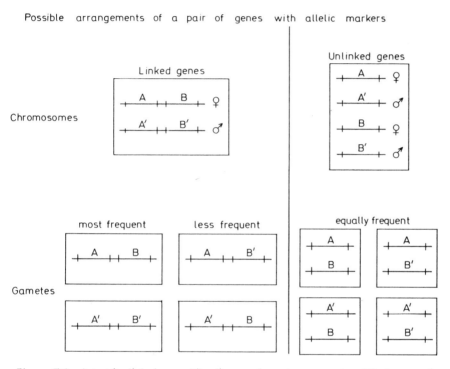

Figure 7.3 A test for linked genes. The diagram shows two genes, A and B of maternal origin, each with allelic forms A′ and B′ of paternal origin. It is possible to determine if A and B are linked or unlinked by the distribution of the allelic forms in the gametes. With linked genes, occasional recombinants give a pattern of markers not found in either parental chromosomes. The frequency of occurrence of these recombinants is a measure of the distance between the genes. Adjacent genes have a very low recombination frequency

linkage studies. In man, a similar analysis shows that the κ-chains C-gene is unlinked from the γ and α heavy chain C-genes[16]. Linkage studies with λ- and μ-chains cannot be done, as there are no allelic markers in these chains (see Table 7.1).

The picture which emerges from these studies is of three separate chromo-somes, each containing the C-genes for κ, λ or heavy chain respectively. This is probably true for all mammals. When there is more than one C-gene for a particular chain, as in the case of heavy chains, and when markers are available, it has been possible to show that these C-genes are very close to each other and probably occur as a tandem array of genes. For instance, rabbits heterozygous for allelic markers in the C-sections of γ and a-chains produce haploid cells carrying only two of the four possible combinations (Figure 7.3). Extensive family studies using inbred mice have failed to detect a recombination between heavy chain C-genes. This gives a recombination frequency between these genes of probably less than 0.05 %[22, 24].

The lack of frequent recombinants makes it difficult to establish the order of the genes in the heavy chain C-gene cluster. One pertinent source of information comes from the existence of unusual human heavy chains in apparently normal individuals[25]. The best studied case of these unusual chains appears to be the result of a deletion involving part of the γ_3 and γ_1 C-genes[26]. The resulting heavy chains carry antigenic determinants characteristic of the Fc part of the γ_1 C-section, and also determinants characteristic of the Fd part of the γ_3 C-section. No amino acid sequence studies on this protein have been reported. Nevertheless, as γ_2 and γ_4 are still expressed in these individuals, it has been suggested that γ_1 and γ_3 C-genes are adjacent and in protein terms with γ_1 to the carboxy-terminal side. The order of the other genes in the heavy chain cluster in humans is still speculative. The order shown in Figure 7.4 is the most generally accepted and is compatible with the combinations of allelic markers most frequently found in different populations[15].

Man		V-genes	C-genes
Light chains	κ	$\overline{Ia}$ $\overline{Ib}$ $\overline{II}$ $\overline{III}$	—
	λ	$\overline{I}$ $\overline{II}$ $\overline{III}$ $\overline{IV}$	$\overline{Arg}$ $\overline{Lys}$ $\overline{Gly}$
Heavy chains		$\overline{I}$ $\overline{II}$ $\overline{III}$	$\overline{\gamma4}$ $\overline{\gamma2}$ $\overline{\gamma3}$ $\overline{\gamma1}$ $\overline{a1}$ $\overline{a2}$ $\overline{\mu2}$ $\overline{\mu1}$ $\overline{\delta}$ $\overline{\epsilon}$

Mouse		V-genes	C-genes
Light chains	κ	$\overline{I}$ $\overline{II}$ $\overline{III}$ $\overline{IV}$ $\overline{V}$ $\overline{VI}$ $\overline{VII}$ $\overline{VIII}$ etc.	—
	λ	$\overline{I}$ $[\overline{II}]$	$\overline{I}$ $\overline{II}$

Figure 7.4 Possible arrangement of the minimum number of genes for human Ig and mouse light chains. The genes on each horizontal line are thought to lie on the same chromosome. In mice the minimum of kappa V-genes is probably well above 8 and the existence of a second lambda V-gene is uncertain (see text)

None of the Ig chain genes have been found linked to any other gene. Of particular importance is that they are *not* linked to the histocompatibility locus (H-2 in mouse or HL-A in man).

7.2.2 V-genes

V-genes code for the V-sections of the immunoglobulin chains. The amino acid sequences of the V-sections have well defined patterns. Thus the V-sections of all κ-chains have features in common which clearly distinguish them from the V-sections of λ and heavy chains. Similarly, λ and heavy chain V-sections can be distinguished from each other (see Chapter 6). This is true for all the species for which sufficient information is available. This observation leads to the conclusion that there are at least three sets of V-genes; one for κ, one for λ and one for heavy chains[27-29].

7.2.2.1 Human V-genes

Each of the three sets of V-genes usually contains more than one gene. The evidence for this comes from the comparison of a large number of V-section sequences belonging to each set. This shows that the sequences can be arranged into subgroups, the sequences in each subgroup having features in common that distinguish them from sequences in other subgroups[30, 31]. These features include the total number of residues in the V-section (e.g. all $V_{\kappa I}$-sections contain 107 while $V_{\kappa III}$ contain 108), and many subgroups specific amino acids[27]. These subgroups are sometimes very well defined, but not always[29, 34]. In human κ-chains three well defined subgroups have been described: $V_{\kappa I}$, $V_{\kappa II}$, $V_{\kappa III}$[30]. $V_{\kappa I}$ has been further subdivided into two very similar subgroups, $V_{\kappa Ia}$ and $V_{\kappa Ib}$[35]. It is generally accepted that if the subgroups are well defined, as in the case of human κ-chains, there is at least one V-gene for each subgroup and the minimum number of genes can be taken as the number of subgroups. Three subgroups have been postulated for λ-chains[32, 36, 37], but these are less well defined[29, 34] and there is at least one protein (Sh) which does not correspond to any subgroup. This could be a representative of a further subgroup. In the case of human heavy chains there appear to be three reasonably well defined subgroups, V_{HI}, V_{HII} and V_{HIII}.

7.2.2.2 Variability within a subgroup

The proteins which belong to a given subgroup have identical amino acid residues in the majority of their positions and these common residues have been used to define basic sequences[27]. Individual proteins may depart from this basic sequence to give rise to variants in an otherwise invariant position (*low frequency variants*). These variants could arise by point mutations at the somatic level or by mutations of the germ-line V-genes. Within a given subgroup, two or even three alternative residues occur with similar frequency in some positions along the chain. These *repeated variants* are critical in the possible further division of the subgroups[67]. They are also the basis for drawing evolutionary trees within a subgroup. For instance, they have been used to argue that the best evolutionary tree for the κI-subgroup requires a minimum of three κI V-genes[29]. Some of the repeated variants could represent alleles of V-genes, and if so would be important genetic markers. The other type of variants occurs in positions of high variability ('hot spots'). These seem to occur in clusters referred to as hypervariable regions, and are particularly interesting as they seem to be the residues most directly responsible for the specificity of the antibody combining sites. It is now clear that the origin of these variants in genetic terms is critical to the controversy on the origin of antibody diversity. These variants represent a striking non-random feature. They could arise by selection of random mutants, or by non-random mutation, or by a combination of both processes operating on either germ-line or soma-line genes.

7.2.2.3 Species variations of V-section subgroups

In other species the sequence data are less complete. The results show many similarities to, as well as very interesting differences from, the human chains discussed above. One striking observation has been that the number of sub-groups is species specific. This is particularly well illustrated by mouse light chains. In the case of κ-chains, it appears that there are so many subgroups[41] that so far insufficient sequences have been determined to accurately estimate the minimum number present. Thirty sequences of the first 23 amino acids have been arranged into 19 subgroups, of which at present, ten are defined by only a single protein[42]. Attempts to estimate the number of subgroups from this data by statistical methods are bound to be inaccurate, as no account can be made of the fact that certain subgroups are rarely expressed. In the few cases where the complete sequence of the V-section is known, the mouse κ-sequences differ from each other by as much, or almost as much, as they differ from the human κ-chain sequence, regardless of which human subgroup is used for comparison[43]. In contrast, the λ-chain V-sections are remarkably similar[44, 45]. Of the twelve V-sections associated with $C_{\lambda I}$, eight are identical, and the others differ from this sequence by not more than three amino acid replacements located in the hypervariable region[46]. This means that there is only one subgroup, and there are no compelling reasons for more than a single germ-line gene for this V-section. Only one λ-chain is known containing the $C_{\lambda II}$-section[13]. Its V-section, although very similar to the V-section of the other mouse λ-chains, contains eight amino acid replacements, at least two, and probably four of which lie outside the hypervariable regions. This suggests the existence of a second V-gene in mice involved with the λ-chains.

In rabbits ca. 20 κ-chains of homogeneous antibodies have been sequenced for the first 20–30 residues[47-49]. These sequences have been arranged into six subgroups, although one is defined by only a single protein[49]. In rat, 11 of the 13 κ-chains sequenced so far up to residue 30 fall neatly into only three subgroups, two of which resemble the human κI-subgroup[50]. The λ-chains of pigs contain a largely homogenous sequence up to residue 20. This sequence displays some features which clearly distinguish it from λ-chains of other species[156]. This again illustrates the variation between species in the number and character of the V-genes. The available sequences from the V-section of heavy chains of cat and dog have so far produced no evidence for more than one subgroup in these species[51]. It has been suggested that the heavy chain of these species contains only one V_H-gene.

7.2.2.4 V-genes as tandem sets

Since the sequences which define the subgroups are derived from myeloma proteins it is crucial to show that the subgroups occur in Ig molecules of normal individuals. If the subgroups are present in all individuals, this proves that the subgroups are not alleles of a single locus, for if they were, they would segregate (Figure 7.1). Technically this is difficult to do, but by chemical means it has been clearly shown that $V_{\kappa Ib}$ and $V_{\kappa III}$ are the expression of non-allelic genes[12, 52]. Although the data is less complete for the other V_κ subgroups and the V_H[39] and V_λ[53] subgroups, the results support the idea that in each set the subgroups are the expression of tandem non-allelic genes.

In summary, it is generally accepted that there are three clusters of V-genes: V_κ-, V_λ- and V_H-genes. The number of genes in each cluster can vary considerably from species to species. The minimum number of genes in each cluster required to explain the protein sequence data varies from one to several, and in some cases may turn out to be as many as one hundred.

7.2.2.5 V-gene genetic markers

A different source of information for V-genes comes from genetic markers. Rabbit heavy chains are the only Ig chains which have well-defined markers in their V-genes (a locus allotypes, Table 7.2). Amino acid sequence studies (see Chapter 6) have shown considerable differences between the V_H-sections which correlate with the three allotypes, $a1$, $a2$ and $a3$[54, 55]. Such multiple differences are usually associated with different subgroups; but unlike subgroups, only one of the allotypes occurs in a haploid set of chromosomes. They behave as true alleles in extensive family studies[7, 9, 56]. There are technical difficulties in detecting small amounts of one of the allotypes in the presence of the other two, making this evidence not as rigorous as its importance warrants. However, it is generally accepted that these allotypes represent a single or a small number of closely linked V_H-genes. Not all the Ig molecules in rabbits carry the a locus allotypes, which indicates that there is an additional gene or genes (a negative) for the V_H-sections[57, 58]. This gene(s) occurs in all rabbits and therefore is not an allele of the a locus.

A spot has been described in a fingerprint of a tryptic digest of the light chains of some strains of mice which was not observed in other strains[59]. This appeared to be a genetic marker of the V_κ-section since the presence or absence of this spot was inherited in a simple Mendelian fashion. This chromatographic spot does not seem to represent a pure peptide and the significance of this marker is still not fully understood.

7.2.3 Linkage of V-genes to C-genes

The genetic markers in the V-section and the C-section of rabbit heavy chains have been used to study the linkage of the corresponding genes (Figure 7.3). It was found that the V_H-genes and C_H-genes were closely linked. In studies involving allotypes in the V_H-genes (a locus) and the C_λ-genes (d and e loci) two separate recombinants were found[60, 61]. Although the number of recombinants is small the data suggest a recombination frequency of *ca.* 0.4%. This means that the V-genes are not adjacent to the C-genes but are fairly close. Since the C-genes for the heavy chain and the two light chains are unlinked, the V_H-genes should also be unlinked from the kappa (*b* locus) and lambda (*c* locus) genes. In all cases this has been found to be true[56].

Linkage between the V- and C-genes is also suggested by two other observations. First, rabbit κ-chains of different *b* locus allotype show differences in average N-terminal amino acid sequence[62] while the *b* locus allotypes had been previously shown to be correlated with amino acid changes in the C-sections[63, 64]. This can be interpreted as allelic forms of both V-genes and C-genes which have segregated together. In other words, V_κ is closely linked to C_κ. An alternative explanation is that the differences in the average N-terminal sequence result from a tandem set of V_κ-genes, which are expressed in different proportions depending on the C-section allotype. Second, mice can respond to certain antigens to produce antibody of a particular idiotype, and this has been shown to be under the control of a gene linked to the C_H locus[65, 66]. As idiotypes are thought to represent very specific structural features of the V-section, this data suggests that the V_H- and C_H- genes are also linked in mice.

The reason for the close linkage of V- and C-genes is not known, but it is possible that it is important for the mechanism of integration. If this is the case, the kappa and lambda V-genes for light chains will also be closely linked to their respective C-genes.

7.2.4 Summary

The minimum number of genes required for human Ig molecules, and their most likely distribution, is summarised in Figure 7.4. It shows sections in three chromosomes each carrying two tandem sets of genes, one set for V-genes and one for C-genes. The chromosomes carrying the light chain genes of mouse are also shown to illustrate the species differences in the minimum number of V-genes. It is not clear to us if $C_{\lambda I}$ and $C_{\lambda II}$ should be placed on the same chromosome. This is because it is uncertain if the postulated $V_{\lambda II}$-gene is a separate gene. If it is, and cannot integrate with $C_{\lambda I}$, then the sets of λI- and λ-II-genes would probably be unlinked and may even occur on different chromosomes.

7.3 INTEGRATION OF V- AND C-GENES

The arrangement of genes shown in Figure 7.4 makes a special mechanism for the integration of V- and C-genes unavoidable. Thus with human κ-chains, there is good evidence for a single C-gene and multiple V-genes, and the products of different V-genes are found associated with the product of a single C-gene. As would be expected, the two allelic forms of the C_κ-gene are found with about equal frequency associated with the different V-section subgroups (see Table 7.5). In the case of multiple C-genes, all the V-section subgroups are found associated with the different C-genes. For example, the three V_H subgroups are found in different classes and subclasses of human heavy chains[68]. In rabbits, the genetic markers in the V_H-genes are found in γ-, a-, μ- and ε-chains[69-72]. However, it is possible that not all the V-genes from the heavy chains can be paired with equal efficiency to every heavy chain C-gene. This could explain some anomalous sequence data[73] as well as the existence of subclass specific antibodies[74, 75].

Table 7.5 Distribution of the InV allelic marker characterised by residue 191 in the different subgroups of κ-chains[148]. Additional data from Refs. 35, 67, 149, 150, 151, 152 and 153

Subgroup	No. of individual chains containing as residue 191	
	Val	Leu
κIa	3	2
κIb	5	1
κII	3	2
κIII	3	1

The process of integration does not take place during or after protein synthesis[76-78] (Chapter 8). It is generally assumed that it is achieved by rearrangement of the linear order of the genes in the DNA although an alternative hypothesis involving a branched network of the DNA structure has been proposed[79]. In fact, there is at present no proof that integration does occur at the DNA level. One line of suggestive evidence comes from the structure of the heavy-chain disease proteins isolated from rare forms of malignant lymphomas[80]. The amino acid sequence of the best studied of these proteins shows that it has arisen from a deletion of most of the V-section and an adjacent part of the C-section[81]. Unfortunately this does not prove that the deletion took place after integration as deletions between non-integrated but linked C- and V-genes could produce the same result. A remarkable feature of these abnormal proteins is that the deletion generally ends at the same position. This is a glutamic acid residue, which is found in all human γ-subclasses, homologous to residue 216 of protein Eu. This is illustrated in Figure 7.5, which also shows that the beginning of the deletion is not restricted to one position. The size of the deleted fragment is, therefore, variable[80].

Whatever the mechanism, the process of integration involves genes on the same chromosome, i.e. the integration is *cis* and not *trans*. The evidence for this comes from studies on rabbits heterozygous for both V- and C-gene markers on the H chains[82, 83]. The majority of the Ig molecules in such rabbits carry only two of the four possible combinations of markers. There is a small but probably significant percentage of recombinant molecules[84]. It would appear, therefore, that the integration mechanism is such that 'mistakes' leading to *trans* integration are not completely excluded. There are many possible mechanisms for the predominantly *cis* integration of V- and C-genes, for example by recombination between sister chromatids or by a deletion.

The 1 % of trans rearrangement could be the result of increased breakage and repair of the DNA during these events. An alternative mechanism is the formation of an episome involving the DNA from one site which re-enters the chromosome at a second site. The predominantly *cis* integration might be achieved by having the relevant genes from only one of the pair of chromosomes available at the time of integration. In fact, it is well known that in antibody-forming cells of animals heterozygous for any Ig allotype only one of the two available alleles is expressed[85,86]. Apart from the X chromosome this phenomenon of allelic exclusion has only been described for Ig genes and

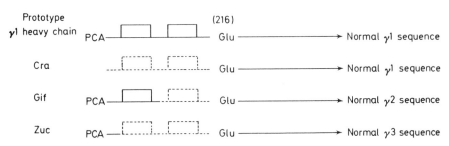

Figure 7.5   Nature of the deletion in three 'heavy-chain disease' proteins. Broken lines indicate the portion of the heavy chain absent from proteins Cra, Gif, and Zuc. Although the deletions are of different size they all end at the glutamic acid residue which is homologous to residue 216 of the γ1 heavy chain prototype (protein Eu[154])

appears to bear no resemblance to the inactivation of the second X chromosome in female cells. It is not clear at which stage of cell maturation allelic exclusion occurs, nor the mechanism of this precise gene inactivation.

With the heavy chains, in addition to the integration of V- and C-genes, another remarkable event occurs. For a long time it has been argued that cells can change the class of immunoglobulin that they synthesise without changing its antibody specificity[87]. Assuming integration occurs at the DNA level, this implies that a V-gene adjacent to a C_μ-gene is translocated to become adjacent to a C_γ-gene. There is now considerable evidence for this type of switch. A patient has been described whose serum contains two different myeloma proteins, one IgM, the other IgG. The light chains of both molecules appear identical. On chemical analysis it was found that the V-sections of the two different heavy chains appeared identical[88]. The possibility that by chance the same V_H-gene is used in two independent different clones is negligible since no two identical V-sections have been reported so far in human myeloma. In other experiments it has been shown that an anti-idiotype antisera which reacts with IgG molecules will also react with IgM molecules found in earlier bleeds[89]. As anti-idiotype antisera are thought to recognise specific V-sections, this implies that the same V-section can be found on IgM and IgG molecules. It is also possible to show that a switch of immunoglobulin class occurs at the cellular level. Cells can be found with IgM receptors on their surface and IgG molecules inside[90].

In summary, there are two, possibly different, translocation events. The first involves the bringing together of V- and C-genes and the expression of a single protein chain. The second, which occurs during the development of the immune response, brings the V_H-gene adjacent to another C_H-gene. This second event occurs after allelic exclusion has taken place.

7.4 GENETICS OF THE IMMUNE RESPONSE

One of the major problems in the study of V-section genes is the lack of genetic markers. Since these genes are responsible for antibody specificity it should be possible to approach this problem by studying the genetic control of the immune response to a particular antigen.

The response of individual animals to antigens varies in the amount of antibody produced, in the chemical nature of their combining sites and in the heterogeneity of the response. The differences in response to specific antigens can often be shown to be genetically inherited. The analysis of such experiments is complicated by the many steps involved in the induction and maintenance of the immune response. Antibody production usually requires specific recognition of antigen by both T and B cells (see Chapter 10). So far there is no evidence that the primary structures of the B-cell antigen receptors are in any way different from the Ig molecules and therefore the same genes probably code for both. It is a reasonable assumption that the receptor of antigen on T cells is analogous to the B-cell antigen receptor inasmuch as it consists of V-sections and C-sections, but their chemical identity is very controversial[91-93]. Inheritable differences of V-genes could lead to differences in response. Among the mutations affecting V-genes the most obvious is the complete absence of a particular V-gene (deletion mutant), or a change in its nucleotide sequence resulting in the failure of this gene to generate chains with any correct antigen-binding site (aberrant mutants). Other mutations could be either in the sites directly involved with interaction between antigen and antibody (contact mutants) or in changes which indirectly affect the topography of the active site (modulation mutants). Defective V-genes could also result from mutations which affect the mechanism of integration (integration mutants) or affect the interaction of the V-sections of heavy and light chains (interaction mutants). On the other hand, the available pool of somatic V-genes could be affected in many ways by other germ-line genes. Finally, it is likely that genes other than the V-genes themselves will influence the level of the response to specific antigens. For example, as the expression of V-genes which can react with self determinants is suppressed (tolerance), response to an antigen will depend on the range of self determinants. The nature of the self components varies from strain to strain. Thus, an antigen which cross-reacts with a self component of one strain, is likely to give a different level of response in another strain lacking that self component.

7.4.1 Inheritance of idiotypes and monoclonal responses

There are several categories of determinants of the V-sections which can be recognised by antibodies raised in the same or different species. The first are the determinants shared by all V-sections of a particular subgroup (V-section isotypes). The second arise from allelic forms of V-genes. These would be present in all the V-sections derived from a particular V-gene found in certain individuals or strains of inbred animals (V-section allotypes). The third category are determinants characteristic of a particular antibody molecule or myeloma protein (idiotypic determinants[94, 95]).

The idiotypic determinants are usually unique for a specific antibody raised in a single animal (see Chapter 6). It is unusual to find idiotypic determinants carried on antibodies from different individuals. Recently, idiotypic antisera have been raised which recognise antibodies from individuals of the same species, but only if they are genetically related. These observations have been made in highly selected systems. For example, the response of mice to streptococcal polysaccharide is strain dependent[96]. Strain A/J mice produce large amounts of antibodies with restricted electrophoretic heterogeneity typical of a monoclonal response. Monoclonal antibody from one of these mice was used to produce an idiotypic-specific antiserum. This antiserum detected the same idiotypic specificity in other mice of the same strain after they had been immunised with streptococcal polysaccharide but the idiotype was never detected in the two other strains tested. Of five A/J mice analysed in detail, four had identical reactions with the idiotypic antiserum while one had an idiotype similar but not identical. The identity of idiotypic determinants in the antibodies to streptococcal polysaccharide was paralleled by an identical isoelectric focusing pattern, suggesting very similar if not identical V-section sequences in these antibody molecules. The implication of this result is that each mouse of this particular strain is able to produce this unique antibody structure, or a structure very similar to it, after immunisation with this antigen. It is as if a V-gene genetic marker becomes detectable after this particular immunisation procedure. Since this V-gene marker is in one strain but not in others of the same species, one is faced with the somewhat confusing situation where an idiotypic specificity appears as a V-gene allotype. There is no apparent association of this response to the H-2 locus. No family studies have yet been reported on this system and, therefore, it is not known if this response is linked to the C-gene markers.

In a more complicated study, using antibodies to various haptens, the same type of phenomenon has been observed. Thus, an anti-idiotype to a particular anti-hapten antibody recognised molecules with similar antibody activity raised in all mice of the same strain[97]. However, in these experiments the anti-hapten antibodies obtained from different animals were in most cases not absolutely identical.

The use of streptococcal polysaccharide in mice was inspired by the restricted response that this antigen could produce in certain rabbits[98]. In some cases the response appeared monoclonal and such monoclonal antibodies were used to raise anti-idiotypes. In family studies[99, 100], a specific idiotype could be traced, but it showed complex genetics indicative of multigenic phenomena. The anti-idiotype antisera reacted weakly with normal rabbit serum of the same V_H allotype but not at all with serum from rabbits with different allotypes. The monoclonal responses seen in unrelated rabbits did not have identical idiotypes or electrophoretic mobilities. Amino acid sequence studies on such antibodies have been reported[49].

7.4.1.1 Responsiveness linked to Ig genes

There are two cases of genetically controlled differential responses to specific antigens which appear to concern V-genes. Different inbred strains of mice immunised with dextrans containing $a1-3$ glycosyl linkages give characteristic low or high responses. In high responders, the majority of the antibody produced is of lambda type and reacts with a particular idiotypic antirserum. High response is dominant and is linked to the heavy-chain allotype, although in strain studies it is obvious that recombinants have occurred[66].

The second example involves the ability of different strains of mice to make antibody to phosphoryl choline. This response is also genetically controlled but in a more complicated manner. It is found that in certain strains of mice, but not in others, the majority of antiphosphoryl choline antibody reacts with a specific idiotypic antiserum. The ability to make such molecules is dominant and by family studies is shown to be linked to the heavy chain allotypes[65]. However, a second independently-segregating gene was required in order to explain all the results. In both these examples the simplest interpretation of the data, and, in particular, of the linkage to the C_H allotypes, is that there is a mutant in the V-genes for heavy chains. The exact nature of this V-gene mutant is an open question.

7.4.2 Immune-response genes linked to the major histocompatibility locus

The functions of other genes which control the response to specific antigens are far less certain. The first specific immune response gene to be identified was the PLL gene in guinea-pigs[101] which controls the response to poly-L-lysine (PLL) and to haptens such as dinitrophenol (DNP) conjugated to PLL. Since

Table 7.6 An example[105] to illustrate linkage to H-2 and dominance of an IR1 gene

All mice of strain	H-2	Response
DBA/1	q	High
SJL	s	Low
(DBA/1 × SJL)F1	q/s	High
(DBA/1 × SJL)F1 × SJL	{if q/s	High
	{if s	Low

Immune response was to the synthetic antigen (Phe,G)–A—L, which has the structure:

$$
\begin{array}{cc}
O & O \\
| & | \\
| & | \leftarrow \text{Poly-D,L-Ala} \\
\end{array}
$$

$---$ Poly-L-lysine $---$

Poly(Phe,Glu)

O

then the response to many specific antigens has been shown to be controlled by genes which, in mice, fall into three immune response (IR) loci: IR1, IR2 and IR3[102-104]. The most fully investigated are the IR1 locus of mice and the IR locus of guinea-pigs, which have three striking features in common.

(a) Both loci are found very closely linked to the genes which control the major histocompatibility antigens of the species[105,106]. In mice these antigens are coded for by two separate regions, H-2D and H-2K. The Ss and S1p locus, which controls the level and presence of a serum substance, lies between the

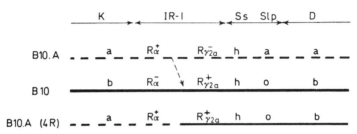

Figure 7.6 Schematic representation of the H-2 region of chromosomes from congenic mouse strains B10.A (H-2ᵃ), B10(H-2ᵇ) and B10.A (4R) (H-2ᵃ/H-2ᵇ crossover). K and D refer to the K and D regions of H-2, Rα and Rγ2a refer to the IR1 genes which control the response to IgA and IgG2a myeloma proteins from BALB/C mice. The Ss, S1p locus controls the level and nature of a serum protein. The pattern of response to IgA and IgG2a shows that the crossover in B10.A (4R) occurs between two IR1 genes. Data taken from Ref. 108

H-2D and H-2K regions. Analysis of mice with recombinant H-2 alleles places the IR1 locus to the left of the Ss locus and to the right of any known H-2K antigen[107]. In fact, recently a recombinant has been found which occurred within the IR1 locus[108] (Figure 7.6). In guinea-pigs there is no information on the fine structure of this region.

(b) All responses controlled by genes in the IR1 and guinea-pig IR loci show dominance in heterozygous animals[101,109]. In other words, in a cross between a high responder and a low responder, the resulting offspring responds as a high responder (see Table 7.6). This strongly suggests, but does not prove, that the failure to respond is not caused by tolerance or partial tolerance to a particular antigenic determinant. The analysis of tetraparental mice produced by fusing eight cell cleavage-stage embryos from low and high responders, shows that some of the chimeric mice are high responders and produce antibody molecules with the low responder allotype[110]. These results make it even less likely that the failure to respond is caused by tolerance.

(c) IR1 and guinea-pig IR low or non-responder strains can be made capable of a good response if the specific antigen is attached to a known immunogenic molecule[111,112], and by other means[113,114]. For example, strain 13 guinea-pigs lack the PLL gene and fail to make antibody to DNP–PLL. However, they respond in a perfectly normal manner to DNP on other carriers such as bovine serum albumin (BSA) and to DNP–PLL attached to BSA. Similarly, in mice high responses have been induced in low responder strains, provided the specific antigen was bound to methylated BSA.

7.4.2.1 Number of genes in the mouse IR1 and the guinea-pig IR loci

It is not known how many genes are involved in either the IR1 or guinea-pig IR locus. However, the guinea-pig IR locus contains at least four genes[102].

(a) The PLL gene which controls the response to polylysine and other positively charged polymers and to haptens attached to them.

(b) The GA gene which controls the response to the linear random co-polymer of L-glutamic acid and L-alanine.

(c) The GT gene which controls the response to the linear random co-polymer of L-glutamic acid and L-tyrosine.

(d) The BSA-1 gene which controls the response to low doses of BSA, haptens on BSA and human serum albumin.

Strain 2 guinea-pigs contain the PLL, GA and BSA-1 genes while strain 13 contains the GT gene. In the random bred Hartley strain, the PLL and GA genes tend to segregate together, but animals are found which respond to GA and not to PLL, and vice versa. This suggests that the PLL and GA genes are separate genes usually arranged as a tandem set. The GT gene on the other hand segregates away from the PLL and GA genes, suggesting that this gene is an allele or pseudo-allele (Figure 7.1) of the GA and PLL genes. The BSA-1 gene appears as an additional gene linked to, but independent from, the PLL and GA genes. Thus in guinea-pigs there is clear evidence for at least three separate genes and one allele or pseudo-allele.

In mice, it has been shown that the IR1 locus controls the response to many synthetic linear or branched polypeptides and weak allogenic antigens or strong protein antigens used at limiting dose[102]. Unfortunately, insufficient data has so far been obtained from random-bred animals to estimate the nature and minimum number of genes required to explain the observed response patterns. The existence of a recombinant between two IR1 genes shows that at least two loci are involved. In general, the number of genes is thought to be large, considering the ease with which they can be demonstrated.

7.4.2.2 Relationship of Ig genes with these genes

It is most unlikely that the IR genes discussed above are the same as the Ig genes. This is indicated by several facts. Failure to produce a given antibody by a strain lacking an IR gene does not mean absence of correct Ig V-genes since the antibodies can be elicited by changing the immunisation procedure. More significantly, in all known cases the Ig genes are unlinked from the major histocompatibility locus. It would be somewhat surprising if genes other than Ig V-genes are involved in specific recognition of antigen. For this reason it has been suggested that IR genes code for a new class of immunoglobulin responsible for antigen recognition on T cells. This controversial problem is discussed in Chapter 10. There are other ways in which IR genes could affect specific antigen recognition. For example, the IR genes may code for surface structures which interfere with the function of antigen receptors made from Ig molecules[115]. Alternatively, the IR genes could affect the range of diversity of Ig V-genes[116]. In fact, there are experiments which suggest that genes in the H2 locus do affect the specificity of the antibodies produced[108, 114].

7.4.3 Other immune-response genes

The specific immune response to many antigens has been shown to be controlled by genes other than those linked to the major histocompatibility locus (for a review see ref. 104). The best studied case[117] involves the response of mice to simple synthetic polymers built on branches of polyproline, on a backbone of polylysine, e.g. (tyrosine-glutamic) polyproline–polylysine, (T,G)-Pro–L. The response is controlled by a dominant autosomal gene which has been called IR3[118].

The other named locus in mouse is IR2[119] which controls the response to erythrocytes of wild mice. This is a recessive autosomal gene which has been shown to be linked not to H-2 but to the H-3 and H-6 minor histocompatibility loci. In addition, animals within a species show a range of abilities in their response to a variety of unrelated antigens. By selective breeding, it is possible to make lines of high and low responders showing that this non-specific property of the immune response is also under genetic control. The best studied case[120] shows complex segregation typical of a multi-gene system. Although the systems referred to in this section have not been discussed in any detail, it should be kept in mind that the elucidation of the function of the genes involved may lead to a greater understanding of the intricacies of the control and induction of the immune response.

7.5 ORIGIN OF ANTIBODY DIVERSITY

7.5.1 The extent of antibody diversity

In order to discuss the origin of antibody diversity, the first task is to define the number of antibody structures an animal can produce as well as the number of antibody specificities it needs to survive in a hostile environment. Since the work of Landsteiner[121], it has been quite clear that antibody response is highly specific. In addition to the large number of antigens recognised by antibodies, the normal response to a simple determinant elicits antibody molecules with a wide range of amino acid sequences as far as the V-section is concerned. This could imply that a very large number of unique antibody molecules can be made. On the other hand, the remarkable cases of cross-reaction shown by homogeneous antibody molecules to completely unrelated haptens, raises the possibility that the number of antibody structures may be relatively restricted[122]. In response to a particular antigen, the immunoglobulins produced may contain some molecules which could have been elicited by other antigens. As these cross-reacting molecules are at low concentration and the number of possible antigens is large, they will be difficult to detect. It is, at present, impossible to judge the importance of this cross-reaction. For this, and other reasons, estimates of the number of antibody structures necessary to explain the immune system have varied from 10^4 to an indefinite number, although the most common estimates are from 10^6 to 10^8.

Attempts have been made in several ways to measure the actual number of antibody structures. Idiotypic antisera directed against myeloma proteins generally fail to detect molecules carrying the same idiotypic determinants in normal Ig. An alternative approach is to estimate the number of different antibody structures which can react with a particular antigen. If a mouse receives a single injection of antigen a large number of different antibodies are made. This heterogeneous response can be analysed by transferring a small number of spleen cells into irradiated recipient mice and rechallenging with antigen. The number of transferred cells can be adjusted so that the response is often monoclonal in the recipient mice[123]. The monoclonal antibodies can be characterised by isoelectric focusing, a very sensitive technique for detecting changes in the amino acid sequence of proteins. In this way the response of four mice to a hapten antigen has been compared[124]. A large number of different antibody structures were found, but occasionally (five out of 337) the same antibody structure, as revealed by isoelectric focusing, occurred in different mice. It was calculated that the response to the hapten 3-nitro-4-hydroxy-5-iodophenylacetyl (NIP) draws from a pool of 3000–30 000 different antibody molecules with a peak probability of 8000. This calculation relies on the resolving power of the isoelectric-focusing technique. It is assumed that this is high, and no account is taken of the possibility of repeats being due to the inability of the apparatus to discriminate between non-identical molecules with very similar or identical isoelectric patterns. The upper limit of the size of the pool of antibodies to NIP may in fact be reasonably near to the resolving power of the apparatus. Since the antibody molecules are made of two chains, and of several classes and subclasses, the actual number of V-sections is very much less. By how much it is reduced depends on the extent of random association of light and heavy chains. If the association were completely random, then there would be $P \times Q$ different antibody structures from P light chains and Q heavy chains. It seems likely that not all possible combinations will form a functional site. The number of individual chains to make $P \times Q$ antibodies is therefore likely to be more than P and Q. Of the 8000 anti-NIP antibodies, 5000 were calculated to be of a single subclass and to require a minimum of $\sqrt{5000}$, i.e. 70 V-genes for each chain. Bearing in mind that all the assumptions make this an absolute minimum estimate (and could be a gross underestimate), 140 V-genes for anti-NIP activity in an inbred strain of mice is a surprisingly large number.

A further approach to this problem is to attempt to estimate the different number of light or heavy chains that a species can make, rather than the number of whole Ig structures. Using immunofluorescent techniques to detect plasma cells containing a unique lambda V-section determinant, it was found that 1 in 25 000 cells producing a lambda chain reacted with this reagent[125]. This experiment suggests that the minimum number of lambda V-sections in humans is 25 000.

7.5.2 Germ-line diversification

One of the most interesting features of the genes which code for immunoglobulins is that as shown in Figure 7.7 all of them are probably derived from a single ancestral gene[126, 127]. This would have coded for a sequence of ca. 100

amino acids with one intrachain disulphide bridge. All the Ig genes possibly evolved from this ancestral gene by using general processes of gene duplication. Examples of such processes have been observed in other proteins as well as Ig chains. One gives rise to a duplicated DNA sequence, coding for a single polypeptide chain of approximately double size. A second also forms a duplicated DNA sequence but in this case each sequence codes for a polypeptide chain. Initially these two chains would be identical but with time each will accumulate its own specific mutants. Both forms of gene duplication probably occur by a mismatched crossover event (see Figure 7.2) but in the first case the genetic information for stopping and starting protein synthesis is not duplicated. A third form of gene duplication is believed to be the result of multiplication of whole chromosomes[128]. This probably was the process responsible for the development of non-linked but structurally related systems such as κ- and λ-chains.

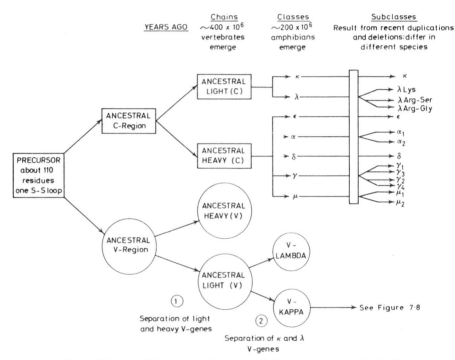

Figure 7.7 Possible scheme for the evolution of immunoglobulins[34]. 1 and 2 indicate stages of evolution at which duplication of whole chromosomes has occurred.

An important development in the understanding of the evolution of immunoglobulins was the realisation that one of the earliest duplications involved the formation of the V- and C-genes of the ancestral chain[34, 129]. This event, followed by further duplications and mutation, led to the multiple and variant forms of the sections (Figure 7.7). The evolutionary scheme shown in Figure 7.7 is based on the hypothesis that the time elapsed for the divergence of two identical genes is proportional to the minimum number of mutational steps required to convert one sequence into the other[130, 155]. This evolutionary rate is different for different proteins but appears to be reasonably constant for each one.

An obvious consequence of gene duplication through mismatched crossover is that it leads to expansion at the expense of deletion (Figure 7.2). If the deletion has selective advantage, then a contraction of the genome will become established. Gene contraction and expansion does occur in the immune system and this is well illustrated by the recent evolution of the C-section genes[34]. The evolution of the V-sections also shows evidence of expansion and contraction but there is disagreement as to the extent and stability of the expansion. An example of V-gene expansion is the κIa- and

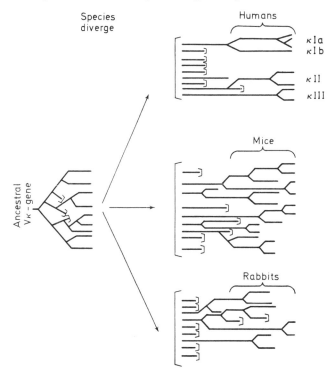

Further variants introduced by either somatic mutation or recent massive expansion followed by selection of suitable mutants.

Figure 7.8   Possible scheme for the evolution of V_κ genes. A scheme of this type explains the general similarities and the specific differences between subgroups in different species

κIb-subgroups in humans. As the basic sequences of these two sub-groups differ only in few amino acids this duplication must have occurred much more recently than the duplication necessary to separate κI from κII and κIII. Examples of the loss of V-genes are not easy to demonstrate. Cat and dog heavy chains appear to express only one V_H-subgroup which is closely related to V_{HIII} found in man[51], while rabbits express V_H- sections more distantly related to man[54]. As we have said earlier, the number of V-gene subgroups varies from species to species and obviously the extent of gene expansion and contraction varies in the different species as well.

7.5.2.1 Restrictions to germ-line expansion

How many genes code for a single basic sequence? If there are more than one, then they must be extremely similar. If this were not so, the well-defined boundaries between the subgroups would disappear. This means that when there are multiple genes for each subgroup they must have been formed by a very recent gene expansion of a single gene. Germ-line theories of antibody diversity require a large number of germ-line genes for each subgroup. The only way that this can be achieved is by massive recent expansion. The difficulties of this type of expansion, which is the basis of modern germ-line theories of antibody diversity[131, 132], are twofold. First it gives rise to a number of identical copies from which the variants, which are essential for the immune system, have to develop by mutation and selection in a relatively short time. The second difficulty arises from the genetic instability of a system containing large numbers of identical genes, as such systems tend to eliminate genes[133-135]. This is well illustrated in frogs where the frequency of occurrence of mutants (3.7%) with diminished numbers of ribosomal genes is remarkably high[136, 137]. This suggests the need for a strong selective pressure to keep a large number of identical, or nearly identical, genes. The important point is that the positive pressure to keep a large number of genes will depend on the immediate usefulness of the genes. In the immune system, multiple copies will have a selective advantage only after they have developed useful variants, while multiple ribosomal genes are required to be identical and have immediate selective advantage by sheer number alone. Some of these difficulties could be simplified if the mutants in the expanded genes were not random but occurred preferentially in hypervariable regions. This will of course, make the development of mutants a more efficient process.

When we discussed the V_H-genes of rabbits we argued that the Mendelian behaviour of their allotypes (a-locus), indicated the presence of a small number of genes. This is indeed the most serious argument against germ-line theories, as one would expect recombinants between the postulated large sets of genes, thus destroying their allelic behaviour. This difficulty can be overcome if lack of recombination in this locus is postulated[29]. This seems to require expansion by a mechanism other than mismatched crossing over. Incidentally, as expansion and contraction is probably the result of mismatched crossover of germ-line genes, other consequences of recombinational events are likely to be found in evolutionary studies of V-genes.

7.5.3 Somatic diversification

The processes involved in duplicating DNA, although extremely accurate, are not free of errors. Consequently, somatic mutation must occur in every individual during development. The importance of these mutants in developing an antigen recognition system is hotly disputed. The extreme view, held in a pure germ-line theory, is that these mutants are of no consequence and should be ignored in the same way as the somatic mutants, which exist in all other structural gene products, are ignored. Most mutants of structural genes will not give a selective advantage to the mutated cell, and their products will be completely masked by the unmutated forms. With the immune system, antigen selects antigen-sensitive cells to proliferate. If mutants occur which can be triggered by antigen, then these mutants will proliferate faster than the unmutated cells. For this reason, one must expect that the proportion of somatic mutants in V-sections will be higher than in other proteins. The number of new mutant forms in a population of cells depends on the mutation rate of the gene in question and on the number of cell divisions. The somatic mutation rate per gene in mammalian cells has not been measured. The difficulty lies in discriminating between mutants which affect the amino acid sequence of the product of a single gene, and mutants in other genes which affect the expression of the gene in question. This difficulty can be partially overcome by using differences in the electrophoretic mobility of a particular protein as a method of detecting mutants in the corresponding gene. This technique has been used to measure the mutation rate for a few enzymes in *Drosophila*, and the highest values are of the order of 10^{-5} mutants per gene cell division[138]. This value is of the same order of magnitude as the mutation rate found in other less-well-defined mammalian systems. Preliminary studies to measure the mutation rate of 'electrophoretic' mutants of immunoglobulin genes in myeloma cells in tissue culture gives a value consistent with 10^{-5}–10^{-6} mutants per gene per cell division[139]. A simple calculation shows that somatic mutation with antigen selection must play a role in increasing antibody diversity. Assume 10^9 lymphocytes divide each day (say 1 % of the total lymphoid cells of an adult man) then 10^3–10^4 mutants will appear for each V-gene. That is at least 10^4–10^5 new V-gene sequences per day, as in man there are at least ten V-genes as defined by V-section subgroups. Even if very few of these mutants affect the combining site, this number of new V-sections cannot be ignored.

7.5.3.1 *Shortcomings of somatic diversification*

Somatic mutation models using the minimum number of germ-line V-genes have no difficulty in explaining the maintenance of diversity seen, for example, in the breaking of tolerance in adult animals. The number of new V-sequences generated each day is a function of three variables: the number of divisions in the relevant population of cells; the mutation rate; the number of V-genes in each cell. The numbers of relevant cell divisions depends on the number of lymphoid cells at any given moment. Consequently, when the population of lymphoid cells is small, for example, in small animals and, in particular, during embryonic development, the rate of formation of new V-sequences will be affected.

Arguments of this type have led to the development of models which do not depend on ordinary somatic mutation alone. For a long time, somatic recombination between the V-genes was favoured by many authors. Some attractive models[140, 141] could be easily tested and repeatedly failed such tests[27, 30]. The evidence shows that if recombination does occur between V-genes of different subgroups, then it occurs very rarely and so far no recombinant forms have been found, even between the very similar κIa and κIb subgroups[142]. Somatic recombination is still held by some authors to be of critical importance in generating diversity[143], but the proposed recombinational events must occur within a set of V-genes all of the same subgroup. It is suggested that the similarity between the genes of such a set is preserved by frequent crossing-over in the germ-line (co-evolution)[28]. This explains the proposed similarity between the genes of one set, but it is not clear how the essential dissimilarities in the hypervariable regions are preserved.

Special somatic selective pressures have been suggested as an alternative way to establish a functional immune system in embryogenesis. Selection of mutants leads to an apparent increase in the rate of somatic mutation. Selective pressures can be used either to encourage division of certain mutants (for example, by antigen, as discussed for the adult animal), or by the progressive elimination of unmutated forms allowing the mutants to accumulate rapidly. In one model it has been suggested that the germ-line genes have evolved to code for antibodies which react with the histocompatibility antigens of the species[116]. During development, all cells expressing V-genes directed against self antigens would at first be driven into proliferation and then eliminated if they still react with self antigens, leaving behind mutants formed during this proliferative phase. The attractive feature of this model is the dependence of V-section diversity on histocompatibility antigens.

A special mechanism to generate diversity in early development may not in fact be necessary and the inevitable normal process of somatic mutation with antigen selection may be sufficient. It is clear that the magnitude of the problem depends on the number of germ-line V-genes and also on the time available to develop a functional system. The problem is further simplified if the mutants are not random, but occur in hot spots which correspond to the hypervariable regions[27, 144]. In general, when the time available is short, there is likely to be evolutionary selection for animals carrying either a large number of V-genes[145], or V-genes with increased mutational frequency in their hypervariable regions, or both.

Models of this type are not entirely free of difficulties. To us, the most serious of these difficulties is how to account for the inheritance of idiotypes. With a pure somatic mutation process, the chance of finding antibody molecules with identical sequence should be very low. Identical idiotypes do not necessarily mean identical sequences, nor do identical isoelectric focusing patterns. As all models require a certain number of germ-line genes, there are bound to be some inheritable identical sequences in germ-line antibodies. One would expect in certain cases a selection for germ-line genes which code for antibodies against common pathogens of the species. This has the double advantage of providing powerful protection against these pathogens, and also early exposure to antigen which further stimulates cell division to increase the accumulation of mutants. In cases where there is strong selective pressure through antigen, monoclonal antibodies may be produced which are very similar, but not identical, to germ-line antibodies. It is possible to imagine very similar or even identical sequences being generated by a few coincidental divergent mutational events of a germ-line gene.

In evolution, there is selection for systems which can readily adapt to changing circumstances. We feel that the generation of antibody diversity is such a system. The final balance of the variables discussed above, at any moment and in each species, will not be the same, and like all evolutionary processes is likely to be in a dynamic equilibrium.

References

1. Hilschmann, N. and Craig, L. C. (1965). *Proc. Nat. Acad. Sci. USA*, **53**, 1403
2. Baglioni, C., Alescio Zonta, L., Cioli, D. and Carbonara, A. (1966). *Science*, **152**, 1519
3. Milstein, C. (1966). *Proc. Roy. Soc. (London)*, B, **166**, 138
4. Ritter, H., Ropartz, C., Rousseau, P. Y., Rivat, L. and Walter, H. (1966). *Blut*, **13**, 373
5. Hunger, H. and Herzog, P. (1965). *Vox. Sang.*, **10**, 635
6. Prokop, O. and Anastosow, B. (1966). *Dtsch. Gesundh. Wes.*, **21**, 1028
7. Oudin, J. (1960). *J. Exp. Med.*, **112**, 125
8. Armerding, D. (1971). *Europ. J. Immunol.*, **1**, 39
9. Mage, R. (1971). *Progress in Immunology*, Vol. 1, 47 (B. Amos, editor) (New York: Academic Press)
10. Ein, D. (1968). *Proc. Nat. Acad. Sci. USA*, **60**, 982
11. Hess, M., Hilschmann, N., Rivat, L., Rivat, C. and Ropartz, C. (1971). *Nature New Biol.*, **234**, 58
12. Gibson, D., Levanon, M. and Smithies, O. (1971). *Biochemistry*, **10**, 3117
13. Schulenberg, E. P., Simms, E. S., Lynch, R. G., Bradshaw, R. A. and Eisen, H. N. (1971). *Proc. Nat. Acad. Sci. USA*, **68**, 2623
14. Appella, E. (1971). *Proc. Nat. Acad. Sci. USA*, **68**, 590
15. Natvig, J. B. and Kunkel, H. G. (1972). *Advan. Immunol.*, in the press.
16. Grubb, R. (1970). *The Genetic Markers of Human Immunoglobulins* (Berlin, Heidelberg, New York: Springer-Verlag)
17. Natvig, J. B., Michaelson, T. E. and Kunkel, H. G. (1971). *J. Exp. Med.*, **133**, 1004
18. Dubiski, S. (1969). *Protides of the Biological Fluids*, **17**, 117
19. Mandy, W. J. and Todd, C. W. (1970). *Biochem. Genet.*, **4**, 59
20. Hanly, W. C., Knight, K. L., Gilman Sachs, A., Dray, S. and Lichter, E. A. (1972). *J. Immunol.*, **108**, 1723
21. Kelus, A. S. and Pernis, B. (1971). *Europ. J. Immunol.*, **1**, 123
22. Potter, M. and Lieberman, R. (1967). *Cold Spring Harbor Symp. Quant. Biol.*, **32**, 187
23. Potter, M. and Lieberman, R. (1967). *Advan. Immunol.*, **7**, 91
24. Herzenberg, L. A., McDevitt, H. O. and Herzenberg, L. A. (1968). *Ann. Rev. of Genetics*, **2**, 209
25. Steinberg, A. G., Muir, W. A. and McIntire, S. A. (1968). *Amer. J. Human Genetics*, **20**, 258
26. Kunkel, H. G., Natvig, J. B. and Joslin, F. G. (1969). *Proc. Nat. Acad. Sci. USA*, **62**, 144
27. Milstein, C. and Munro, A. J. (1970). *Ann. Rev. Microbiology*, **24**, 335
28. Gally, J. A. and Edelman, G. M. (1972). *Ann. Rev. of Genetics*, **6**, 1
29. Smith, G., Hood, L. and Fitch, W. (1971). *Ann. Rev. Biochem.*, **40**, 969
30. Milstein, C. (1967). *Nature (London)*, **216**, 330
31. Niall, H. D. and Edman, P. (1967). *Nature (London)*, **216**, 262
32. Langer, B., Steinmetz-Kayne, M. and Hilschmann, N. (1968). *Hoppe-Seyler's Z. Physiol. Chem.*, **349**, 945
33. Kohler, H., Shimizu, A., Paul, C., Moore, V. and Putnam, F. W. (1970). *Nature (London)*, **227**, 1318
34. Milstein, C. and Pink, R. L. (1970). *Progr. Biophys. Molec. Biol.*, **20**, 209 (J. A. V. Butler and D. Noble, editors) (Oxford: Pergamon)
35. Milstein, C. P. and Deverson, E. V. (1971). *Biochem. J.*, **123**, 945

36. Garver, F. A. and Hilschmann, N. (1971). *FEBS Lett.*, **16**, 128
37. Putnam, F. W., Titani, K., Wikler, M. and Shinoda, T. (1967). *Cold Spring Harbor Symp. Quant. Biol.*, **32**, 90
38. Press, E. M. and Hogg, N. M. (1970). *Biochem. J.*, **117**, 650
39. Wang, A. C., Fudenberg, H. H. and Pink, J. R. L. (1971). *Proc. Nat. Acad. Sci. USA*, **68**, 1143
40. Kaplan, A. P., Hood, L., Terry, W. D. and Mitzger, H. (1971). *Immunochemistry*, **8**, 801
41. Hood, L. E., Potter, M. and McKean, D. J. (1970). *Science*, **170**, 1207
42. Potter, M. (1972). *Physiological Reviews*, **52**, 631
43. Svasti, J. and Milstein, C. (1972). *Biochem. J.*, **128**, 427
44. Appella, E. and Perham, R. N. (1967). *Cold Spring Harbor. Symp. Quant. Biol.*, **32**, 37
45. Weigert, M. G., Cesari, I. M., Yonkovich, S. J. and Cohn, M. (1970). *Nature (London)*, **228**, 1045
46. Cesari, I. M. and Weigert, M. (1973). *Proc. Nat. Acad. Sci. USA*, in the press
47. Hood, L., Eichmann, K., Lackland, H., Krause, R. M. and Ohms, J. J. (1970). *Nature (London)*, **228**, 1040
48. Appella, E., Chersi, A., Roholt, O. A. and Pressman, D. (1971). *Proc. Nat. Acad. Sci. USA*, **68**, 2569
49. Braun, D. G. and Jaton, J. C. (1973). *Immunochemistry*, in the press
50. Secher, D. S., Querinjean, P., Bazin, H. and Milstein, C. (unpublished observation)
51. Kehoe, J. E. and Capra, J. D. (1972). *Proc. Nat. Acad. Sci. USA*, **69**, 2052
52. Milstein, C., Milstein, C. P. and Feinstein, A. (1969). *Nature (London)*, **221**, 151
53. Tischendorf, F. W., Michelitsch, B., Ledderhose, G. and Tischendorf, M. M. (1971). *J. Molec. Biol.*, **61**, 261
54. Mole, L. E., Jackson, S. A., Porter, R. R. and Wilkinson, J. M. (1971). *Biochem. J.*, **124**, 301
55. Fleischman, J. B. (1971). *Biochemistry*, **10**, 2753
56. Kelus, A. S. and Gell, P. G. H. (1967). *Progress in Allergy*, **11**, 141
57. David, G. S. and Todd, C. W. (1969). *Proc. Nat. Acad. Sci. USA*, **62**, 860
58. Vice, J. L., Gilman-Sachs, A., Hunt, W. L. and Dray, S. (1970). *J. Immunol.*, **104**, 550
59. Cunningham, B. A., Gottlieb, P. D., Pflumm, M. N. and Edelman, G. M. (1971). Progress in Immunology, Vol. 1, 3 (B. Amos, editor) (New York: Academic Press)
60. Mage, R. G., Young-Cooper, G. O. and Alexander, C. (1971). *Nature New Biol.*, **230**, 63
61. Kindt, T. J. and Mandy, W. J. (1972). *J. Immunol.*, **108**, 1110
62. Hood, L., Waterfield, M. D., Morris, J. and Todd, C. W. (1971). *Annal. N.Y. Acad. Sci.*, **199**, 26
63. Appella, E., Rejnek, J. and Reisfeld, R. A. (1969), *J. Molec. Biol.*, **41**, 473
64. Lamm, M. E. and Frangione, B. (1972). *Biochem. J.*, **128**, 1357
65. Sher, A. and Cohn, M. (1972). *Europ. J. Immun.*, **2**, 319
66. Blomberg, B., Gekeler, W. R. and Weigert, M. (1972). *Science*, **177**, 178
67. Schiechl, H. and Hilschmann, N. (1971). *Hoppe-Seyler's Z. Physiol. Chem.*, **352**, 111
68. Pink, J. R. L., McNally, M. P., Wang, A. C. and Fudenberg, H. H. (1972). *Immunochemistry*, **9**, 84
69. Todd, C. W. (1963). *Biochem. Biophys. Res. Commun.*, **11**, 170
70. Feinstein, A. (1963). *Nature (London)*, **199**, 1197
71. Pernis, B., Torrigiani, G., Amante, L., Kelus, A. S. and Cebra, J. J. (1968). *Immunology*, **14**, 445
72. Kindt, T. J. and Todd, C. W. (1969). *J. Exp. Med.*, **131**, 343
73. Bennett, C. (1968). *Biochemistry*, **7**, 3340
74. Yount, W. J., Dorner, M., Kunkel, H. G. and Kabat, E. (1968). *J. Exp. Med.*, **127**, 633
75. Anderson, B. R. and Terry, W. D. (1968). *Nature (London)*, **217**, 174
76. Lennox, E. S., Knopf, P. M., Munro, A. J. and Parkhouse, R. M. E. (1967). *Cold Spring Harbor Symp. Quant. Biol.*, **32**, 249
77. Fleischmann, J. B. (1967). *Biochemistry*, **6**, 1319
78. Knopf, P. M., Parkhouse, R. M. E. and Lennox, E. S. (1967). *Proc. Nat. Acad. Sci. USA*, **58**, 2288
79. Smithies, O. (1970). *Science*, **169**, 882

80. Cooper, S. M., Franklin, E. C. and Frangione, B. (1972). *Science*, **176**, 187
81. Frangione, B. and Milstein, C. (1969). *Nature (London)*, **224**, 597
82. Landucci-Tosi, S., Mage, R. G. and Dubiski, S. (1970). *J. Immunol.*, **104**, 641
83. Kindt, T. J., Mandy, W. J. and Todd, C. W. (1970). *Biochemistry*, **9**, 2028
84. Landucci-Tosi, S. (1972). Personal communication
85. Weiler, E. (1965). *Proc. Nat. Acad. Sci. USA*, **54**, 1765
86. Pernis, B. (1967). *Cold Spring Harbor Symp. Quant. Biol.*, **32**, 333
87. Nossal, G. J. V., Szenberg, A., Ada, G. L. and Austin, C. M. (1964). *J. Exp. Med.*, **119**, 485
88. Nisonoff, A., Wilson, S. K., Wang, A. C., Fudenberg, H. H. and Hopper, J. E. (1971). Progress in Immunology, Vol. 1, 61 (B. Amos, editor) (New York: Academic Press)
89. Oudin, J. and Michel, M. (1969). *J. Exp. Med.*, **130**, 619
90. Pernis, B., Forni, L. and Amante, L. (1971). *Annal. N.Y. Acad. Sci.*, **190**, 420
91. Vitetta, E., Bianco, C., Nussenzweig, V. and Uhr, J. W. (1972). *J. Exp. Med.*, **136**, 81
92. Marchalonis, J. J., Cone, R. E. and Atwell, J. L. (1972). *J. Exp. Med.*, **135**, 957
93. Crone, M., Koch, C. and Simonsen, M. (1972). *Transplant. Rev.*, **10**, 35
94. Oudin, J. (1966). *Proc. Roy. Soc. London*, *B*, **166**
95. Kunkel, H. G., Mannik, M. and Williams, R. S. (1963). *Science*, **140**, 1218
96. Eichmann, K. (1972). *Europ. J. Immunol.*, **2**, 301
97. Kuettner, M. G., Wang, A. and Nisonoff, A. (1972). *J. Exp. Med.*, **135**, 579
98. Krause, R. M. (1970). *Advan. Immunol.*, **12**, 1
99. Eichmann, K. and Kindt, T. J. (1971). *J. Exp. Med.*, **134**, 532
100. Eichmann, K., Braun, D. G. and Krause, R. M. (1971). *J. Exp. Med.*, **134**, 48
101. Levine, B. B., Ojeda, A. and Benacerraf, B. (1963). *J. Exp. Med.*, **118**, 953
102. Benacerraf, B. and McDevitt, H. O. (1972). *Science*, **175**, 273
103. McDevitt, H. O. and Benacerraf, B. (1969). *Advan. Immunol.*, **11**, 31
104. Mozes, E. and Shearer, G. M. (1972). Current Topics in Microbiology and Immunology, Vol. 59, in the press. (Berlin: Springer-Verlag)
105. McDevitt, H. O. and Chinitz, A. (1969). *Science*, **163**, 1207
106. Ellman, L., Green, I., Martin, W. J. and Benacerraf, B. (1970). *Proc. Nat. Acad. Sci. USA*, **66**, 322
107. McDevitt, H. O., Deak, B. D., Shreffler, D. C., Klein, J., Stimpfling, J. H. and Snell, G. D. (1972). *J. Exp. Med.*, **135**, 1259
108. Lieberman, R., Paul, W. E., Humphrey, W. and Stimpfling, J. H. (1972). *J. Exp. Med.*, **136**, 1231
109. McDevitt, H. O. and Sela, M. (1965). *J. Exp. Med.*, **122**, 517
110. McDevitt, H. O., Bechtol, K. B., Grumet, F. C., Mitchell, G. F. and Weymann, T. G. (1971). Progress in Immunology, Vol. 1, 495 (B. Amos, editor) (New York: Academic Press)
111. McDevitt, H. O. (1968). *J. Immunol.*, **100**, 485
112. Green, I., Paul, W. E. and Benacerraf, B. (1966). *J. Exp. Med.*, **123**, 859
113. Ordal, J. C. and Grumet, F. C. (1972). *J. Exp. Med.*, **136**, 1195
114. Levin, H. A., Levine, H. and Schlosman, S. F. (1971). *J. Exp. Med.*, **133**, 1199
115. Shevach, E. M., Paul, W. E. and Green, I. (1972). *J. Exp. Med.*, **136**, 1207
116. Jerne, N. K. (1971). *Europ. J. Immunol.*, **1**, 1
117. Jaton, J. C. and Sela, M. (1968). *J. Biol. Chem.*, **243**, 5616
118. Mozes, E., McDevitt, H. O., Jaton, J. C. and Sela, M. (1969a). *J. Exp. Med.*, **130**, 493
119. Gasser, D. L. (1969). *J. Immunol.*, **103**, 66
120. Biozzi, G., Stiffel, C., Monton, D., Bouthillier, Y. and Decreusefond, C. (1971) Progress in Immunology, Vol. 1, 529 (B. Amos, editor) (New York: Academic Press)
121. Landsteiner, K. (1936). *The Specificity of Serological Reactions*. (Springfield, Ill.: Thomas, C. C.)
122. Eisen, H. N. (1971). Progress in Immunology, Vol 1, 243. (B. Amos, editor) (New York: Academic Press)
123. Askonas, B. A., Williamson, A. R. and Wright, B. E. G. (1970). *Proc. Nat. Acad. Sci. USA*, **67**, 1398
124. Kreith, H. W. and Williamson, A. R. (1973). *Europ. J. Immunol.*, **3**, 141
125. Pernis, B. (1967). *Cold Spring Harbor Symp. Quant. Biol.*, **32**, 333
126. Hill, R. L., Lebovitz, H. E., Fellows, R. E. and Delaney, R. (1967). Nobel Symposium on γ-Gobulins, p. 109 (J. Killander, editor) (Stockholm: Almqvist and Wiksell)

127. Singer, S. J. and Doolittle, R. F. (1966). *Science*, **153**, 13
128. Ohno, S. (1970). Evolution by Gene Duplication (Berlin: Springer-Verlag)
129. Dreyer, W. J., Gray, W. R. and Hood, L. (1967). *Cold Spring Harbor Symp. Quant. Biol.*, **32**, 353
130. Zuckerkandl, E. and Pauling, L. (1965). Evolving Genes and Proteins, p. 97 (V. Bryson and H. J. Vogel, editors) (New York: Academic Press)
131. Hood, L. and Talmage, D. W. (1970). *Science*, **168**, 325
132. Hood, L. and Prahl, J. (1971). *Advan. Immunol.*, **14**, 291
133. Ritossa, F. M. and Spiegelman, S. (1965). *Proc. Nat. Acad. Sci. USA*, **53**, 737
134. Britten, R. J. and Kohne, D. E. (1968). *Science*, **161**, 529
135. Walker, P. M. B. (1968). *Nature (London)*, **219**, 228
136. Miller, L. and Gurdon, J. B. (1970). *Nature (London)*, **227**, 1108
137. Miller, L. and Knowland, J. (1970). *J. Molec. Biol.*, **53**, 329
138. Tobari, Y. N. and Kojima, K. (1972). *Genetics*, **70**, 397
139. Cotton, R. G. H., Secher, D. S., Milstein, C. (1973). *Europ. J. Immunol.*, **3**, 135
140. Smithies, O. (1969). *Cold Spring Harbor Symp. Quant. Biol.*, **32**, 161
141. Crick, F. H. C. (1967). *Cold Spring Harbor Symp. Quant. Biol.*, **32**, 169
142. Milstein, C. P. (1973). *FEBS Lett.*, **30**, 40
143. Edelman, G. M. and Gally, J. A. (1967). *Proc. Nat. Acad. Sci. USA*, **57**, 353
144. Mäkelä, O. and Cross, A. M. (1970). *Progr. Allergy*, **14**, 145
145. Burnet, F. M. (1967). *Cold Spring Harbor Symp. Quant. Biol.*, **32**, 1
146. World Health Organisation (1965). *Bull. W.H.O.*, **33**, 721
147. Lieberman, R. and Humphrey, W. (1972). *J. Exp. Med.*, **136**, 1222
148. Milstein, C., Milstein, C. P. and Jarvis, J. M. (1969). *J. Molec. Biol.*, **46**, 599
149. Cunningham, B. A., Gottlieb, P. D., Konigsberg, W. H. and Edelman, G. M. (1968). *Biochemistry*, **7**, 1983
150. Köhler, H., Shimizu, A., Paul, C. and Putnam, F. W. (1970). *Science*, **169**, 56
151. Watanabe, S. and Hilschmann, N. (1970). *Hoppe-Seyler's Z. Physiol. Chem.*, **351**, 1291
152. Braun, M., Leibold, W., Barnikol, H. U. and Hilschmann, N. (1972). *Hoppe-Seyler's Z. Physiol. Chem.*, **353**, 1284
153. Eulitz, M., Gotze, D. and Hilschmann, N. (1972). *Hoppe-Seyler's Z. Physiol. Chem.*, **353**, 487
154. Edelman, G. M., Cunningham, B. A., Gall, E. W., Gottlieb, P. D., Rutishauser, U. and Waxdal, M. (1969). *Proc. Nat. Acad. Sci. USA*, **63**, 71
155. *Atlas of Protein Sequence and Structure* (1972). Vol. 5 (M. O. Dayhoff, editor) (Silver Spring: The National Biomedical Research Foundation)
156. Novotný, S., Dolejš, L. and Franěk, F. (1972). *Europ. J. Biochem.*, **31**, 277

8
Biosynthesis of Immunoglobulins

A. R. WILLIAMSON
National Institute for Medicine Research, London

8.1 INTRODUCTION

An eventual understanding of immune responses in molecular terms is the main motive behind studies on immunoglobulin biosynthesis. For several years, such studies drew on precedents and advances in the understanding of protein biosynthesis in other eukaryotic systems. Increasingly, however, biosynthetic studies of immunoglobulins are providing new clues about controls which may prove to be operative in gene expression in other differentiated cell systems. Despite the complexities of immune responses, antibody formation may prove to be one of the better systems for probing the molecular mysteries of differentiation.

8.2 SYNTHESIS OF THE LIGHT AND HEAVY POLYPEPTIDE CHAINS

8.2.1 Introduction

The light and heavy chains of immunoglobulins each appear to be controlled by two structural genes. As discussed in Chapter 7, this necessitates the integration of the information from these two genes. Study of the biosynthesis of light (L) and heavy (H) chains was initially motivated by the need to discover at which stage integration occurs; this could be at the level of DNA, messenger RNA or intermediate polypeptide fragments. The evidence discussed in this section clearly places integration at the DNA level.

Three types of systems have been studied. (a) Plasma cell tumours (myeloma tumours) of both human and murine origin. Each tumour represents the expansion of a single clone of plasma cells and the characteristic secreted immunoglobulin product may be of any class or subclass. In mice a large number of transplantable myeloma lines have been established[1], these cell lines can also be maintained in tissue culture. (b) Human lymphoid cell lines[2,3]. These lines are established in tissue culture from the peripheral blood or bone marrow of patients or subjects and can be maintained over long periods of time. These cell lines secrete immunoglobulin, in the absence of deliberate antigenic stimulus. The rate of secretion is variable between cell lines and is always much lower than for myeloma cells. (c) Immune lymphoid tissue. This can be obtained from many experimental animals, usually after hyperimmunisation. A heterogenous population of cells is obtained producing a diverse range of immunoglobulin molecules.

Despite various imaginative hypothetical schemes[4,5] for the generation of antibody diversity during transcription or translation of L and H chains there is no evidence that diversity arises at these steps. Fidelity is maintained in the flow of information from gene to polypeptide. The systems developed for the study of immunoglobulin synthesis provide valuable tools for gaining an understanding of transcriptional and translational control in eukaryotic cells.

Three lines of evidence show that integration of V and C gene information must take place at the level of the gene. Firstly, each L and H chain is synthesised as a single polypeptide chain with a single N-terminal initiation point (Section 8.2.2). Secondly, L and H chains are made on separate polyribosome structures the respective sizes of which are compatible with the translation of complete L and H chain messenger-RNA molecules (Section 8.2.3). Lastly, large molecular weight mRNA molecules have been isolated and translated *in vitro* into complete L and complete H chains (Section 8.2.4).

8.2.2 A single initiation point for translation of each chain

Polypeptide chains are synthesised sequentially from amino-terminus to carboxy-terminus. A systematic demonstration of this point is afforded by the experimental design of Naughton and Dintzis[6]. The approach involves brief pulse labelling of the polypeptides using radioactive amino acids. Newly completed chains are found to be more highly labelled in their C-terminal peptides with a gradient of specific activity declining towards the N-terminus. This experiment was performed with immunoglobulin synthesising cells in order to ascertain whether complete L and H chains are translated from one initiation point or whether each L and H chain is assembled by covalent linkage of two independently-synthesised polypeptide chains.

H Chain synthesis has been studied in both rabbit immune lymphoid tissue[7,8] and in mouse myeloma cells[9]. For the H chain a partial answer could be obtained by using papain cleavage of labelled immunoglobulin molecules. In this way Fleischman[7] showed that the Fc and Fab portions of rabbit IgG were not synthesised separately. Using a mouse myeloma Knopf, Parkhouse and Lennox[9] separated Fc and Fd fragments of pulse labelled H chains and found that their specific activities agreed with predictions made for the sequential synthesis of complete H chains. They could not fit their data to a model in which H chains were assembled from constant sized pools of variable or constant sequences. In a study of the specific activity of the peptides obtained by cyanogen bromide cleavage of pulse-labelled rabbit H chains, Fleishman[8] showed a gradient of labelling from C-terminus to N-terminus in agreement with the single N-terminal initiation point model.

For light-chain synthesis a mouse myeloma cell line secreting only L chains was the ideal system[10]. The specific activity of tryptic peptides of pulse-labelled L chain could be arranged in sequence giving a good fit with the single initiation point model.

While none of the evidence above is easily interpreted on any model other than the sequential synthesis of complete L and H chains, it is not, of itself, conclusive. However, in extensive biosynthetic studies no unequivocal evidence has been found for the hypothetical variable and constant polypeptide chains. The occurrence of variable fragments of L chain in human urine has been shown to be due to catabolism[11]. There is a single report[12] claiming the detection of a rapidly turning over pool of a polypeptide chain corresponding to the variable region of a mouse lyeloma L chain. Discrepancies in this report have been discussed elsewhere[13]. In the absence of further data or independent verification, this claim must be set aside.

8.2.3 Polyribosomes synthesising individual L and H chains

There is no genetic linkage between the structural genes for L and H chains (see Chapter 7). Consequently, one would expect to find separate classes of polyribosomes synthesising L and H chains. If monocistronic messengers are involved, as is the rule in eukaryotic cells, then the maximum size of the polyribosomes is interpretable in terms of the functional length of the L and H chain mRNA molecules. The actual length of the mRNA is greater than the translated length (see Figure 8.2, Section 8.2.4).

The independent synthesis of light and heavy chains on different-size classes of polyribosomes has been demonstrated in immune lymphoid tissue[14-18] and myeloma cells[12, 19-24]. Identification of the specific polyribosomes was performed either by acrylamide gel electrophoresis of the nascent chains[12, 20, 22, 23] or by the use of antisera specific for L or H chains[12, 17, 19, 21-24].

The concensus of the various studies is that L chain synthesis occurs on polyribosomes sedimenting not greater than *ca.* 200 S while H chains are made on larger polyribosomes sedimenting up to *ca.* 300 S. The number of ribosomes per polyribosome can be estimated from the sedimentation coefficient but the best estimate comes from direct counting in the electron microscope. De Petris[25] examined polyribosomes of mouse myeloma tumour 5563, taking from a sucrose gradient the most rapidly sedimenting fractions previously shown with specific antisera to be synthesising H and L chains[19, 21]. L-Chain-synthesising polyribosomes contained four–five ribosomes while H-chain polyribosomes contained 11–18 ribosomes; these counts were in agreement with the calculations based on sedimentation rate[21]. The number of ribosomes simultaneously translating the H-chain mRNA agrees well with the 16 ribosomes (as illustrated in Figure 8.1) expected by analogy with globin-synthesising polyribosomes. L-Chain mRNA would be expected to carry seven ribosomes at maximal loading (Figure 8.1). The lower number found experimentally could be due to technical difficulty in defining the upper size limit of L-chain-synthesising polyribosomes; it is also possible that the number of ribosomes translating L-chain mRNA might be less than the expected maximum.

L- and H-chain synthesising polyribosomes are located on the membrane of the endoplasmic reticulum (shown schematically in Figure 8.1). Immunoglobulin-secreting cells usually have an extensive net-work of rough endoplasmic reticulum such as is seen in other secretory cells. Free and membrane-bound ribosomes are separable by discontinuous sucrose density gradient centrifugation. The nascent chains can then be separated either with their t-RNA still attached[26] or by release with [³H]puromycin[27]; in either case this circumvents the problem of contaminating completed immunoglobulin in the subsequent immunological characterisation of the nascent chains.

Using these methods nascent L and H chains are found only on membrane-bound ribosomes. As discussed in later sections, the membrane-bound character of L- and H-chain synthesising polyribosomes predetermines the

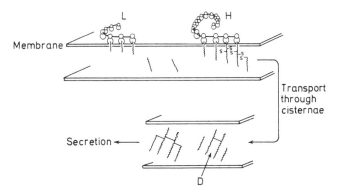

Figure 8.1 Biosynthesis and assembly of immunoglobulin G. The separate polyribosomes synthesising L and H chains are located on the endoplasmic reticulum. Nascent chains grow vectorially and are released into the cisternae where assembly of four-chain molecules is completed. D, dimer of H chains which is an intermediate in assembly of many immunoglobulins (see Table 8.1). (From Williamson[124], by courtesy of Academic Press)

post-synthetic processing (Section 8.5.2), addition of carbohydrate (Section 8.5.3) and ultimate secretion (Section 8.5.4) of completed immunoglobulin molecules.

8.2.4   Messenger RNA for L and H chains

The isolation of separate mRNA molecules coding for complete L chains and complete H chains provides the best evidence for the integrated transcription of the respective V and C gene pairs. The calculated sizes for mRNA molecules coding for complete L and H chains are shown in Figure 8.2. These theoretical sizes are shown superimposed on the best current estimate for the actual size of the L and H chain RNA molecules. In the cytoplasm both L and H chain messages contain additional nucleotide sequences. These additional sequences include a stretch of poly(A)-rich sequence located at the 3′ end of the message. These findings are consistent with present knowledge of mammalian mRNA, based mainly on the properties of mRNA coding for globin chains.

Various expected properties of L- and H-chain mRNA molecules have been used to effect separation of messenger activity from bulk RNA. Messenger activity is assayed in heterologous protein-synthesising systems. The first demonstration of biologically-active L-chain mRNA was made by Stavnezer and Huang[28] using an RNA fraction obtained only on the basis of size. Starting from the total RNA of a κ-chain-producing mouse myeloma tumour (MOPC 41) these investigators took a 9–13 S fraction of RNA and assayed its messenger activity in a cell-free system prepared from rabbit reticulocytes. Newly synthesised L chain was identified by immunoprecipitation and peptide analysis. A similar fraction of RNA (10–12 S) isolated from a mouse myeloma (MOPC 21) producing an $IgG_1\kappa$ has been shown to direct the synthesis of L chains in a cell-free system derived from Krebs II ascites tumour cells[29].

Swan, Aviv and Leder[30] achieved a partial purification of L chain mRNA by first isolating membrane-bound polyribosomes and then fractionating the extracted polyribosomal RNA by chromatography on an oligo(dT)cellulose column. The fraction of RNA containing poly(A)-rich sequences showed L-chain mRNA activity in the ascites tumour cell-free system. Sucrose density-gradient analysis of this messenger RNA fraction showed two peaks of

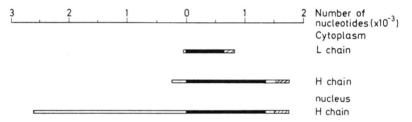

Figure 8.2 Coding length and experimentally determined length of L- and H-chain mRNA molecules. ▆▆▆, predicted coding length; ▭, additional nucleotide sequences based on current best estimate of molecular weights[30, 32, 35]; ▨▨, poly(A)-rich sequence

messenger activity; both the major peak at 13 S and the minor peak at 19 S when added to the cell-free system, stimulated synthesis of L chains. In this study and in the study of MOPC 21 L-chain mRNA it appears that the initial translation product of the mRNA is a precursor of L chain which is slightly longer than native L chain. This precursor is discussed further in Section 8.5.2. The major L-chain mRNA fraction ($S_{20,w}$,13) is estimated to contain *ca.* 850 nucleotides[30]. This is 200 nucleotides longer than is required to code for the complete L chain. A small part of this additional sequence is apparently translated to give the precursor L chain; for the MOPC 21 L-chain mRNA this would place an extra sequence of at least 45 nucleotides at the 5' end of the messenger RNA. The majority of extra sequence is accounted for by poly(A)-rich sequences which appear to be characteristic of most eukaryotic mRNA molecules. The presence of poly(A)-rich sequences on both L- and H-chain mRNA molecules has been shown by the isolation of A-rich RNA from mouse myeloma 5563 cells using chromatography on a poly-U Geon 425 column[31]. The isolated RNA fractions were assayed for messenger activity by micro-injection into *Xenopus laevis* eggs or oocytes. Both L- and H-chain synthesis is obtained using the poly(A)-rich containing RNA from either the cytoplasm or the nucleus of the myeloma cells. The poly(A)-rich sequence present in these preparations appeared to average *ca.* 150–200 nucleotides in length.

H-Chain mRNA has been obtained in greater than 90% purity from mouse myeloma 5563 cells. For this isolation, Stevens and Williamson[32] made use of the specific affinity of 5563 myeloma protein (H_2L_2) for H-chain mRNA from 5563 cells. This affinity has been demonstrated in the course of studies on the translational control of immunoglobulin production[33, 34]. It has been postulated that the intracellular pool of H_2L_2 molecules controls H chain production by a feed-back mechanism in which the crucial step is an interaction between H_2L_2 molecules and H-chain mRNA (see Section 8.7.2). This weak interaction can apparently be stabilised by adding antibody specific for H_2L_2. H-Chain mRNA is then precipitated together with the H_2L_2–anti H_2L_2 complex. When the RNA recovered from this precipitate is translated in *Xenopus laevis* oocytes, it produces H chains without any detectable L chains being made. The absence of L-chain synthesis provides a good criterion for the purity of H-chain mRNA and the specificity of the isolation procedure. Using this method, H-chain mRNA is isolated from the cytoplasm of 5563 cells in two forms, one with terminal poly(A)-rich sequence and one with little or no terminal poly(A)-rich sequence; it is possible that the loss of poly(A) occurs during phenol extraction. The H-chain mRNA appears to be *ca.* 2000 nucleotides long which gives an excess of 650 nucleotides over the necessary coding length for H chain (Figure 8.2). H-chain mRNA isolated from the nucleus of 5563 cells is contained in a polynucleotide at least 4300 nucleotides long containing a poly(A)-rich sequence of 150–200 nucleotides. Kinetic experiments show that this large nuclear form of the mRNA is, in fact, a precursor of the cytoplasmic H-chain mRNA[35]. This is consistent with evidence from other eukaryotic cells suggesting that large heterogeneous nuclear RNA is the precursor to cytoplasmic mRNA. The processing of this mRNA precursor has been followed for the SV_{40} RNA transcript[36] but the H-chain mRNA provides the first case where a defined message can be isolated from both the nucleus and cytoplasm and the interconversion demonstrated.

A promising route for the specific isolation of pure L-chain mRNA is the use of immuno-precipitation of the polyribosomes synthesising the L chain[37]. Antibodies against L chain will interact with the nascent chains thus precipitating the polyribosomes. This method had been used analytically (see Section 8.2.3) but has to be refined to be used preparatively. The use of purified $F(ab')_2$ fragments of an IgG fraction of anti-L-chain antiserum yields a polyribosome precipitate from which undegraded RNA can be extracted. This method has yielded a messenger-like RNA for L chain of MOPC 149. This RNA is 11–12 S but has not yet been tested for messenger activity[37].

8.3 SYNTHESIS OF J CHAIN AND SECRETORY COMPONENT

8.3.1 Introduction

In addition to L and H chains two other polypeptides are found in certain immunoglobulins. These additional polypeptides are J chain and secretory component. J chain is found only on polymeric forms of IgA and on IgM.

There is only one J chain per polymeric molecule whether that molecule is a dimeric IgA or a pentameric IgM. Monomeric immunoglobulins including the monomeric form of IgA in serum lack J chain[38, 39].

Secretory component is found on IgA dimers present in external secretions (colostrum, milk, saliva, gastric juices) but not on IgA in serum or on other immunoglobulins which have been found in external secretions[40].

8.3.2 J chain

J Chains are synthesised by the same plasma cells producing the L and H chains of the immunoglobulin and appear to be added to the polymers just prior to their secretion. This was established by Parkhouse[41] for two IgM secreting murine plasma cell tumours (MOPC 104E and TEPC 183) and for IgA secreting tumour (MOPC 315). The cells were incubated with radioactive amino acids for 4 h and labelled J chain was found to be present in secreted IgM or in the dimeric IgA The proportion of label in J chain suggested the presence of one uniformly labelled J chain per polymeric molecule. Monomeric IgA secreted by the MOPC 315 cells did not contain labelled J chain. It has also been shown by Halpern and Coffman[42] that, in four other IgA secreting murine plasmacytoma cell lines, J chain is present only on secreted polymeric IgA and not on either intracellular or secreted monomeric IgA. Since intracellular IgA or IgM are almost entirely in the monomeric form, it appears that J chain is added to the secreted immunoglobulin at the time of polymerisation. One chain line (S 117) secreted only monomeric IgA and this contained no J chain.

Free J chain has not been demonstrated either intracellularly or secreted by any cell line. It would, however, be difficult to detect free J chain without specific anti-serum which has yet to be used. The role of J chain is still unclear. A possible involvement of J chain in polymerisation is discussed in Section 8.4.3.

8.3.3 Secretory component

Each dimeric molecule of secretory IgA contains a covalently linked secretory component. This component may consist of two identical polypeptide chains each having a mol. wt. of *ca.* 25 000 (see Chapter 6). The absence of secretory component from serum IgA dimers suggests a role for the component in the actual secretion process. This putative role must be specific for IgA since IgG and IgM are also found in external secretions but do not contain secretory component.

The subject of secretory IgA has been recently reviewed in detail[40]. A definitive picture of the biosynthetic processes is lacking but the best model available for testing is shown in Figure 8.3. Secretory component does not appear to be made in the same cells which are making IgA for secretion. Certainly none of the IgA synthesising myeloma cell lines produce secretory component. The site of synthesis of secretory component is most probably epithelial cells of the secretory organ. IgA destined for secretion is thought to be made by plasma cells local to the secretory organ and to be compart-mentalised from serum IgA. This latter point is still not definitely proven.

The most likely site for the assembly of secretory component with IgA dimers is inside the epithelial cells synthesising secretory component. Dimeric IgA could enter the epithelial cell by pinocytosis at the internal face of the plasma membrane and acquire secretory component by fusion of IgA containing vesicles with those containing newly-synthesised secretory component. The completed molecule would then be secreted at the external face of the plasma membrane. (Figure 8.3).

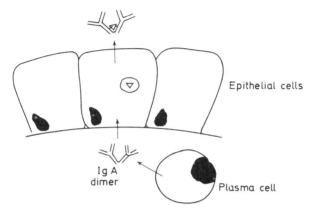

Figure 8.3 Possible model for the synthesis of IgA and secretory component, their assembly and external secretion. IgA dimers are probably made in plasma cells in the secretory organ. Secretory component ($\triangledown$) is probably made in epithelial cells[40, 43]

Ideas which have been advanced to explain the need for secretory com-ponent include the attraction of secretory IgA on the cells synthesising that IgA to the local secretory organs, the facilitation of secretion of IgA via the epithelium and the stabilisation of secreted IgA in the relatively-hostile external milieu.

8.4 ASSEMBLY OF COMPLETE IMMUNOGLOBULIN MOLECULES

8.4.1 Introduction

To function effectively as antibodies immunoglobulins have evolved as multichain proteins with two or a multiple of two combining sites. Each site is defined by the amino acid sequence of both a V_L and a V_H region thus enhancing the available diversity of antibodies. The evolution of the immuno-globulins has thus necessitated that the L and H chains interact to form a stable protomer which must also form a stable four chain H_2L_2 molecule. The protomer is formed by virtue of non-covalent interactions between the

C_L region and the constant region of the F_d half of H chain. Two protomers interact non-covalently via the F_c regions of the two H chains. In most immunoglobulins the structure is stabilised by interchain disulphide bonds. The following two sections deal with the order of interchain disulphide bond formation (Section 8.4.2.1) during biosynthetic assembly of various immunoglobulins. For IgA and IgM polymerisation or superassembly of four chain molecules can take place. Biosynthetic polymerisation (Section 8.4.3) involves weak non-covalent interactions between the H_2L_2 monomers; the molecule is held intact by disulphide bonds.

8.4.2 Four-chain molecules

The most readily demonstrable intermediate in the assembly of four-chain H_2L_2 molecules is free L chain[44]. Newly completed L chains are released from polyribosomes into an intracisternal pool of free L chains. These free L chains can be shown by kinetic and pulse-chase experiments to be in precursor-product relationship with completed H_2L_2 molecules[45]. An intracellular pool of free L chains is common to all immunoglobulin-synthesising cells so far examined. Usually the pool is maintained at a constant size by turnover of L chains. However, in cases of unbalanced L and H chain production (see Section 8.7) there may be secretion of excess L chains. It can be shown that even in such cells new L chains mix with the large L-chain pool which serves as a source of L-chains for H_2L_2 assembly[46].

Only small amounts of free H chains are present in any of the plasma cells so far examined. Free H chain does not appear to be a major intermediate in assembly of H_2L_2.

8.4.2.1 Inter-chain disulphide bond formation

The basic rule for the formation of any disulphide bond either within or between polypeptide chains is that the appropriate cysteine sulphydryl groups are brought together by the folding of the polypeptide chain or chains into a stable conformation. The newly-synthesised polypeptide chain rapidly assumes its most stable conformation; where possible this may precede chain completion. Consequently, we can assume the formation of intrachain disulphide bonds prior to the assembly of H and L chains into H_2L_2 molecules.

A quaternary structure stabilised by non-covalent interactions should be formed between H and L chains or H and H chains prior to covalent linkage by inter-chain disulphide bonds. Experimentally it is easier to identify covalently linked intermediates in assembly of multichain proteins than to identify non-covalently linked intermediates. Polyacrylamide gel electrophoretic analysis of intracellular pulse-labelled immunoglobulin polypeptides is performed in the presence of sodium dodecyl sulphate which dissociates non-covalent interactions between subunits. This analysis is performed after various short times of pulse labelling and the relative amounts of the three possible covalent intermediates H_2, H_2L and HL are determined.

The major intermediates found for a range of immunoglobulin classes in several species are shown in Table 8.1. The pattern of intermediates is determined by the order of formation of the two types of disulphide bond, either between H chains or between H and L chains. The last column in Table 8.1 shows the products of mild reduction of the various immuno-globulins; these products reflect the differential lability of the two types of disulphide bonds. In general, it can be seen that the disulphide bond most stable to reduction is the first one to form biosynthetically. The formation of interchain disulphide bonds will depend on the reducing conditions of the intracellular environment. That the more stable disulphide bond forms first, suggests that reducing conditions at the site of assembly are sufficient to

Table 8.1 Major pathways of interchain disulphide bond formation

Immunoglobulin		Covalent intermediates in biosynthesis			Products of mild reduction*
Species	Class	H_2L	H_2	HL	
Mouse	IgG_1	+	+		N.D.
Mouse	IgG_{2a}	+	+		H_2,L
Mouse	IgG_{2b}	+	+	+	N.D.
Mouse	IgA		+		H_2,L
Mouse	IgM			+	H_2L_2,HL
Rabbit	IgG			+	HL
Human	IgG	+	+		H_2L,H_2,HL
Human	IgM			+	N.D.
Human	IgA_2		+		H_2,L

Biosynthetic intermediates and products of reduction with 10^{-2} M 2-mercaptoethanol or 5×10^{-4} M dithioery-throtol were separated and identified by polyacrylamide gel electrophoresis in the presence of sodium dodecyl sulphate. Table compiled from data previously reviewed[13] with the addition of more recent data on the reduction of human IgG[47].
*N.D. = no determination.

prevent oxidation of the more labile cysteine pair. Absolute reducing con-ditions within the microsomes are not known but the high sulphydryl require-ment for protein synthesis *in vitro* suggests that similar reducing conditions prevail *in vivo* in the local ribosomal environment. The sequential formation of disulphide bonds may be due to the migration of the non-covalently assembled molecule from the site of synthesis to a less reducing environment.

For mouse IgG_{2b} there is a random order of interchain disulphide bond formation[48] which could be due either to the fact that the stabilities of the two types of disulphide bond are similar or to the fact that the conditions required to reduce either type of bond are sufficiently distant from the microsomal redox conditions.

Mouse IgA and human IgA_2 exist in serum as H_2, L_2 with no L–H disulphide bonds but with a disulphide linked L chain dimer. For two murine IgA myeloma proteins (MOPC 315 and 5647)[49,50] it has been shown that intra-cellular and freshly-secreted protein is in the form of L, H_2, L. Monomeric L chains are bound non-covalently to H_2 and the dimerisation of these L chains is a slow process occurring after secretion[49].

8.4.2.2 Non-covalent chain interactions

The order of initial non-covalent interaction between the four polypeptide chains cannot be assumed to be indicated by the order of covalent linkage of the chains since the latter depends on the independent parameters discussed above. It is difficult to define the order of non-covalent assembly because any method used to examine the system may perturb the equilibrium. A probable pathway of non-covalent assembly which may hold generally for immunoglobulin biosynthesis has been put forward on the basis of the physical properties of free H chains[13]. Native H chains isolated from either rabbit[51] or human[52, 53] IgG exist at neutral pH as dimers. These dimers are stabilised by non-covalent interactions between both F_d and F_c regions but there exists an equilibrium as shown in Figure 8.4a with a tendency to form

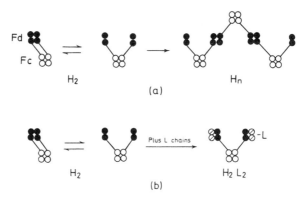

Figure 8.4 (a) The association equilibria of isolated heavy chains under neutral conditions *in vitro*. H chains exist as dimers (H_2) and polymer (H_n). Dimers non-covalently linked via Fd and Fc regions are in equilibrium with dimers only linked via the Fc regions; the latter conformation tends to give rise to polymers. Scheme redrawn from Björk and Tanford[51], by courtesy of *Biochemistry*. (b) Proposed non-covalent assembly of heavy and light chains *in vivo*. Newly completed heavy chains dimerise via both Fd and Fc regions. Association could be initiated through Fd regions, prior to completion of translation of the Fc regions. Light chains will interact with the form of H_2 involving only Fc regions, thus shifting the equilibrium in that direction. In the presence of a pool of light chains assembly of non-covalently linked four chain structures would be a rapid process. (From Bevan *et al.*[13], by courtesy of Pergamon Press)

polymers through F_d interactions. This suggests the biosynthetic assembly pathway shown in Figure 8.4b. It is envisaged that newly-completed H chains exist as dimers; this dimerisation could be initiated between F_d regions of nascent H chains prior to completion of F_c regions. The completed dimer would exist in two forms and L chains would interact with that form held only through F_c interactions, thus shifting the equilibrium in that direction. Comparison with Table 8.1 shows that with this model for human IgG the order of non-covalent and covalent assembly agree. On the other hand, for rabbit IgG the order of non-covalent assembly should be the opposite of the order of disulphide bond formation to comply with the physical properties of rabbit H chains.

8.4.3 Polymeric immunoglobulins

For IgM and IgA the assembly process is not necessarily complete at the four-chain stage. IgM is normally found in mammalian sera as a 19 S covalently-linked pentamer of the basic H_2L_2 structure. IgA is found mainly as monomers and dimers with lesser amounts of higher polymers. In both bases the polymeric forms contain disulphide linked J chain. Within IgM and IgA secreting cells the immunoglobulin is found predominantly if not exclusively as H_2L_2 (i.e. IgMs or IgA monomers).

In both murine[46,54] and human cells[55] IgMs has been shown to be the precursor for polymer formation. Multimeric forms of IgM were not found inside murine IgM-secreting cells and only trace amounts of IgMs are detectable in the secreted IgM. Thus it was suggested than an efficient polymerisation of IgMs occurs at, or just prior to, the time of secretion[54]. Intracellular 19 S IgM has been detected in the bone marrow cells of patients with Waldenstrom's macroglobulinaemia showing that in some cases polymerisation may precede secretion[55].

IgA does not polymerise to a uniform extent. The degree of polymerisation varies from one myeloma tumour to another, but is a characteristic, stable property of a given myeloma[56,57]. In all cases the monomeric form of IgA predominates intracellularly[49,50,57] although in certain tumours small amounts of oligomer have been found inside the cell[42].

The control of the polymerisation process is not yet understood. Non-covalent interactions between IgMs subunits are weak but should govern the formation of the disulphide bonds which maintain the integrity of the pentamer under physiological conditions. Since J chain is only found on polymeric molecules it is tempting to invoke a role for J chain in polymerisation. Such a role is yet to be proven. The stoichiometry of one J chain per 19 S IgM does not permit any symmetrical model for the binding of J chain. One possible model is to have J chain initiate polymerisation by combining with a single subunit. The intracellular IgMs subunits do not exhibit a free sulphydryl in the position required for polymerisation and this is probably due to mixed disulphide formation with a low molecular weight sulphydryl compound. Removal of this block might control polymerisation and this unblocking step could involve J chain and/or the enzyme-catalysing disulphide interchange[58].

8.5 POST-TRANSLATIONAL MODIFICATIONS AND SECRETION

8.5.1 Introduction

Completely-assembled immunoglobulin molecules are either secreted from the cell or incorporated into the plasma membrane. This externalisation is predestined by the site of synthesis of immunoglobulin on membrane-bound polyribosomes. The secretion of immunoglobulin from the cell is dealt with in Section 8.5.4. Prior to leaving the cell the newly-synthesised immunoglobulin chains undergo various modification. There is evidence for the synthesis of L chains in a precursor form which is several amino acids longer at the N-terminus than L chains found in serum immunoglobulin (Section 8.5.2). The precursor form of L chain has raised an interesting suggestion for a mechanism to determine the secretory fate of immunoglobulin (Section 8.5.4.)

All immunoglobulins are glycoproteins. This they share in common with most other secretory proteins and carbohydrate addition has been suggested, without proof, to be an obligatory step in secretion[59]. Oligosaccharides are added to the polypeptide chain by membrane-bound glycosyl transferases (Section 8.5.3) to which immunoglobulin is necessarily exposed *en route* to secretion via the Golgi apparatus.

8.5.2 Post-translational alteration of amino acid sequence

An intracellular precursor form of assembled IgG has been shown by isoelectric focusing analysis of pulse-labelled murine myeloma (5563) cells. This precursor molecule has two more basic groups (approximate pK_a 7.5) than the serum myeloma protein[60]. These groups appear to be lost sequentially (Figure 8.5a). Both H and L chains of this protein have pyrrolidone carboxylic acid (PCA) N-terminii and it was speculated that the extra basic charges could be due to N-terminal amino groups prior to formation of PCA. PCA probably arises by cyclisation of an N-terminal glutamine (or glutamic acid). Evidence from a murine myeloma (Adj PC5) suggests that the cyclisation occurs on completed H chains[61].

Cell-free synthesis of L chains has shown that for two different murine myeloma L chains the initial translation product is a slightly longer precursor polypeptide chain. Translation of the partially purified mRNA for MOPC 41 L chain in a cell-free system derived from Krebs II ascites tumour gives four products, one corresponding to secreted MOPC 41 L chain, two shorter polypeptides related to L chains but incomplete, and one longer polypeptide chain which is apparently a precursor with an additional 6–8 amino acids on the L chain[30]. A precursor of MOPC 21 L chain which contains an additional 14–15 amino acids has been detected in cell-free translation of the L chain mRNA[62]. In this case, addition of the active RNA fraction to a Krebs II cell-free system resulted in synthesis of authentic L chain. In a rabbit reticulocyte lysate cell-free system, however, only the larger precursor L chain was made; addition of Krebs II ascites cell supernatant factor to the reticulocyte system generated authentic L chain. The additional amino acids in the precursor appear to be at the N-terminus of the *L* chain and addition of labelled formylmethionine $tRNA_F$ to the cell-free system labels only the precursor molecule. Thus L chain synthesis appears to be initiated by methionine $tRNA_F$ which appears to be the general initiator for eukaryotic proteins[62].

The conversion of the precursor polypeptide into L chain is probably rapid *in vivo*. The precursor alone is made in a cell-free system using poly-ribosomes from the myeloma cells but using microsomes only L chains are found as the product[62] (Figure 8.5b).

8.5.3 Addition of carbohydrate

The carbohydrate present on immunoglobulin consists of a number of oligo-saccharide chains attached at specific sequences along the H chain and occasionally on the L chain. The proportion of carbohydrate ranges from 3–12% by weight. Oligosaccharide chains are attached via a 'bridge-sugar' which can be either *N*-acetylglucosamine or *N*-acetylgalactosamine.

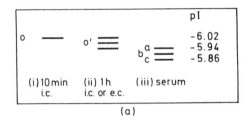

(a)

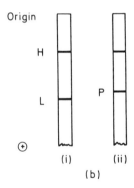

Figure 8.5 (a) Precursor of immunoglobulin G 5563 and its conversion into serum 5563 protein shown by isoelectric focusing. [^{14}C]-labelled myeloma protein spectrum after labelling in 5563 cells for (i) 10 min, intracellular protein; (ii) 1 h, either intracellular or extracellular protein. The isoelectric spectrum of myeloma protein in serum of tumour bearing mice is shown in (iii). The isoelectric points of bands 0, a and c are shown at right. (From Awdeh *et al.*[60], by courtesy of the Biochemical Society)

(b) Precursor of MOPC 21 L chain synthesised *in vitro*. Immunoglobulin chains synthesised in cell-free systems using: (i) microsomes from P3 cells; (ii) microsome-derived polyribosomes from P3 cells. ^{35}S-labelled product separated by SDS-polyacrylamide gel electro-phoresis. (From Milstein *et al.*[62], by courtesy of Macmillan)

In all the cases where the bridge is N-acetylglucosamine the attachment sequence on the protein is probably Asn-X-$^{Ser}_{Thr}$ [63-65] and the link is made by the enzyme UDP-N-acetylglucosamine-asparagine transferase. The sequence Asn-X-$^{Ser}_{Thr}$ is necessary but not sufficient for attachment of the bridge-sugar. This sequence occurs in several Bence-Jones proteins without carbohydrate being found there[66]. Most striking is a case in which the Bence-Jones protein contained carbohydrate while the L chain of identical sequence isolated from the accompanying IgG myeloma lacked carbohydrate[67]. It appears that the sequence must be present in a position on the completed molecule such that is is accessible to the glycosyl transferase. The implication is that the addition of carbohydrate begins after tertiary and quaternary structure is finalised. In contrast, studies on the incorporation of [³H]glucosamine into immuno-globulin in various cell fractions has been interpreted as showing the attach-ment of the bridge sugar to the nascent immunoglobulin chains on the poly-ribosomes[68]. This evidence is not conclusive.

Several studies on the incorporation of various radioactive monosaccharides into immunoglobulins in either mouse myeloma cells or normal rabbit lymphoid cells have shown the step-wise growth of the oligosaccharide chains[120-123]. The rate of appearance of each sugar on intracellular and extracellular immunoglobulin is compared in the presence and absence of an inhibitor of protein synthesis. The results indicate that glucosamine and mannose are added closest to the time of translation and were also added later together with galactose; sialic acid and fucose (and galactose in the case of mouse IgM) are added shortly before secretion of the immuno-globulin.

The addition of sugars is not programmed by coded information and so there is a margin for variation in carbohydrate content between otherwise identical molecules secreted by a given cell. This is reflected in the micro-heterogeneity of serum immunoglobulin. One example which illustrates this is that of a human G-myeloma and its associated Bence-Jones protein which was found to differ from the L chain of the intact IgG only in sialic acid content. The L chain contained one sialic acid per molecule, while the Bence-Jones protein existed in various forms containing from one to six molecules of sialic acid per polypeptide chain[64]. Another dramatic example is the finding that rabbit IgG molecules show asymmetry at the C-2 oligo-saccharide. This carbohydrate chain is attached to threonine via N-acetyl-galactosamine in the hinge region of one H chain but not the other in each IgG molecule[69, 70]. Discounting the selective removal of carbohydrate from one of the chains this asymmetry is further evidence that the bridge sugar is added after the quaternary structure is established.

Glycosyl transferase enzymes catalysing the addition of N-acetylglucos-amine, galactose, and fucose have been partially purified[68]. Nucleotide mono- or di-phosphate sugars are used as donors and carbohydrate-depleted immunoglobulin as acceptor molecules. The transferase enzymes are firmly bound to the membranes of the endoplasmic reticulum, both rough and smooth (Figure 8.6). In the cell-free system the immunoglobulin substrate becomes membrane bound after accepting the labelled sugar[71]. The trans-ferases lose specificity in cell-free preparations using an exogenous acceptor immunoglobulin since there is labelling of peptides other than those accepting carbohydrate *in vivo*. However, the fact that incorporation of sugars into acceptor immunoglobulin can be competitively inhibited by other carbohydrate depleted proteins (e.g. fucin, bovine submaxillary mucin) suggests that the same glycosyl transferase, serves to synthesise the carbohydrate of most,

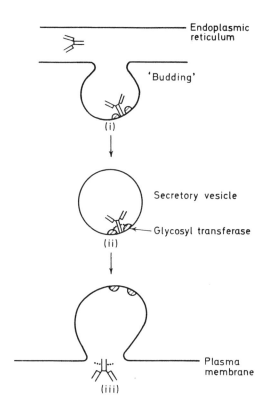

Figure 8.6 Model for intracellular transport, and secretion of IgG. (i) Postulated energy dependent 'budding' of IgG containing vesicles; (ii) stepwise growth of oligosaccharide chains catalysed by membrane-bound glycosyl transferases; (iii) postulated reverse pinocytotic secretion across plasma membrane

if not all, of the cells glycoproteins[72]. The simplest conclusion would be that the glycoprotein nature of immunoglobulins has arisen as a result of their exposure to glycosyl transferases during secretion rather than the addition of carbohydrate being required for secretion. The function which has evolved for the carbohydrate remains to be elucidated.

8.5.4 Intracellular transport and secretion

Immunoglobulin secreting cells exhibit the extensively developed endo-plasmic reticulum typical of other protein secretory cells. L and H chains are synthesised on membrane-bound polyribosomes (see Section 8.2.3 and Figure 8.1) and are vectorially released into the cisternae of the endoplasmic reticu-lum. The vectorial growth of L and H chains into the cisternae is best shown by releasing the nascent polypeptide chains prematurely with [³H]puromycin and identifying H and L chain peptides by immune precipitation[73]. Growth of the chains into the cisternae presages a similarly oriented vectorial release; this release of newly completed immunoglobulin chains has been shown in a cell-free amino acid incorporating system using microsomes derived from rat lymph nodes[74].

Our picture of immunoglobulin secretion (Figure 8.6) generally conforms to earlier evidence on the mode of secretion of proteins by pancreatic[75] and liver cells[76]. Newly synthesised and assembled immunoglobulin passes from the rough endoplasmic reticulum to the smooth endoplasmic reticulum and is secreted via the Golgi apparatus. Intracellular transport of immuno-globulin has been demonstrated by carbohydrate labelling coupled with cell fractionation[77-80] and electron microscopic autoradiography[81]. The mechanism of transport is not known. An energy requiring step can be shown by blocking with inhibitors of respiration, oxidative phosphorylation[82] or by temperature reduction[33]. This step could be the budding of membranes (Figure 8.6) to form immunoglobulin containing smooth vesicles of the Golgi. However, there is no apparent dense packaging of immunoglobulin into secretory granules prior to secretion; on the contrary secretion appears to be a steady continuous process. It has been suggested that the secretory mechanism involves discharge of immunoglobulin from the small vesicles of the Golgi apparatus by reversed pinocytosis at the plasma membrane[81, 83]. However, immunoglobulin secretion is not blocked by cytochalasin-B[84] a drug which blocks many microfilament-related contractile systems including pinocytosis and phagocytosis in macrophages.

A major factor predetermining that immunoglobulins will be secreted from the cell is the site of H and L chain synthesis on membrane-bound ribosomes. This raises the intriguing question of how certain mRNA mole-cules come to be selectively translated by membrane-bound ribosomes. One explanation postulates a non-translated nucleotide sequence in mRNAs coding for secretory proteins and having an affinity for membrane or mem-brane-bound ribosomes. An alternative idea invokes the nascent polypeptide chain in the selective formation and stabilisation of membrane-bound polyribosomes. With the finding that some L chains are synthesised in a precursor form with an additional N-terminal oligopeptide[30, 62] (Section 8.4.2), the latter model has been revived. There is contradictory evidence suggesting on the one hand that newly-synthesised ribosomal subunits bind directly to the membrane with subsequent attachment of the 40S ribosome–mRNA complex[85] and on the other that polyribosomes are bound to the membranes after protein synthesis is initiated[86]. A third speculation suggests specific translation initia-tion factors which select mRNAs for secretory proteins and direct the binding of the initiation complex to membrane bound 60 S ribosomes[85].

8.6 CONTROL OF GENE EXPRESSION

8.6.1 Introduction

The number of known structural genes coding for the immunoglobulin chains is increasing at the present time (see Chapter 7). Expression of this plethora of genes is under many specific controls. These are discussed in the following paragraphs, although little is known at a molecular level. This should be a fruitful area for future investigations since knowledge of internal control and external manipulation of the immune response has many potential medical applications.

8.6.2 Changes in gene expression during the cell cycle

Evidence for differential production of immunoglobulin at various stages of the cell cycle comes from experiments on human lymphoid cell lines maintained in continuous culture. The cell lines studied had a normal diploid chromosome number[87]. Synthesis of immunoglobulin in cells synchronised by thymidine-colcemid or by double thymidine block was found to be maximal during late G_1 and early S phases of the cell cycle[3, 88, 89] (Figure 8.7). It is

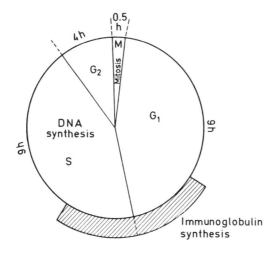

Figure 8.7 Cell cycle of immunoglobulin producing human lymphoid cell showing the period from late G1 to early S phase during which immunoglobulin is synthesised[88]

not clear whether this cyclic production of immunoglobulin is regulated at a transcriptional or translational level since the life time of mRNA for H and L chains is yet to be determined.

By contrast in murine myeloma cells (P3 culture line derived from MOPC 21 tumour) synchronised by double thymidine block there is an almost constant rate of incorporation of [³H]lysine into immunoglobulin[90]. These and other murine myeloma cells are heteroploid and from the view point of these experiments this is probably the most important way in which these cells differ from the human lymphoid cell lines. Klevecz has shown that cyclical enzyme synthesis occurs in synchronised diploid Chinese hamster cells but not in a heteroploid hamster cell line (G3)[91]; he predicted that this might be a general distinction between diploid and heteroploid cells.

Normal, as opposed to malignant, plasma cells are terminal non-dividing cells which may be arrested in G_1 thus ensuring a high rate of antibody production[3].

8.6.3 Changes in gene expression during clonal development

The synthesis of two different immunoglobulins by a single clone of human lymphoid cells in culture[3, 125, 126] is an exception to the rule of restriction to a unique product. While the simultaneous production of two immuno-globulins may be rare there is evidence for the sequential production of different immunoglobulins within the development of a single clone.

The most compelling molecular evidence comes from a case of double myeloma, an $IgG_2\kappa$ and IgM present simultaneously in one patient (Til). These two proteins share idiotypic determinants, have identical κ-chains and have identical V_H region amino acid sequence in the γ_2- and μ-chains[92, 93]. A second case of double myeloma has been analysed and the IgG and IgM were found to share idiotypic determinants[94]. Approximately 1 % of myeloma sera have two different myeloma proteins; further comparisons will be instructive. When patient Til came under clinical observation the IgG_2 and IgM proteins were being produced by separate plasma cells. The possibility that these two sets of plasma cells arose by independent neoplastic events is remote. The shared V_H region indicates that both sets of plasma cells arose from a single precursor cell having the potential to express both C_γ and C_μ genes. We cannot know whether at any time during clonal development C_γ and C_μ were simultaneously expressed or whether the potential was fulfilled by sequential expression. The possibility of simultaneous expression of C_γ and C_μ in the same cell is raised by the demonstration, with fluorescent antisera, of rabbit lymphocytes containing cytoplasmic IgG and having IgM on their surface[95]. These doubly straining cells, may, of course, represent a transition between IgM and IgG production. Sequential expression of C_H genes during clonal development in ontogeny is well documented in both the chicken[96, 97] and the mouse[98]. In chickens both IgM and IgG production are eliminated by treatment with anti-μ chain antibodies *in ova* followed by bursectomy at hatching[96]. Germ-free mice treated from birth with anti-μ chain antibodies resembled bursectomised chickens in having depressed serum levels of all immunoglobulins, greatly reduced numbers of immunoglobulin bearing cells and being incapable of mounting normal immune responses[98]. A model for differentiation of the genetic potential for antibody secretion during clonal development in the chicken is shown in Figure 8.8. This model only deals with the differential expression of C_H genes. During clonal expansion these sequential expressions of each C_H gene may occur with one and the same V_H gene or there may be a different V gene expressed at each change in C_H expression[97]. The expression of one V_H gene (and one V_L gene) throughout clonal expansion is indicated by the Til myeloma proteins. The sequential expression of one V_H with two or more C_H genes requires the postulate of a switch mechanism. The switch could be at the level of V_H–C_H integration

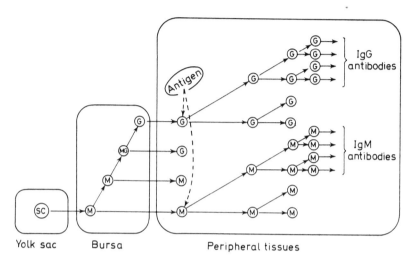

Figure 8.8 Model of lymphoid cell differentiation in chickens. The production of IgM or IgG antibodies is indicated by M or G or both. The sequential appearance of M and G in the bursal cells is antigen independent. (From Cooper *et al.*[97], by courtesy of Plenum Press)

with the transposition of the V_H gene[93]; this model excludes simultaneous expression of one V_H with two C_H genes. Alternatively V_H integration may originally involve a copy-choice mechanism[99] which could link the same V_H to any or all C_H genes[13]; this model can explain both sequential expression of one V_H with two or more C_H genes (phenotypic switch) or the simultaneous expression of the same V_H gene with different C_H genes. A hint that the latter situation might occur comes from the data of Pernis, Forni and Amante[95] on cells containing cytoplasmic IgG and having surface IgM. In heterozygous rabbits the allotype at both a and b loci were identical for cytoplasmic and surface immunoglobulin of all cells examined[95]. Rabbit γ- and μ-chains share only a_1, a_2, a_3 allotypes which are V-region markers[127].

8.6.4 Gene expression in hybrid cells

Hybridisation of immunoglobulin producing cells is a potentially powerful system for the analysis of gene expression. Use of this system has been limited to date. Hybrids produced between mouse myeloma cells and fibroblasts usually cease to produce immunoglobulin[13, 100]. One exception to this was hybridisation of anti-DNP secreting MOPC 315 murine myeloma cells with L cells which produced hybrids with detectable secretion of a DNP-binding protein[101].

Mohit[102] has hybridised a Balb/c myeloma (RPC 5) with a $C_{57}Bl/6n$ lymphoma (EL$_4$) and selected 13 clonal hybrid cell lines. The parental RPC 5 cells produced IgG_{2a} and excess κ-chains. Eleven of the hybrid clones produced free κ-chains but no detectable IgG_{2a}. The other two clones produced IgG_{2a} and free κ chains in excess; these hybrid cells had higher chromosome numbers than the eleven lines lacking γ-chain production. The loss of γ-chain synthesis could, therefore, be attributed to chromosome loss. This supports the idea that γ- and κ-chain genes are on separate chromosomes.

8.7 REGULATION OF IMMUNOGLOBULIN BIOSYNTHESIS

8.7.1 Introduction

Assembly of complete immunoglobulin molecules requires an equal number of L and H chains. It would appear to be most economical for the cell to produce L and H chains in approximately equal numbers. The balance of production and also the absolute level of synthesis of each chain could be regulated at several levels: transcription, mRNA processing, mRNA transport or various stages during translation. The simplest assumption is that transcriptional rates for H and L chain genes are balanced and that this provides equal numbers of each chain. Recent evidence discussed below Section 8.7.2 suggests that the maintenance of a normal balance may be a more complex process. With controls at various stages, defects in immunoglobulin production might be located at any of these stages as discussed in Section 8.7.3.

8.7.2 Maintenance of normal balanced synthesis

In high-rate immunoglobulin secreting cells it would appear to be normal to have a balanced synthesis of L and H chains[13]. Most studies of antibody-secreting cells have shown such a balance and a balance is also seen in many plasmacytoma cells[13]. The idea that balance might be maintained solely by transcriptional control has to be abandoned in the light of experiments on murine myeloma cells (5563) in culture showing translational controls. It was found that the translation of H-chain mRNA is regulated by direct feed-back repression by the intracellular H_2L_2 pool[33].

The role of H_2L_2 pool-size was shown by increasing the intracellular H_2L_2 pool by incubating the cells at a lower temperature (25 °C) thus blocking secretion but permitting continued synthesis of H and L chains. The increase in the H_2L_2 pool depresses the rate of H chain synthesis, but not L chain synthesis upon return of the cells to 37 °C. When the H_2L_2 pool is depleted, by blocking protein synthesis with cycloheximide which allows secretion to continue, the subsequent rate of H chain synthesis is increased. This implies that under normal conditions the rate of H chain synthesis can be repressed to at least 60 % of its potential maximal rate.

Control of H chain synthesis by H_2L_2 is effected by a specific interaction between H_2L_2 molecules and H-chain mRNA[34]. Although this is a weak interaction the specificity is attested by the fact that it has been utilised to purify H-chain mRNA[32] (see Section 8.2.4). Regulation of gene expression in eukaryotic cells by steroid hormones has been postulated to occur at the level of translation; it is thought that a repressor molecule (presumably a protein) binds to mRNA and the steroid hormone can reverse this binding[103]. The interaction of H_2L_2 with H-chain mRNA provides a defined system for testing translational control models involving protein–nucleic acid interactions.

Control mechanisms at the levels of transcription, processing and transport of mRNA must also be examined. Knowledge gained using plasma cells constitutively producing immunoglobulin can then be used to probe the more difficult problem of the induction of antibody synthesis.

8.7.3   Defects in biosynthetic control

A useful technique for investigating regulatory mechanisms is to examine situations in which control has been lost at some particular step. Many of the biosynthetic studies described in this chapter have been performed in neoplastic plasma cell tumours either maintained by transplantation in mice or as long-term continuous cultures. Since the differentiated function of immunoglobulin production is of no value for the continued proliferation of the cells, non-producing mutants are not at a selective disadvantage and may be selected for readily. Many defective lines of plasma cell tumours have arisen spontaneously and involve either an altered balance of gene expression or internal deletions or other mutations in structural genes leading to defects in covalent and/or non-covalent assembly.

In cases of unbalanced production of L and H chains the tendency has always been found to be towards an increased L:H ratio. Situations ranging from a slight excess of L chain to a complete repression of H chain production have been reported[128]. When there is predominant or sole production of L chains these may be secreted by the cell and, for a tumour growing *in vivo* L chain appears in urine and is known as Bence-Jones protein.

With transplantable murine myeloma tumours defective sublines are obtained only when they over-grow the original tumour line. Using myeloma cells in culture, Coffino, Laskov and Scharff[104] were able to use cloning techniques to select for mutant cells; the rate of appearance of cells having lost the ability to make H chain was found to be 10^3 per cell per generation for the MPC-11 cell line[105]. This high rate suggests that there are many different events which can lead to loss of H chain synthesis. These mutants provide ample material for biochemical experiments.

While H chain suppression is not uncommon, L chain suppression has been seen rarely, if ever. Apparent absence of L chains is seen in 'heavy-chain disease' in humans. Defective a, γ- or μ-chains appear in the urine of H-chain disease patients. Partial sequence analysis of the defective chains has revealed that each has an internal deletion comprising part of the V region and part of the C region[106-108]. These deletions strongly suggest that V and C genes were integrated in the cell in which the mutation occurred. The defective chains are true synthetic products of the patient's myeloma cells which do not appear to make any L chains[109, 110].

The defective α-chains found in urine are shorter than normal α-chains are also probably deletion mutants involving both V and C regions; these defective chains could not be combined with any L chains tested[111].

Mutant chains may also cause a defective pattern of assembly of H and L chains. Several myeloma tumours secrete half molecules (HL) with no detectable H_2L_2[128]. In two such cases the half molecules contain α-chains which are shorter, and contain fewer cysteines than normal α-chain[112, 113]. Failure of HL to form H_2L_2 in these cells is most readily attributable to an H chain deletion leading to a loss of the tendency of the H chains to dimerise.

One plasmacytoma (MPC 11) has been found to secrete molecules in all stages of assembly: HL appeared to be blocked by non-covalent attachment of L chains which are present in excess[114].

Defects in the polymerisation of IgM can result in the secretion of IgMs into serum. This is seen in certain antibody deficiency syndromes and lymphoproliferative disorders as well as in patients with systemic lupus erythematosis and ataxia telangiectasia[115-118]. This IgMs is secreted as such and is not a degradation product of 19s IgM[119]. The nature of the block in polymerisation and the relationship of this biosynthetic defect to the various disease with which it is associated are presently unknown.

References

1. Potter, M. (1967). *Methods in Cancer Research*, **2**, 105
2. Takahashi, M., Tanigaki, N., Moore, G. E., Yagi, Y. and Pressman, D. (1968). *J. Immunol.*, **100**, 1176
3. Buell, D. N., Sox, H. C. and Fahey, J. L. (1971). *Developmental Aspects of the Cell Cycle*, 279. (I. L. Cameron, G. M. Padilla and A. M. Zimmerman, editors) (New York: Academic Press)
4. Potter, M., Apella, E. and Geisser, S. (1965). *J. Molec. Biol.*, **14**, 361
5. Campbell, J. (1967). *J. Theoret. Biol.*, **16**, 321
6. Naughton, M. A. and Dintzis, H. M. (1962). *Proc. Nat. Acad. Sci. USA*, **48**, 1822
7. Fleischman, J. B. (1963). *J. Immunol.*, **91**, 163
8. Fleischman, J. B. (1967). *Biochemistry*, **6**, 1311
9. Knopf, P. M., Parkhouse, R. M. E. and Lennox, E. S. (1967). *Proc. Nat. Acad. Sci. USA*, **58**, 2288
10. Lennox, E. S., Knopf, P. M., Munro, A. J. and Parkhouse, R. M. E. (1967). *Cold Spring Harbor Symp. Quant. Biol.*, **32**, 249
11. Cioli, D. and Baglioni, C. (1968). *J. Exp. Med.*, **128**, 517
12. Schubert, D. and Cohn, M. (1970). *J. Molec. Biol.*, **53**, 305
13. Bevan, M. J., Parkhouse, R. M. E., Williamson, A. R. and Askonas, B. A. (1972). *Progr. Biophys. Molec. Biol.*, **25**, 131
14. Norton, W. L., Lewis, D. and Ziff, M. (1965). *Proc. Nat. Acad. Sci. USA*, **54**, 851
15. Scharff, M. D. and Uhr, J. W. (1965). *Science*, **148**, 646
16. Becker, M. J. and Rich, A. (1966). *Nature (London)*, **212**, 142
17. Voss, E. W. and Bauer, D. C. (1967). *J. Biol. Chem.*, **242**, 4495
18. Kuechler, E. and Rich, A. (1969). *Nature (London)*, **222**, 544
19. Askonas, B. A. and Williamson, A. R. (1966). *Proc. Roy. Soc. (London), Ser. B.*, **166**, 232
20. Shapiro, A. L., Scharff, M. D., Maizel, J. V. and Uhr, J. W. (1966). *Proc. Nat. Acad. Sci. USA*, **56**, 216

21. Williamson, A. R. and Askonas, B. A. (1967)., *J. Molec. Biol.*, **23**, 201
22. Schubert, D. (1968). *Proc. Nat. Acad. Sci. USA*, **60**, 683
23. Schubert, D. and Cohn, M. (1968). *J. Molec. Biol.*, **38**, 273
24. Namba, Y. and Hanoaka, M. (1969). *J. Immunol.*, **102**, 1486
25. De Petris, S., (1970). *Biochem. J.*, **118**, 385
26. Cioli, D. and Lennox, E. (1971). Personal communication
27. Bevan, M. J. (1972). *Ph.D. Thesis*, Univ. of London
28. Stavnezer, J. and Huang, R-C. C. (1971). *Nature, New Biol.*, **230**, 172
29. Brownlee, G. G., Harrison, T. M., Mathews, M. B. and Milstein, C. (1972). *FEBS Lett.*, **23**, 244
30. Swan, D., Aviv, H. and Leder, P. (1972). *Proc. Nat. Acad. Sci. USA*, **69**, 1967
31. Stevens, R. H. and Williamson, A. R. (1972). *Nature (London)*, **239**, 143
32. Stevens, R. H. and Williamson, A. R. (1973). *Proc. Nat. Acad. Sci. USA*, **70**, 1127
33. Stevens, R. H. and Williamson, A. R. (1973). *J. Molec. Biol.*, in press
34. Stevens, R. H. and Williamson, A. R. (1973). *J. Molec. Biol.*, in press
35. Stevens, R. H. and Williamson, A. R. (1973). *Nature*. Submitted for publication
36. Wall, R. and Darnell, J. (1971). *Nature, New Biol.*, **232**, 73
37. Delovitch, T. L., David, B. K., Holme, G. and Sehon, A. H. (1972). *J. Molec. Biol.*, **69**, 373
38. Halpern, M. S. and Koshland, M. E. (1970). *Nature (London)*, **228**, 1276
39. Mestecky, J., Zikan, J. and Butler, W. T. (1971). *Science*, **171**, 1103
40. Tomasi, T. B. and Grey, H. M. (1972). *Progress in Allergy*, **16**, 81
41. Parkhouse, R. M. E. (1972). *Nature, New Biol.*, **236**, 9
42. Halpern, M. S. and Coffman, R. L. (1972). *J. Immunol.*, **109**, 674
43. Heremans, J. F. and Crabbe, P. A. (1967). in *Gamma Globulins Nobel Symposium*, Vol. 3, 129 (J. Killander, editor)
44. Askonas, B. A. and Williamson, A. R. (1966). *Nature (London)*, **211**, 369
45. Williamson, A. R. and Askonas, B. A. (1968). *Arch. Biochem. Biophys.*, **125**, 401
46. Parkhouse, R. M. E. (1971). *Biochem. J.*, **123**, 635
47. Virella, G. and Parkhouse, R. M. E. (1973). *Immunochemistry*, **10**, 213
48. Baumal, R., Potter, M. and Scharff, M. D. (1971). *J. Exp. Med.*, **134**, 1316
49. Bevan, M. J. (1971). *Europ. J. Immunol.*, **1**, 133
50. Parkhouse, R. M. E. (1971). *FEBS Lett.*, **16**, 71
51. Björk, I. and Tanford, C. (1971). *Biochemistry*, **10**, 1271
52. Stevenson, G. T. (1968). *Bibl. Haematol.*, **29**, 537
53. Stevenson, G. T. and Dorrington, K. J. (1970). *Biochem. J.*, **118**, 703
54. Parkhouse, R. M. E. and Askonas, B. A. (1969). *Biochem. J.*, **115**, 163
55. Buxbaum, J., Zolla, S., Scharff, M. D. and Franklin, E. C. (1971). *J. Exp. Med.*, **133**, 1118
56. Fahey, J. L. (1963). *J. Clin. Invest.*, **42**, 111
57. Abel, C. A. and Grey, H. M. (1968). *Biochemistry*, **7**, 2682
58. Fuchs, S., DeLorenzo, F. and Anfinsen, C. B. (1967). *J. Biol. Chem.*, **242**, 398
59. Eylar, E. H. (1966). *J. Theoret. Biol.*, **10**, 89
60. Awdeh, Z. L., Williamson, A. R. and Askonas, B. A. (1970). *Biochem. J.* **116**, 241
61. Stott, D. I. and Munro, A. J. (1972). *Biochem. J.*, **128**, 1221
62. Milstein, C., Brownlee, G. G., Harrison, T. M. and Mathews, M. B. (1972). *Nature, New Biol.*, **239**, 117
63. Sox, H. C. and Hood, L. (1970). *Proc. Nat. Acad. Sci. USA*, **66**, 975
64. Spiegelberg, H. L., Abel, C. A., Fishkin, B. G. and Grey, H. M. (1970). *Biochemistry*, **9**, 4217
65. Milstein, C. P. and Milstein, C. (1971). *Biochem. J.*, **121**, 211
66. Edelman, G. M. and Gall, E. W. (1969). *Ann. Rev. Biochem.*, **38**, 415
67. Edmunson, A. B., Sheber, F. A., Ely, K. R., Simmonds, N. B., Hutson, N. K. and Rossiter, J. L. (1968). *Arch. Biochem. Biophys.*, **127**, 725
68. Sherr, C. J., Schenkein, I., and Uhr, J. W. (1972). *Ann. N.Y. Acad. Sci.*, **190**, 250
69. Hinrichs, W. A. and Smyth, D. G. (1970). *Immunol.*, **18**, 759
70. Fanger, M. W. and Smyth, D. G. (1972). *Biochem. J.*, **127**, 767
71. D'Amico, R. P. and Kern, M. (1968). *J. Biol. Chem.*, **243**, 3425
72. D'Amico, R. P. and Kern, M. (1970). *Biochem. Biophys. Acta*, **215**, 78
73. Bevan, M. J. (1971). *Biochem. J.*, **122**, 5

74. Vassalli, P., Lisowska-Bernstein, B., Lamm, M. E. and Benacerraf, B. (1967). *Proc. Nat. Acad. Sci. USA*, **58**, 2422
75. Jamieson, J. D. and Palade, G. E. (1967). *J. Cell. Biol.*, **34**, 577 and 597
76. Campbell, P. N. (1970). *FEBS Lett.*, **7**, 1
77. Melchers, F. (1969). *Biochemistry*, **8**, 938
78. Melchers, F. (1971). *Biochemistry*, **10**, 653
79. Uhr, J. W. and Schenkein, I. (1970). *Proc. Nat. Acad. Sci. USA*, **66**, 952
80. Choi, Y. S., Knopf, P. M., and Lennox, E. S. (1971). *Biochemistry*, **10**, 659 and 668
81. Zagury, D., Uhr, J. W., Jamieson, J. D. and Palade, G. E. (1970). *J. Cell Biol.*, **46**, 52
82. Jamieson, J. D. and Palade, G. E. (1968). *J. Cell Biol.*, **39**, 589
83. Uhr, J. W. (1970). *Cellular Immunol.*, **1**, 228
84. Parkhouse, R. M. E. and Allison, A. C. (1972). *Nature, New Biol.*, **235**, 220
85. Baglioni, C., Bleiberg, I. and Zauderer, M. (1971). *Nature, New Biol.*, **232**, 8
86. Rosbach, M. (1972). *J. Molec. Biol.*, **65**, 413
87. Huang, C. C. and Moore, G. E. (1969). *J. Nat. Cancer Inst.*, **43**, 1119
88. Finegold, I., Fahey, J. L. and Dutcher, T. F. (1968). *J. Immunol.*, **101**, 366
89. Takahashi, M., Yagi, Y., Moore, G. E. and Pressman, D., (1969). *J. Immunol.*, **103**, 834
90. Cowan, N. J. and Milstein, C. (1972). *Biochem. J.*, **128**, 445
91. Klevecz, R. R. (1969). *Science*, **166**, 1536
92. Wang, A. C., Wang, I. Y. F., McCormick, J. N. and Fudenberg, H. H. (1969). *Immunochem.*, **6**, 451
93. Wang, A. C., Wilson, S. K., Hopper, J. E., Fundenberg, H. H. and Nisonoff, A. (1970). *Proc. Nat. Acad. Sci. USA*, **66**, 337
94. Penn, G. M., Kunkel, H. G. and Grey, H. M. (1970). *Proc. Soc. Exp. Biol. Med.*, **135**, 660
95. Pernis, B., Forni, L. and Amante, L. (1971). *Ann. N.Y. Acad. Sci.*, **190**, 420
96. Kincade, P. W., Lawton, A. R., Bockman, D. E. and Cooper, M. D. (1970). *Proc. Nat. Acad. Sci. USA*, **67**, 1918
97. Cooper, M. D., Lawton, A. R., and Kincade, P. W. (1972) in *Contemporary Topics in Immunobiology*, Vol. 1, 33 (M. G. Hanna, editor) (New York: Plenum Press)
98. Lawton, A. R., Asofsky, R., Hylton, M. B. and Cooper, M. D. (1972). *J. Exp. Med.*, **135**, 277
99. Dreyer, W. J., Gray, W. R. and Hood, L. (1967). *Cold Spring Harbor Symp. Quant. Biol.*, **32**, 353
100. Coffino, P., Knowles, B., Nathenson, S. G. and Scharff, M. D. (1971). *Nature, New Biol.*, **231**, 87
101. Periman, P. (1970). *Nature (London)*, **228**, 1086
102. Mohit, B. (1971). *Proc. Nat. Acad. Sci. USA*, **68**, 3045
103. Tomkins, G. M., Gelehrter, T. D., Granner, D., Martin, D., Samuels, H. H. and Thompson, E. B. (1969). *Science*, **166**, 1474
104. Coffino, P., Laskov, R. and Scharff, M. D. (1970). *Science*, **167**, 186
105. Coffino, P. and Scharff, M. D. (1971). *Proc. Nat. Acad. Sci. USA*, **68**, 219
106. Prahl, J. W. (1967). *Nature (London)*, **215**, 1386
107. Frangione, B. and Milstein, C. (1969). *Nature (London)*, **224**, 597
108. Terry, W. D. and Ohms, J. (1970). *Proc, Nat. Acad. Sci. USA*, **66**, 558
109. Ein, D., Buell, D. and Fahey, J. L. (1969). *J. Clin. Invest.*, **48**, 785
110. Buxbaum, J., Franklin, E. C. and Scharff, M. D. (1970). *Science*, **169**, 770
111. Seligmann. M., Milhaesco, E., Hurez, D., Mihaesco, C., Preud-Homme, J. L. and Rambaud, J. C. (1969). *J. Clin. Invest.*, **48**, 2374
112. Seki, T., Apella, E. and Itano, H. A. (1968). *Proc. Nat. Acad. Sci. USA*, **61**, 1071
113. Mushinski, J. F. (1971). *J. Immunol.*, **106**, 41
114. Laskov, R., Lanzerotti, R. and Scharff, M. D. (1971). *J. Molec. Biol.*, **56**, 327
115. Stobo, J. D. and Tomasi, T. B. (1967). *J. Clin. Invest.*, **46**, 1329
116. Solomon, A. and Kunkel, H. G. (1967). *Amer. J. Med.*, **42**, 958
117. Griggs, R. C., Strober, W. and McFarlin, D. E. (1969). *Arch. Neurol.*, **21**, 303
118. Rothfield, N. F., Frangione, B. and Franklin, E. C. (1965). *J. Clin. Invest.*, **44**, 62
119. Solomon, A. and McLaughlin, C. L. (1970). *J. Clin. Invest.*, **49**, 150
120. Cohen, H. J. and Kern, M. (1969). *Biochim. Biophys. Acta*, **188**, 255
121. Schenkein, I. and Uhr, J. W. (1970). *J. Cell Biol.*, **46**, 42
122. Melchers, F. (1970). *Biochem J.*, **119**, 765

123. Parkhouse, R. M. E. and Melchers, F. (1971). *Biochem. J.*, **125,** 235
124. Williamson, A. R. (1969). *Essays in Biochem.*, **5,** 139
125. Takahashi, Y., Yagi, Y., Moore, G. E. and Pressman, D. (1969). *J. Immunol.*, **103,** 834
126. Bloom, A. D., Choi, K. W. and Lumb, B. J. (1971). *Science*, **172,** 382
127. Kindt, T. J., Mandy, W. J. and Todd, C. W. (1970). *Biochemistry*, **9,** 2028
128. Potter, M. (1972). *Physiol. Revs.*, **52,** 631

9
Histocompatibility Antigens

Part 1
A Chemical Approach to Transplantation Antigens

R. A. REISFELD
Scripps Clinic and Research Foundation La Jolla, California
and
B. D. KAHAN
Northwestern University Medical Center, Chicago

9.1 INTRODUCTION

The study of histocompatibility antigens is one of the most challenging tasks in biology today which deals with a fascinating biological and chemical phenomena—the uniqueness of the individual. Through their ability to elicit transplantation immunity against tissue grafts, histocompatibility (H) antigens as genetically-segregating cell-surface markers provide an excellent tool to study this biological phenomenon. In this regard, the individuality system reflecting tissue and organ compatibility is particularly amenable to study, as it offers one of the most fertile areas for the immunologist due to the ready and unequivocal biological assay, the destruction of foreign tissue grafts. However, the significance of tests depending upon the transplantation of tissues, i.e. assays of histocompatibility, extends far beyond the unnatural challenge of duping the host to accept foreign cells. The basic issues in biological recognition and response, as well as in cell-surface membrane structure and physiology are elucidated by investigations of the substances eliciting transplantation immunity. The gene systems which determine histocompatibility, their gene products, a set of unique chemical markers of individuality and the mechanisms of antigenic recognition and immune responsiveness can be studied in transplantation systems.

The nature of transplantation antigens has been under study for some time. Thus, in 1930 Loeb[1] had suggested that grafts were destroyed by a local toxic reaction induced by the effects of products released from the graft upon elements of the host. The experiments of Gibson and Medawar[2] with inbred strains of mice demonstrated that transplantation rejection was mediated by the immune system. Subsequent ('second set') grafts derived from the original donor were rejected by the host in accelerated fashion. Thus, grafting engenders a systemic specific resistance against donor tissues[3]. Simonsen et al.[4] confirmed this phenomenon with canine renal allografts. Of great import were two subsequent experiments performed by Medawar and his colleagues in which they showed that all of the foreign factors eliciting an immune response against skin grafts are also present on lymphoid cells. First, immunisation of prospective hosts with spleen cells yielded a second-set destruction of donor-type skin grafts. Second, Billingham, Brent and Medawar[5], proved that alteration of the host's response by exposure to allogenic spleen cells in neonatal life resulted in a permanent infirmity in response toward the donor-type skin grafts. This experiment conclusively demonstrated that there were no local factors which could interfere with the survival of grafts and reaffirmed the overriding importance of the immune system in determining transplant survival.

Medawar[6] then proposed that specific genes, the histocompatibility genes, control the production of cellular factors which upon transplantation into a foreign host elicit an immune reaction resulting in graft destruction. The factors eliciting the reaction have been the subject of considerable inquiry due to their central importance in the genesis of transplant immunity.

9.2 SEROLOGICAL IDENTIFICATION OF HUMAN HISTOCOMPATIBILITY (HI-A) ANTIGENS

9.2.1 Genetics of the HL-A system

Only a brief discussion of the genetic aspects of the HL-A system is presented here as a detailed treatment of this subject appears in Chapter 9, Part 2.

Extensive serological investigations of human histocompatibility antigens carried out on a large international scale in population and family studies have greatly contributed to an understanding of the genetics of the HL-A system in man. This development was, of course, linked closely to extensive prior work in the rodent by virtue of the deep commitment of the field of transplantation to the study of the murine model. The HL-A system was described as being controlled by a bipartite locus constructed of two segregant series each containing a number of specificities[7]. This antigenic system was found to be the most polymorphic one in man exhibiting a large degree of allelism with each segregant series determining a single one of a number of allelic antigenic specificities. In other words, the first or LA series contained one of the allelic series 1,2,3,9,10,11 and the second or FOUR series contained one of the 5,7,8,12 or 13 series[8]. The genetic determinants for HL-A antigens are localised on a single pair of autosomal chromosomes. The alleles in each segregant series are mutually exclusive, i.e. any one individual can have at most 4 different HL-A antigens, 2 LA and 2 FOUR antigens. Segregation analyses from considerable family data agree with the 2 segregant series concept and imply that the parental LA and FOUR antigens are heritable either in coupling if they belong to the same haplotype or in repulsion if they belong to different haplotypes (for reviews see Refs. 8 and 9).

9.2.2 Serological assay techniques

The various assays utilised to detect H-antigens fall into two major categories, i.e. biological and serological. Biological tests evaluate (a) the fate of tissue grafts on sensitised subjects; (b) elicitation of humoral antibody, (c) induction of a state of delayed hypersensitivity to injected H-antigens; and (d) the response of leukocytes when reacted with allogeneic cells in tissue culture. Although these tests are most meaningful to study immunogenicity, they are time consuming and cumbersome. Serological assays, however, are simple and rapid as they measure the extent to which an antibody can complex specifically with its alloantigenic determinants. Since H-antigens stimulate the production of humoral alloantibody, cytotoxic alloantisera have been used widely in microlymphocytotoxic tests to detect antigenic determinants either identical or closely associated with those mediating transplantation immunity.

Among a number of serological assays utilised, such as leukoagglutination[10, 11], lymphocytotoxicity[12-14], complement-fixation[15-17], antiglobulin consumption[18], mixed agglutination[19] and immune adherence[20], two have been most widely used, i.e. leukoagglutination and lymphocytotoxicity. The former proved less effective since it is less sensitive and thus many alloantisera react as if they were monospecific. However, lymphocytotoxicity has proven to be a most effective test, especially for the serological analysis of HL-A antigens since the miniaturisation of this method by Terasaki and McClelland[13]. The microcytotoxic test requires only minute amounts of reagents, e.g. 2μl antiserum and only 2000 target cells, thus overcoming the problem of limited supplies of highly-specific alloantibody and increasing sensitivity as the latter is inversely proportional to the number of target cells[21, 22]. The cytotoxic test relies upon alterations in the permeability of cell membranes effected by the action of complement on target cells reacted previously with specific cytotoxic alloantibodies. Cell death resulting from specific interaction is measured either by uptake of supravital dyes[23], the release of fluorescent materials[24, 25], changes in cell morphology[13] or the release of radiolabel from target cells[26].

Table 9.1 summarises the principal steps in the microlymphocytotoxic test. A modified micromethod for another assay technique utilising platelet complement fixation is shown in Table 9.2. The two techniques are at present used most commonly for HL-A typing, especially in conjunction with histocompatibility testing. The largest number of HL-A antigens can be detected using lymphocytotoxicity as it seems even more difficult to find antisera useful for the complement fixation assay than for the lymphocytotoxicity technique. However, complement fixation has an advantage in quantitative work such as investigating gene dose effects where it could be shown that homozygous platelets have twice as many antigenic sites as heterozygous ones. The two procedures have been critically discussed in a recent review[9].

Table 9.1 The microcytotoxicity test

Target cells: Human peripheral lymphocytes or human cultured lymphoid cells
HL-A alloantisera: Alloantisera from multiparous women or from subjects immunised with blood transfusions or transplants.
Complement: Selected rabbit serum for peripheral lymphocytes. Absorbed or suitably diluted rabbit serum for cultured human lymphoid cells

Sera (2 µl) + cells (2000) are incubated under mineral oil for 30 min at room temperature. Rabbit complement (3 µl) is added and the incubation is continued for 60 min at room temperature. Eosin 5% (2 µl) is added and after 2 min the reaction is stopped by the addition of 2 µl of formalin 33%. The percentage of dead cells is determined under phase-contrast microscopy.

Table 9.2 Platelet complement fixation technique*

Component	Amount µl
Antiserum	2
Platelet suspension (500 000 µl⁻¹)	2
Human complement (2 H 100 units (2 µl)⁻¹)†	2
Sensitised sheep red blood cells (200 000 µl⁻¹)‡	2

* The test is carried out in Falcon Microtest Tissue Culture Plates ♯3034
† Mix and incubate 1 h at 37 °C
‡ Mix and incubate 30 min at 37 °C; centrifuge and determine titre with serology ready box

9.2.3 Immunological cross-reactivity of histocompatibility antigens

The sharing of antigenic determinants even by widely separated phylogenetic groups was first observed by Ehrlich and Morgenroth[27] and later became widely recognised through the work of Landsteiner[28]. In the studies at the turn of the century, rabbits immunised with ox erythrocytes produced not only anti-ox but also anti-goat and anti-sheep haemolysins. Forssman[29] then described his classic studies of the production of sheep haemolysins by immunising rabbits with guinea-pig tissues. These heterologous antigens became known as Forssman antigens which were found to occur in a wide variety of animal cells and micro-organisms[30].

A sharing of surface antigenic determinants was observed in a variety of mammalian cells other than erythrocytes. Thus, Kaplan[31] detected cross-reactions between whole group A streptococci, streptococcal cell walls and human as well as rabbit heart, skeletal and smooth-muscle cells. Numerous studies showed group A streptococci to share a significant number of antigenic determinants with mammalian tissues (for a review see Ref. 32).

9.2.3.1 Cross-reactivity between histocompatibility and streptococcal antigens

Cross-reacting streptococcal antigens clearly affect another form of altered tissue response, i.e. allograft rejection. Thus, a clear cut relationship was demonstrated between antigen(s) of group A streptococci and histocompatibility antigens of several animal species including mouse, rat, guinea-pig, rabbit, dog and rhesus monkey[33]. This was particularly well illustrated by the experiments of Rapaport and Chase[34] which showed that immunisation of guinea-pigs with group A streptococci induced a state of altered reactivity to skin allografts indistinguishable from that observed following pretreatment of the recipients with leukocytes or allogeneic tissues. In a series of elegant experiments, Rapaport[35] demonstrated altered reactivity, i.e. hyperacute rejection responses to renal allografts in dogs pretreated with group A type 12 streptococcal cells. Hypersensitivity states to this class of bacterial antigens apparently mediated the hyperacute rejection of these tissue transplants. These data support the hypothesis of Simmons et al.[36] that bacterial infections may trigger renal allograft rejection crises and the observations of Hume et al.[37] that altered reactivity states to bacterial antigens may seriously affect the survival of kidney transplants in man.

A direct consequence of the cross-reactivity of histocompatibility antigens of the above-mentioned animal species with antigens present in group A streptococcal cells may be that each of these species, in turn, share histocompatibility antigen(s) with other members of the group. This has been examined by two different experimental approaches. The first utilises in vivo studies with active sensitisation of recipients by heterologous transplantation antigens while the second approach makes use of in vitro serological methods. Thus, soluble blood group A and B substances isolated from pigs and horses can induce in human recipients a group-specific state of allograft sensitivity indistinguishable from that observed after pretreatment of the host with either donor-specific or group-specific histocompatibility antigens[32].

9.2.3.2 Cross-reactivity within the HL-A system

Cross-reactivity also occurs within the HL-A system as indicated by in vitro and in vivo experiments (Table 9.3). Thus, serological investigations have shown that human lymphocytes, human cultured lymphoid cells or platelets bearing a given HL-A specificity can absorb from operationally-monospecific alloantisera antibodies to other HL-A determinants (for a review see Ref. 38). Furthermore, streptococcal M1 proteins can block the cytotoxicity of histo-compatibility typing sera directed against different HL-A specificities[39]. These data were confirmed by studying the DNA synthesis of human lymphocytes stimulated by M1 proteins in short-term tissue culture[40]. The M1 stimulation is inhibited by HL-A alloantisera of different specificity, possibly by their masking of the mitogenic site on the M1 protein so as to prevent interaction between M1 and specific lymphocyte receptors necessary to induce a prolifer-ative response. Furthermore, HL-A antigens solubilised from cultured lym-phoid cells can specifically inhibit anti-HL-A alloantisera directed against determinants cross-reacting with those present on the cells used for extraction[41]. Cross-reacting HL-A specificities seem to be of clinical relevance as skin

Table 9.3   Cross-reactivity within the HL-A system*

First Segregant Series	HL-A1, HL-A3, HL-A10, HL-A11, W 32, W 29, W 31
	HL-A2, HL-A9, HL-A28
Second Segregant Series	HL-A5, HL-A12, R*, LND, HL-A17, CM*
	HL-A7, HL-A13, AA, FJH, BB
	HL-A28, HL-A14

* Schematic representation of cross-reactivity among HL-A specificities. Cross-reactivity may occur among all specificities within one segregant series.

grafts and kidney transplants[42] survive longer when HL-A incompatibility is within a group of cross-reacting antigens rather than between different groups.

The experimental data thus far indicate cross-reactivity to occur only between allelic gene products of a single HL-A segregant series and not be-tween those of the two different series[43-45]. Some data suggest the possibility that within each segregant series exist groups of families of cross-reacting HL-A specificities[46], whereas other work shows that cross-reacting groups do not form clusters but are interconnected[45].

Cross-reactions between antigens within the HL-A system have also been shown to extend to isoantigens of other species as those reported between rabbits and mice[47] and mice and rats[48]. There is also a sharing of antigens between HL-A and ChL-A, the histocompatibility system of chimpanzees[49], the lymphocytes of which can be typed with anti-HL-A alloantisera[50]. Close similarities were found between HL-A and ChL-A specificities as chimpanzee alloantisera can detect HL-A 1, HL-A 11, 4a and 4b in the human population and antisera against these same specificities give like reaction patterns with chimpanzee antisera in the chimpanzee population (for a review see Ref. 49). The HL-A system has also been shown to cross-react with the mouse histo-compatibility system. Sera from rabbits immunised with soluble HL-A anti-gens reacted in the cytotoxic test not only with human lymphocytes but also with murine lymphocytes from different strains[51]. H-2 Antigens solubilised from murine L1210 lymphoid cells could specifically inhibit the cytotoxic activity of anti-HL-A rabbit heteroantisera with a level of activity similar to that observed in the inhibition test with monospecific H-2 alloantisera.

In conclusion, cross-reactivity between HL-A determinants and bacterial antigens is of great clinical interest and may provide a key to understand the susceptibility to certain diseases. Antigens shared between man and bacteria might favour the parasite since the host is unable to have an adequate immune response against the shared antigens. If this is the case, the polymorphism of the HL-A system may actually be an important safeguard to preserve the human species. The study of cross-reactivity between the HL-A system and histocompatibility systems of other species is of both theoretical and practical interest as it may provide insight into the phylogeny of histocompatibility antigens in many species. Such knowledge facilitates the selection of animals for the production of heterologous antisera which are specific for HL-A alloantigenic determinants. Thus, HL-A antisera can be produced without resorting to the potentially hazardous isoimmunisation of human volunteers. The cross-reactivity within each of the two segregant series of the HL-A system is of clinical relevance since skin grafts and kidney transplants[42] have longer survival times when HL-A incompatibility occurs within a group rather than between different groups of cross-reacting antigens.

9.3 EXTRACTION OF SOLUBLE HISTOCOMPATILIBITY ANTIGENS

The impetus to obtain soluble histocompatibility antigens came initially from the observations of Medawar[52] that these antigens, in non-particulate form, can induce a degree of immunological unresponsiveness resulting in prolonged allograft survival. Extensive histocompatibility testing in families and populations which led to the genetic concepts of the H-2 and HL-A systems ultimately produced renewed interest in the isolation and physico-chemical characterisation of the gene products of the H-2 and HL-A loci. It was mandatory to isolate water-soluble antigens as presently available chemical methods for the analysis of proteins and conjugate proteins can only cope with these materials in soluble form. A number of methods have been applied in an attempt to solubilise histocompatibility antigens which are embedded on the cell surface within a large number of chemically complex and, in part, hydrophobic substances. These include pressure-decompression homogenisation, treatment with detergents, digestion with proteolytic enzymes, application of low-frequency sonic energy and extraction with complex and simple salts.

9.3.1 Nitrogen pressure decompression

Nitrogen pressure-decompression homogenisation of mammalian tissue as initially described by Hunter and Commerford[53] was applied by Manson et al.[54] as it was thought least deleterious for the subsequent isolation of subcellular particulates. Briefly, a cell suspension is subjected to positive nitrogen pressure for 15–20 min inside a suitable pressure vessel, the contents of which, driven by internal pressure, are then permitted to emerge through a small orifice. Upon exposure to atmospheric pressure, the nitrogen gas forced into solution by pressure (ca. 1000 lb in^{-2}) comes out of solution as microbubbles within the cell cytoplasm with the result that each cell 'explodes' from within resulting in rupture of the surface membrane and release of its internal content in the surrounding medium. When pressure decompression was applied to cultured mouse lymphoblast cells, L5178Y, 5 μg of microsomal lipoprotein (MLP) could be obtained from 2×10^6 cells which constitutes the amount of antigen found to be the minimal sensitising dose required to cause a statistically significant acceleration of the median survival time of test allografts in congenic-resistant mice. It is suggested that MLP is derived from elements of the endoplasmic reticulum in cells such as lymphoblasts or fibroblasts that are processed by nitrogen decompression in a variety of tissues as depicted in Table 9.4[55]. The advantages for the use of this method for transplantation

Table 9.4   Yield of MLP from tissue homogenates by nitrogen decompression*

Species	Tissue	No. of experiments	MLP Average yield (mg g^{-1} wet tissue)
Mouse	L-5178 Y†	33	4.4 ± 1.7
	L-cell†	12	4.5 ± 1.8
	Liver (perfused)	19	11.8 ± 3.3
	Kidney	3	11.7 ± 2.5
	Spleen	28	9.4 ± 1.8
	Thymus	3	5.2 ± 0.5
Rat	Spleen	5	9.8 ± 0.1
Human	W1-L2†	3	7.8 ± 0.1

* From Manson[98]
† Cultured cell line

antigen isolation were delineated by Avis[56]. Accordingly, a high percentage of cell breakage is achieved without any problems of heating at the time of rupture and without breaking of nuclei. There is little likelihood of oxidation as everything takes place in an atmosphere of nitrogen.

9.3.2 Proteolytic enzymes

Histocompatibility antigens have been extracted from human spleenocytes and cultured cells by hypotonic lysis[57] and from murine spleen and tumour cells by papain solubilisation[58, 59]. Antigens obtained in this manner have been purified by cation exchange, Sephadex G-200 or G-150 filtration, cation- and anion-exchange chromatography and disc electrophoresis[58, 60-63].

To obtain membraneous preparations, spleens (150–250 g) are usually minced finely with scissors and are then homogenised at 4 °C in 200 ml cold saline containing antibiotics (cloxacillin 25 mg and ampicillin 25 mg). After

Table 9.5 Protein recovery and specific activities of papain—solubilised human, mouse and rat histocompatibility antigens at various stages of purification*

Purification stage	Human		Mouse		Rat	
	Protein mg	Specific activity units mg⁻¹	Protein mg	Specific activity units mg⁻¹	Protein mg	Specific activity units mg⁻¹
Spleen	100 000	ND†	100 000	ND	100 000	ND
Membrane lipoprotein	3 000	ND	3 000	600	10 000	ND
Papain digest	1 000	400	1 200	75	4 000	400
Sephadex	300	1 000	20	1 200	2 000	250
Cation exchange	150	2 000	8	2 000	500	400
Anion exchange	5	25 000	1.6	5 000	25	5 000
Disc electrophoresis	0.05‡	100 000	0.05	40 000	0.5	25 000

* Modified from Sanderson and Welsh[167]
† ND, not done
‡ Only estimate of protein concentration

van der Waals attractions between apolar groups are relatively weak and hydrogen bonds of the C=O . . . H—N and C=O . . . H—O type are thermodynamically unstable if not protected from water. For this reason,

296	301	313	320	*regions, D and K*
296	301			
296	304	313	320	
299	308	317		
300	311		323	

passage through a stainless steel sieve and two rehomogenisations, the cell suspension is admixed with 20 ml of cold distilled water per 70 ml suspension and stirred at 0–5 °C for 2 h to complete the hypotonic lysis. After removal of cell debris by low speed (500 g, 10 min) centrifugation, the suspension is centrifuged at 10 000 g for 2–3 h, and the resultant pellet then serves as starting material for papain digestion[64]. To solubilise histocompatibility antigens, the above membrane lipoprotein pellet is resuspended in 50 ml 0.01 M Tris buffer, 0.14 M NaCl, pH 8.2. Papain (Worthington; 1 ml of 30 mg ml^{-1} suspension) and 0.1 M systeine (2.5 ml) are added and the mixture stirred for 3 h at 37 °C. Insoluble material is removed by centrifugation at 10 000 g for 2 h, and the resultant supernate represents the crude antigenic extract[64]. The enzymic degradation by papain is usually stopped by the addition of iodoacetamide to a final concentration of 0.01 M. Mann[65] uses a slightly different digestion procedure as he applies 300 mg of crude papain to 300 mg of membrane protein at pH 8.2 and 37 °C for 1 h and then centrifuged at 100 000 g for 2 h to obtain the crude antigen extract as the supernate.

Cation-exchange chromatography on CM-52 cellulose (Whatman) 0.005 M sodium phosphate, pH 5.8, is followed by Sephadex gel filtration in distilled water and then anion-exchange chromatography on DE 52 cellulose using a concave Tris–phosphate gradient consisting of 0.72 volume fractions of 0.05 M, pH 8.0 and 0.28 volume fraction 0.5 M, pH 4.5. In each case the fractions chosen to be pooled for re-chromatography are selected on the basis of their capacity to inhibit the cytotoxic activity of specific alloantisera. Table 9.5 depicts a summary of protein and antigen recovery at the various fractionation steps[64].

Purification of papain-solubilised histocompatibility antigens has also been achieved by analytical polyacrylamide gel electrophoresis simply by slicing out 1.5 mm slices of gel and eluting them with distilled water. Recovery of 100% of inhibitory activity is reported to be achieved by three such extractions[64]. A similar technique, utilising analytical acrylamide electrophoresis to purify papain-solubilised HL-A alloantigens has also been reported by Mann et al.[62] and for H-2 antigens by Shimada and Nathenson[61].

9.3.3 Detergents

The early efforts to solubilise histocompatibility antigens with detergents and phospholipase A from murine sarcoma I cells have been reviewed recently[66, 67]. Although these efforts by Kandutsch and Stimpfling[68] and Graff and Kandutsch[69] generally produced antigenically-active immunogenic moieties; these materials were usually poorly soluble once detergent was removed and were so complex in nature that it was almost impossible to characterise them by physico-chemical means. More recently, Hilgert et al.[70] evaluated the effectiveness of three detergents, Triton X-100, Triton X-114 and potassium cholate to solubilise H-2 antigens from a particulate fraction of sarcoma I. The ^{51}Cr-cytotoxicity assay was used to measure antigenic activities. Both cholate and Triton X-114 was found more suitable than Triton X-100, since they were equally effective when used for shorter periods of time and at lower concentration. However, all these antigen preparations were not water soluble when placed in dilute salt solutions in the absence of detergent.

Human histocompatibility antigens were extracted with deoxycholate from human tissue culture cell lines by Metzgar *et al.*[71]. Briefly, after addition of deoxyribonuclease (1/10 volume, 0.5 mg ml^{-1} in phosphate-buffered saline), deoxycholate was added (1/10 volume of a 5% solution in water) and the mixture incubated for 15 min at 37 °C; MgCl$_2$ (0.08 M) was then added and the mixture incubated for an additional 15 min. The suspension was adjusted to 0.4 M MgCl$_2$ concentration to precipitate deoxycholate and centrifuged at 100 000 g for 1 h; the supernatant was dialysed against phosphate-buffered saline overnight and recentrifuged 100 000 g for 30 min and stored at −75 °C. Antigenic preparations thus prepared specifically inhibited agglutination of leukocytes, mixed agglutinations and cytotoxicity reactions and induced the accelerated rejection of donor skin grafts[72]. The same procedure outlined above was used to extract HL-A antigens from human spleenocytes and the product obtained was compared with that achieved by papain treatment of the same source material. Both preparations specifically inhibited H-AL alloantisera directed against specificities present on the donor cells. Gel filtration of the 2 antigenic preparations on Sephadex G-150 showed two peaks of antigenic activity with the detergent-solubilised extracts, one in the exclusion and one in the inclusion volume, respectively. The papain-solubilised material showed only one activity peak in the inclusion volume. The two activity peaks of the detergent extract were thought to be due to the presence of reaggregated materials[67].

Decyl and dodecyl sulphate was also used to extract murine microsomal lipoproteins which specifically inhibited alloantibody. The antigenic materials were apparently complex lipoproteins as they had sedimentation constants in the range from 15 to 55 which permitted only speculation concerning their actual molecular weight[73].

More recently, non-ionic detergents such as NP-40 were used to solubilise H-2 antigens from murine tumour cells. These materials possessed specific alloantigenic activity and could react with alloantibody at low detergent concentration (0.5%). Although H-2 alloantibodies are non-precipitating, H-2 alloantigens could thus be directly isolated from NP-40 solubilised cell extracts in the form of specific alloantigen–alloantibody complexes by indirect immunological precipitation[74].

9.3.4 Sonication

9.3.4.1 The sonic process

Exposure to low intensity sonic energy liberates a wide variety of active water-soluble components from intracellular, intraorganelle and membraneous locations. Soluble transplantation antigens can be released from mouse, spleen, lung, liver and kidney cells and from their cell membranes; from guinea-pig, spleen, lung, liver, kidney and sarcoma cells; from dog spleen and lymphocytes; from rat spleen and from human adult and foetal spleen, lung, liver and kidney, as well as from cultured lymphoblasts and their exhausted culture media. The purified moiety has antigenic specificity corresponding to the histocompatibility phenotype of the donor. Since they affect the survival of allografts and participate in specific immunologic reactions, these solubilised substances fulfil the criteria of transplantation antigens[66, 75].

(a) *Sonic and ultrasonic energy*—The effects of both sonic (<16 kHz) and of ultrasonic (>16 kHz) energy have been reviewed by Grabar[76] and by Hughes and Nyborg[77]. The main effects of sonic energy are mechanical as the radiation pressures of the sonic wave generate agitation similar to foaming and shearing due to the friction caused by the transport of molecules at rates different than the solvent. The passage of sonic waves results in local pressure reductions causing bubbles of gas and/or vapour to grow and to undergo cavitation. This latter effect is primarily responsible for the disruption of cells and the release of transplantation antigens.

Sonic energy disrupts animal, plant and bacterial cells and degrades or depolymerises macromolecules. The effects of the exposure depends upon the intensity, i.e. the greater the intensity the more pronounced the destruction. Whereas sonic energy fragments anisometric molecules such as DNA by breaking across the phosphate sugar backbone, its effects on proteins depends not only on its intensity but also on the nature of the protein[78]. Ultrasound alters the three-dimensional structure of macromolecules due to hydrogen bond breakage, oxidation of sulphydryl groups, disulphide interchange reactions or direct peptide bond cleavage[79, 80]). Thus, after exposure to 16 kHz waves, ovalbumin becomes insoluble and acquires a new immunologic specificity.

In contrast, application of low frequency sound (9 kHz) for 2 h does not alter the physical properties of bovine serum albumin[81]. Thus, by choosing the intensity and frequency of the sonic generator, one commits himself to the physico-chemical effects in the material subjected to this treatment. Two types of magnetostrictive generators are in wide use: (i) low-intensity diaphragm-mediated 9–10 kHz, 15.5 W cm^{-2} machines manufactured by Raytheon and (ii) ultrasonic 20 kHz 60 W cm^{-2} probe-mediated instruments available from M.S.E. and Branson. While the second type of instrument is quite easy to use and totally destroys cellular particles, the energy it delivers also effectively destroys transplantation antigens. Thus, murine lymphoid cells yielded only a trace of sensitising activity after ultrasonication and ultracentrifugation at 173 000 g[82]. In contrast, low-frequency and low-intensity sonic energy liberates water-soluble, potent transplantation antigens. This finding is consistent with the extensive literature on the application of this form of energy to the extraction of biologically-active materials from animal, plant and bacterial cells (for a review see Refs. 75 and 83).

(b) *Conditions for sonic release of transplantation antigens*—The conditions of sonic exposure for efficient release of transplantation antigens are governed by (i) intensity and frequency, (ii) nature of the medium, (iii) temperature, (iv) length of exposure; and (v) concentration of the cell suspension. In low-intensity sonication, the 250 W power input is converted to a 175 W output with radiofrequency output transduced to physical energy yielding on average 42 W which is distributed on a 15.5 W cm^{-2} stellite diaphragm area. The intensity of the sonic energy and the efficiency of transduction can be determined either with a cavitation meter or a colouric test. Even after prolonged periods of sonic exposure the released antigenic activity is not denatured, an observation confirmed by exposure of purified HL-A antigen to 10 kHz sonication without change of its serological activity[84].

The suspension medium should not interfere with cell dispersion. The latter can be easily measured with a Coulter Counter[85]. The particle size profile reveals the number of clumped (threshold value of 90) *v.* single cells (threshold value of 60). Many cell clumps are undesirable as sonic energy is dissipated to disperse them. One optimal medium with low-viscosity stabilising nuclei, intracellular organelles and membrane vesicles is that of 0.05 M Tris, 0.08 M $MgCl_2$, 0.0025 M KCl and 0.15 M sucrose adjusted to pH 7.45 at 25 °C[83].

The temperature of sonication must be held at 7 °C or less by perfusion of the sonication chamber with an alcohol: water mixture precooled to −10 °C. The number of intact cells is related logarithmically to the length of sonic exposure. Thus, when cell suspensions containing 4×10^7 cultured human lymphoblasts per ml were exposed to sonic energy, maximal release of antigens with HL-A 2 specificity occurred at 5 min. During the period from 0 to 5 min a logarithmic increase in antigenic activity occurred. Thereafter the total antigenic activity released did not change markedly. In practice the point of maximal antigen release corresponds to the disappearance of 90 to 95% of the intact cells[83]. In contrast to adult tissues and cells, foetal lung, liver and spleen cells were more sensitive to sonic energy, releasing their antigenic activity within 2 min[86].

The role of cell concentration is depicted in Figure 9.1. At 5 min sonication 40% of the 778×10^6 guinea-pig lymphoid cells ml^{-1}, 30% of the 148×10^6 cells ml^{-1}, 25% of the 60×10^6 and 3–5% of 2.5–50×10^6 cells ml^{-1} were intact. Similar results were obtained with murine and human cells. Monodisperse suspensions were most efficiently handled at 50×10^6 cell ml^{-1}.

9.3.4.2 *Transplantation antigens released by sonic energy*

(a) *Mouse*—Using a 9 kHz Raytheon Model S102A generator, soluble transplantation antigen was released from murine cells. After sonic treatment, *ca.* 22% of the antigenic activity was present in soluble form[87]. Soluble antigens were prepared from lung, spleen, brain, kidney and liver in order of decreasing potency and doses of 40 μg of soluble material immunised allogenic mice to reject skin grafts[88]. Antigen prepared from mice bearing determinants with $H\text{-}2^a$, $H\text{-}2^q$, $H\text{-}2^d$ and $H\text{-}2^k$ specificities, respectively, induced immunity against skin and subcutaneous tumour implants in hosts differing at combined H-2 and non-H-2 disparities as well as in hosts differing for solely non-H-2 factor(s)[89].

(b) *Rat*—Zimmerman[90] sonicated Lewis × Brown Norway F_1 hybrid male rat splenic cells in the manner described above and obtained an antigen which did not sediment at 150 000 g. Untreated allogenic Lewis rats survived for only 9 days following bilateral nephrectomy and implantation of an F_1 hybrid kidney. However, animals pretreated with 60×10^6 cell equivalents of soluble F_1 antigen on the day of transplantation survived for *ca.* 40 days, while those pretreated with this dose of antigen 1 week prior to transplantation survived as long as 200 days without deterioration of renal function or the use of immunosuppressive agents. Zimmerman[90] proposed that the graft prolongation was due to specific active-graft enhancement, although it has not been possible thus far to produce it by passive transfer of a humoral factor.

(c) *Guinea-pig*—Soluble transplantation antigens were prepared by exposing dissociated spleen, lung, liver and kidney cells of inbred histoincompatible strains 2 and 13 to 10 kHz energy generated by the Raytheon Model DF 101[91]. Fractionation of the 135 000 g active supernate on Sephadex G-200 resulted in the isolation of an antigenically-active fraction (K_D 0.92). Purification by discontinuous electrophoresis in a 7.5% acrylamide gel revealed at least 20 components (Figure 9.2). The antigenic activity was, however, confined to a moiety with a relative mobility compared to that of the tracking dye front of 0.73–0.74. This antigen elicited direct delayed hypersensitivity reactions in hosts presensitised with skin grafts, interacted with immune allogenic

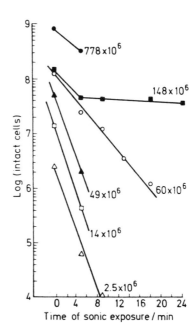

Figure 9.1 Effect of initial lymphocyte concentration on sonic disruption

lymphocytes in local passive transfers into third party guinea-pig or xenogeneic irradiated hamster hosts and stimulated lymphoblastic transformation in tissue culture. Purified soluble antigen induced allogeneic hosts to reject donor-type skin allografts in accelerated fashion[92].

Because of their distinctive biological activities, these antigens were subjected to chemical characterisation. Electrophoretically, the antigenic moiety was homogeneous as it migrated as a single component at acid or alkaline pH values as determined by sensitive radiolabelling techniques (Figure 9.3)[91]. The molecular weight of the antigen was determined to be 15 000 dalton by ultracentrifugal analyses using Yphantis sedimentation-equilibrium methods, by gel filtration on calibrated Sephadex columns and by calculation from the integral amino acid composition. On one occasion either a degradation product or a 'true' monomer of 7000 dalton was detected in a purified preparation subjected to ultracentrifugational analyses in the presence of 6 M guanidine–HCl[93].

Chemical analyses of the purified antigenic moiety of these guinea-pig strains failed to reveal lipid or carbohydrate at levels $>1\%$[94]. The amino acid composition of these strain 2 and 13 antigens was characteristic and reproducible. They contained relatively large amounts of acidic amino acids, consistent with their high electrophoretic mobility at alkaline pH and a large number of serine and threonine residues, suggesting little likelihood of an α-helical configuration. Of interest were the distinct and statistically-significant differences in the content of certain amino acids, i.e. serine, alanine, valine, isoleucine, leucine, between antigens derived from strain 2 and strain 13 animals (Table 9.6). Since the remaining amino acids were present in similar amounts, it

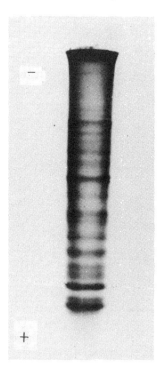

Figure 9.2 Electrophoretic profile of extract from sonically treated guinea-pig spleen cells. Acrylamide gel electrophoresis was performed in 7.5% gels, pH 9.4 at 25 °C

seemed that the allotypic expression of these transplantation antigens was related to protein structure[95].

(d) *Dog*—Wilson and his colleagues[96] extracted water soluble antigens by sonic exposure of dog spleen cells and lymphocytes and demonstrated that pretreatment with antigen produces accelerated rejection, no effect, or prolonged survival depending upon the dose and timing of antigen injections. In bilaterally nephrectomised dogs random renal allografts were rejected at 10 days. Treatment with soluble antigen (105 000 g supernatant) combined with low doses of post-transplant immunosuppressive agents resulted in consistent graft survival of 45 days and occasional prolongation to one year.

(e) *Human organs*—Spleen, lung or kidney cell suspensions were exposed to 10 kHz sonic energy for 5 min. The 130 000 g supernate when passed through Sephadex G-200 yielded an active moiety. This antigen was electrophoresed on acrylamide gels similar to the guinea-pig antigen moiety described above. The active component (R_f 0.78–0.80) elicited hypersensitivity reactions in individuals pre-immunised by leukocyte injection and inhibited the cytotoxic action of alloantisera reactive against HL-A specificities present in the organ donor[97].

Table 9.6 Amino acid compositions of guinea-pig transplantation antigens*

Amino acid†	Strain 2‡ Mol %	Strain 13 Mol %	Difference§ (Strain 2)−(Strain 13)
Lysine	7.94±0.44	8.25±0.81	−0.31
Histidine	2.23±0.18	2.34±0.50	−0.11
Arginine	3.64±0.28	2.96±0.20	+0.68
Aspartic acid	11.84±0.30	11.98±0.49	−0.14
Threonine	6.42±0.02	6.06±0.07	+0.36
Serine	*10.95±0.18*	*18.87±0.04*	*−7.92*
Glutamic acid	16.63±0.71	16.75±0.21	−0.12
Proline	4.30±0.26	4.29±0.81	±0.01
Alanine	11.40±0.08	7.96±0.15	+3.44
Half-cystine	trace	trace	—
Valine	*6.46±0.13*	*5.48±0.20*	*+0.98*
Methionine	0.74±0.22	trace	+0.74
Isoleucine	*4.46±0.16*	*3.32±0.01*	*+1.14*
Leucine	*8.58±0.05*	*7.19±0.03*	*+1.39*
Tyrosine	0.86±0.16	1.66±0.24	−0.80
Phenylalanine	3.74±0.27	2.96±0.13	+0.78
Hexosamine	absent	absent	—

* Values are expressed as mol %
† Glycine was not determined due to residual binding following disc electrophoresis
‡ Mol % of each amino acid with standard deviations calculated from two analyses
§ Difference of means in mol %: 2<13 is negative. 2>13 is positive. Amino acids which differ significantly at the $P<0.01$ level are in italics

There were a number of problems with the antigens isolated from human organs: (i) the antigens lost their activity during 48 h storage at −20 °C, (ii) the antigens could be purified from closely associated contaminants only by electrophoresis in 8 M urea which interfered with its biological activity; and (iii) there were ca. 8% anomalous serological reactions, i.e. CYNAP (cytotoxicity-negative absorption-positive)[98].

(f) *Human lymphoid cell lines*—The utilisation of cultured human lymphoid cells as a source for the extraction of HL-A antigens overcame the problem inherent in the use of human organs listed above. In addition, since a number of cultured long-term cell lines were available yielding large numbers of lymphoblasts, it became possible to determine the yield, assess the reproducibility of the extraction method and to accumulate sufficient amounts of material for chemical analysis.

The antigenic moiety of 135 000 g supernates of sonicated suspensions of 25–40 × 10⁶ lymphoblasts ml⁻¹ was purified by fractional salting out at 0.5 ammonium sulphate saturation, Sephadex G-200 gel filtration and preparative discontinuous acrylamide gel electrophoresis. The active component

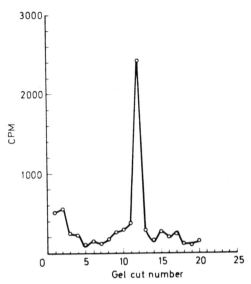

Figure 9.3 Electrophoretic profile of electrophoretically purified guinea-pig transplantation antigens. Antigen had been labelled with ^{125}I to increase the sensitivity of detecting any microheterogeneity

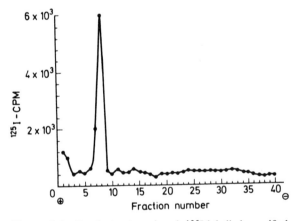

Figure 9.4 Re-electrophoresis of ^{125}I-labelled, purified HL-A antigen solubilised by low-frequency sound treatment of cultured lymphoid cells RPMI 1788 (pH 9.4, 25 °C, 7.5% polyacrylamide gel)

(R_f 0.78–0.80) was shown to be free of contaminants by radiolabelling methods (Figure 9.4). The antigenic moiety inhibited alloantisera in a pattern consistent with the phenotype of the donor from which the cell line was derived. From 45–60% of the inhibitory activity of the 130 000 g supernate was recovered in the purified component with a 25-fold increase in antigenic potency[84].

The antigen had a molecular weight of 34 600 dalton and was 94% mono-disperse as judged from Yphantis sedimentation equilibrium studies. The amino acid composition of alloantigens purified from cell lines derived from donors with different HL-A phenotypes revealed distinct statistically-signifi-cant differences in their content of aspartic acid, serine, proline, alanine and tyrosine. These findings reinforced those noted in strain 2 and 13 guinea-pigs and together suggested that amino acids play an important role in determin-ing alloantigenic specificity in transplantation.

9.3.5 Solubilisation of HL-A antigens with complex and simple salts

Recently additional methods were described for HL-A antigen solubilisation which owe their effectiveness largely to non-covalent bond cleavage. These include (a) complex salts, namely TIS, i.e. a Tris salt of 2-hydroxy-3, 5-di-iodobenzoic acid[65, 99] and (b) simple salts such as potassium chloride[84, 100].

9.3.5.1 *Complex salts*

TIS was reported to release from 7–12% of the total antigenic activity detected on the surface of lymphocytes as compared with 15–20% release obtained from these cells by papain. The papain-solubilised material appeared electro-phoretically complex, whereas the TIS extract seemed more uniform by this criteria[65]. However, TIS is difficult to remove from proteins due to its di-iodo groups which at alkaline pH can readily form covalent bonds with reactive moieties on amino acids, e.g. sulphydryl, phenolic hydroxyl and amino groups. Additional purification is somewhat impaired by this phenomenon. TIS apparently effectively extracts HL-A antigens at a 0.1 M concentration, while it destroys antigenic activity completely at 0.2 M although solubilising 80% of the cell membrane material[65].

9.3.5.2 *Simple salts*

The extraction of cultured human lymphoid cells with 3 M KCl prove to be one of the more promising methods to obtain water-soluble histocompatibility antigens as it can extract soluble HL-A antigens in yields as high as 80%[100]. The major advantage of this method is its simplicity and excellent reproduc-ibility as well as its efficacy in producing relatively high antigen yields. This method has now found additional wide use for (a) the solubilisation of HL-A antigens from spleen cells[101, 102], (b) the extraction of soluble H-2 antigens from peripheral murine leukocytes and from cultured murine leukaemia L1210 cells[103] and (c) the extraction of tumour specific antigens from diethyl nitrosamine-induced guinea-pig sarcomas[104].

(a) *Mechanism of KCl extraction of HL-A antigens*—The mode of action of KCl in solubilising HL-A antigens from the cell surface is generally assumed to be that of a 'chaotropic agent.' In this regard, Hofmeister[105] long ago recognised that ions differ in their efficiency to salt out globulins. Those ions, being most effective in this regard, cause folding, coiling and association of proteins whereas less effective precipitants trigger dissociation and unfolding. These latter ions have been termed 'chaotropic' by Hamguchi and Geiduschek[106]. These investigators thought that such anions break hydrophobic bonds mainly by their disordering effects on the ordered structure of water. The action of chaotropic ions and the role of water structure and hydrophobic bonding in the stabilisation of macromolecules have been discussed in an extensive review by Dandliker and de Saussure[107]. The possible role of KCl in the dissociation of HL-A antigens from lymphoid cell surfaces has been discussed in detail by Reisfeld *et al.*[108]. Briefly, since cell membrane structures are held together mainly by hydrophobic bonds, substances associated with cell surfaces have poor water solubility. The major contribution to their stability in aqueous media is made by hydrophobic attraction forces, largely because van der Waals attractions between apolar groups are relatively weak and hydrogen bonds of the C—O ... H—N and C—O ... H—O type are thermodynamically unstable if not protected from water. For this reason, apolar groups form hydrophic bonds largely because of their thermodynamically unfavourable reaction with water. Once an apolar molecule is transferred from a lipophilic environment to water, there is a decrease in entropy related almost entirely to the highly ordered structure of water. Such a negative entropy change can, in turn, be diminished by increasing any disorder in water structure. This can be accomplished by certain inorganic anions, e.g. SCN^-, ClO_4^-, I^-, Br^- or Cl^-, which possess large positive entropies due to their structure breaking effects on water. These anions act as chaotropic agents and also decrease the polarity of the surrounding water, making it more lipophilic and thus weakening hydrophobic attractions and facilitating the entry of apolar ions into the aqueous phase. Although Cl^- ions are only weak chaotropic agents, they seem highly effective in solubilising HL-A antigens from lymphoid cell surfaces.

(b) *Solubilisation of HL-A antigens by 3 M KCl extraction*—The KCl extraction technique is carried out essentially as described by Reisfeld *et al.*[100]. Thus, cultured human lymphoid cells are washed three times with phosphate-buffered saline (0.15 M) at pH 7.4 and then dispersed by vibration on a Vortex mixer to be resuspended in 0.9% NaCl solution containing 3 M KCl buffered with phosphate (0.015 M) at pH 7.4 (20 ml solvent per 10^9 cells). The suspension is gently agitated on a mechanical shaker for 16 h at 4 °C and then centrifuged at 163 000 g (average) for 1 h. The supernatant, when dialysed at 4 °C against two changes each of 100 volume of saline, forms a gelatinous precipitate containing primarily DNA. This material is easily removed by centrifugation at 1500 g for 20 min. Extraction for 16 h with 3 M KCl proved optimal. Prolonged extraction time, up to 96 h, failed to increase the yield to any marked extent, but no destruction of solubilised HL-A antigenic activity was observed.

Good viability of cultured cells utilised for antigen extraction is most important in order to achieve maximal yields, as batches of cells with less than 50% viability yielded only *ca.* 10% of soluble HL-A antigen with relatively poor immunological potency in contrast with the 50–80% recovery values achieved when the cells had 95–100% viability. Table 9.7 shows some of the

Table 9.7 Yields of soluble HL-A antigen from cultured cell lines

Cell line	HL-A	ID_{50} units/* 10^9 cells	AD_{50} units/† 10^9 cells	Percentage‡ Recovery
RPMI 1788	2	920 000	1 082 350	85
	7	341 000	532 800	64
RPMI 4098	3	1 666 666	1 666 666	100
RPMI 7249	2	350 000	1 250 000	28
	7	35 000	285 000	12
WI-L2	2	2 785 712	3 061 222	91
	5	793 912	980 138	81

* Number of ID_{50} inhibiting doses (µg) per mg of antigen: the ID_{50} inhibition dose represents amount of antigen (µg) necessary to halve the cytotoxic activity of an HL-A alloantiserum in the microcytotoxicity test
† Number of cells required for 50% reduction of the cytotoxic activity of an HL-A alloantiserum
‡ Percentage recovery = (ID_{50} units/10^9 cells)/(AD_{50} units/10^9 cells) × 100

typical yields and immunological potency of soluble HL-A antigens extracted from cultured cells.

The HL-A antigenic activity of crude KCl extracts from cultured lymphoid cells proved to be very stable at $-20\,°C$ over periods up to 2 years. In a few instances, some antigen preparations did, however, lose some antigenic activity. Filtering crude 3 M KCl extracts through millipore filters (0.22 µm) renders the occasionally opalescent antigen crystal clear without destroying any of its serologic reactivity.

(c) *Purification of KCl-solubilised HL-A antigens*—KCl-solubilised HL-A antigens have been purified by preparative acrylamide gel electrophoresis essentially as described by Reisfeld and Kahan[109]. It is feasible to apply as much as 100 mg of crude antigen extract to a Buchler Polyprep 100 column and to obtain *ca.* 1–2 mg of highly purified antigen. Soluble extracts in saline are dialysed against pH 6.7 (0.045 M Tris, 0.032 M H_3PO_4) buffer and applied to the column usually in volumes of up to 10 ml. Electrophoresis is carried out in system 'B' of Rodbard and Chrambach[110] (pH 9.6, 7.5% acrylamide gel) at a constant current of 35 mA. Fractions (8 ml) are collected at a flow rate of 0.8 ml min^{-1} with a Tris–HCl elution buffer (0.138 M Tris, 0.18 M HCl, pH 8.2 containing 5% sucrose). The fractions eluting at a relative mobility of 0.78–0.80 as compared to the dye-buffer front exhibit antigenic activity as they specifically inhibit the cytotoxic reactions of HL-A alloantisera. Upon re-electrophoresis in the same preparative system, the active antigenic moiety consists essentially of a single electrophoretic component when analysed by analytical gel electrophoresis (Figure 9.5). The yield of antigen recovery from the gel column was ascertained by incubating 1 × 10^9 cells cultured in log growth phase (2 × 10^7 cells ml^{-1}) for 4 h with a mixture of [^{3}H] labelled amino acids (2.5 mCi total) in Eagle's minimum essential medium which during a period of 30 min contained only 1 % of its normal complement of amino acids. Under these conditions, *ca.* 15 % of the radiolabel was incorporated into the cells while 2 % was detected in the ultracentrifugal supernate, i.e. the crude antigen extract and 0.04 % in the purified antigen. In the best case, 2 % of the nitrogen and from 45–60 % of the total antigenic activity applied to the acrylamide gel column initially can be recovered in the purified component with a 20-fold increase in antigenic activity, i.e. ID_{50} units mg^{-2} nitrogen[109].

The physico-chemical properties of KCl-solubilised antigens have been investigated to some extent[108, 109], and they were shown to possess size homogeneity as judged from studies utilising Archibald sedimentation equilibrium analyses. The electrophoretically-purified antigenic moiety is monodisperse and has a sedimentation coefficient $S_{20,w}$ of 2.3 and a mol. wt. of 31 000

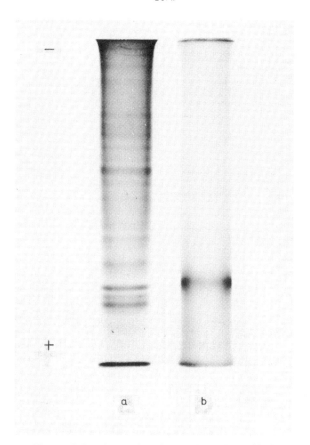

Figure 9.5 Electrophoretic profile of purified HL-A antigens isolated from cell line RPMI 1788. (a) Antigen extract prior to preparative acrylamide gel electrophoresis. (b) HL-A antigenic moiety isolated by preparative electrophoresis and re-electrophoresis

daltons, assuming a partial specific volume of 0.72. The purified antigen possesses not only size uniformity but also electrophoretic homogeneity in polyacrylamide gels at varying pH values and gel porosity. Structural homogeneity is also suggested by tryptic peptide maps showing the number of peptides (24) expected from the arginine (5) and lysine (18) residues found upon amino acid analysis[109] (Figure 9.6).

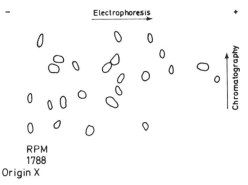

RPM
1788
Origin X

Figure 9.6 Tryptic peptide map of electrophoretically purified HL-A antigen isolated from cultured cells (RPMI 1788) which had been pulse labelled in log growth phase with a mixture of [14C] amino acids. Electrophoresis was performed at pH 3.5

In conclusion, as far as the advantages and disadvantages of the various solubilisation procedures are concerned, it is obvious that not one of them is ideal. All methods presently used are non-specific, i.e. they extract vast amounts of contaminant materials together with relatively very small amounts of antigen making the purification a 'needle in the haystack' problem. The choice of solubilisation procedure depends to some extent on one's objectives. Thus, if the goal is to isolate any kind of protein or glycoprotein fragment with antigenic activity as evidenced, e.g. by serologic reactivity, it seems reasonable to employ enzymatic techniques. For this purpose one can even utilise a relatively non-specific proteolytic enzyme such as papain, provided that it is feasible to more or less reproducibly produce the same chemically defined fragment with a defined antigenic reactivity. For certain purposes, it may be worth while to employ detergents such as NP-40 or deoxycholate which 'solubilise' the plasma membrane but possibly also membranes of intracellular organelles. Actually the micelles bearing antigenic activity which are produced by detergent action may resemble most closely the actual 'membrane representation' of antigenic determinants and can thus be used for certain biological experiments where for some reason whole viable cells are undesirable. Detergents produce, of course, chemically highly complex materials and often enhance the activity of cellular proteolytic enzymes (Manson, personal communication), which complicates the chemical characterisation of antigens solubilised by this method. The use of low-frequency sound to solubilise H-antigens has the disadvantage of requiring specialised equipment and requires considerable time as due to the size of the sonication chamber only

50 ml of cell suspension can be handled at one time. In addition, this procedure results in antigenic extracts containing large amounts of lipids which often interfere with subsequent purification procedures. The advantage of the method is that it is relatively mild and apparently does not break covalent bonds and that it has actually produced soluble transplantation antigens from the cells of many species. The use of hypertonic salt extraction has the advantage of simplicity and relatively high antigen yields. In addition, the mode of action, e.g. 3 M KCl at 4 °C, is essentially that of chaotropic agent effecting the dissociation of non-covalent bonds. It has been demonstrated that this method does not depend for its efficiency on the action of proteolytic enzymes[111]. Specifically, aliquots taken during the 3 M KCl extraction of HL-A antigen from cultured human lymphoid cells showed little or no proteolytic activity when tested at 37 °C against acid-denatured haemoglobin (Table 9.8).

Table 9.8   Time course study of protease activity* during the 3 M KCl
extraction of cultured lymphocytes

	% Protein digested			
	Time of assay/h			
Cell lines	$\frac{1}{2}$	2	8	20
WI-L2	0.3	1.0	0.9	0.7
RPMI 4098	2.4	1.3	0	0

* 0.5% acid-denatured haemoglobulin was used as substrate. Activity was checked after 1 h incubation at 37 °C at each time point

Essentially, the same results were obtained with casein, azocasein and N,N'-[^{14}C]-dimethyl casein as substrates. Salt digestion, when measured in the extract *per se* showed essentially the same values as depicted in Table 9.8.

There was no correlation between antigen yield and reactivity on the one hand and proteolytic activity on the other since during the early phases of extraction ($\frac{1}{2}$–2 h) when proteolytic activity was at its maximum, antigen yield was only *ca.* 10% of that achieved at 16–20 h when proteolytic activity was negligible. Protease inhibitors such as phenyl methyl sulphonyl fluoride (PMSF), di-isopropylfluorophosphate (DFP), iodoacetamide and EDTA had no effect whatsoever on the detectable low grade proteolytic activity. However, pepstatin, a specific inhibitor for cathepsin D, essentially inhibited proteolytic activity, suggesting that this enzyme is responsible for whatever proteolysis was detectable by Lowry and micro-Kjeldahl techniques or by [^{14}C]-labelling of the casein substrate. Thus, it seems that native proteases have little or no effect on the extraction of soluble HL-A antigens with 3 M KCl. There remains at least the possibility to resolve from the membrane mosaic an antigenic unit with its subunit structure relatively intact, perhaps revealing a polypeptide chain structure interlinked with di-sulphide bridges with different chains expressing the various HL-A specificities of a heterozygous individual. Whether this is indeed feasible is presently being determined in our laboratory. A disadvantage of this method is that it releases large amounts of DNA and nuclear protein materials which interfere with purification procedures unless they are removed to a large extent. It is reasonable to assume that when more is known about the physico-chemical nature of histocompatibility antigenic determinants and their mode of attachment to cell membranes, highly specific and effective methods may be developed which are more suitable than the techniques presently in use.

9.4 SEROLOGICAL DETECTION OF SOLUBLE HISTOCOMPATIBILITY ANTIGENS

Soluble HL-A antigens are commonly detected *in vitro* by serological methods based on the ability of these cell surface antigens to combine specifically with cytotoxic HL-A alloantibody and thus to prevent their lytic action on selected target cells in the presence of complement. The reaction mixture thus consists of (a) peripheral or cultured lymphoid cells as target cells, (b) human cytotoxic alloantisera as antibody and (c) fresh rabbit serum as a source of complement. The interaction of antibody and complement which produces functional damage to the cell membrane can be detected by either (i) phase-contrast microscopy, (ii) exclusion of supravital dyes, e.g. eosin; (iii) uptake of a fluorescent dye, e.g. fluorescein diacetate; or (iv) release of intracellular isotopic markers such as ^{51}Cr from labelled cells (for a review see Refs. 38, 64, 66 and 112).

The activity of the soluble antigen is measured as a decreased potency of the cytotoxic alloantibody preincubated with soluble antigen detectable morphologically as an increased precentage of viable target cells or isotopically by diminished release of intracellular markers such as ^{51}Cr.

9.4.1 The blocking assay

In this assay alloantiserum at various selected dilutions is preincubated with 1 μl of twofold progressive dilutions of HL-A antigen[97]. To achieve complete blocking of the antibody, incubation is carried out for 60 min at room temperature after which target cells are added and the mixture is incubated for an additional 60 min. If a supravital dye like eosin is used, then 2 μl of a 5% solution is added to each microdroplet and after 2 min the reaction is stopped by the addition of 1 μl of 36% formalin. Microdroplets under oil are examined for cell survival by inverted phase-contrast microscopy at a magnification of 320×.

The target cells are lymphocytes from subjects typed for all recognised HL-A specificities. One needs at least one target cell for each specificity in order to compare the inhibitory capacity of the soluble alloantigen with the phenotype of the antigenic source material. To avoid erroneous results, operationally monospecific[113] HL-A alloantisera are required. To test the specificity of the assay, it is necessary to demonstrate that each antiserum selected for the homologous antigen is not inhibited by antigenic preparations lacking the specificity against which the alloantibody is directed. This is illustrated in Figure 9.7. Each antiserum has to be used at the highest dilution at which

95% cell death (zero cytotoxicity units) occurs, as this has been found to be most sensitive for the detection of soluble alloantigen. It is useful to perform inhibition reactions at zero cytotoxic units and at both twofold greater and twofold lower concentrations, since the alloantiserum titre can vary from one

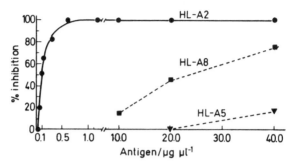

Figure 9.7 Specificity ratio. The inhibitory activity of RPMI 1788 (HL-A 2, 10, 7, 14) against TO-11-03 (homologous anti-HL-A 2 alloantiserum) and Chayra (anti-HL-A 8) and DE-66 (anti-HL-A 5), both indifferent alloantisera, is plotted on an arithmetical scale. Note that only 0.2 μg μl antigen is required to halve the cytotoxic activity of the anti-HL-A sera while at least 20 μg ul^{-1} is required to achieve this with the anti-HL-A 8 sera, indicating a specificity ratio of at least 100

time to the next. Control reactions include alloantiserum incubated with Hank's buffered salt solution (BSS) instead of soluble antigen to check the serum titre. Cell viability is also examined by incubating cells with BSS alone and with complement alone; the experiment is considered invalid whenever the viability of the cells is <95%.

9.4.1.1 Inhibition parameters

A number of parameters were adapted in order to compare data among different laboratories[84, 114]: (a) inhibition dose (ID_{50}) is the dose of antigen required to halve the cytotoxic potency of a specific alloantiserum; (b) avidity coefficient (AC) represents the association constant of the antigen–antibody complex, (c) specificity ratio (SR) is the ratio of ID_{50} of an antigen preparation against an indifferent serum v. the ID_{50} of the same preparation against an antiserum recognising the determinant present on the donor cells.

(a) *Inhibition dosage*—The percentage inhibition is calculated as follows:

$$\% \text{ inhibition} = 100 - \frac{\% \text{ cells killed in presence of inhibitor}}{\% \text{ cells killed in absence of inhibitor}} \times 100$$

The percentage of inhibition of a cytotoxic alloantiserum is plotted on a arithmetic scale against the amount of antigen added to the antiserum. The relationship between the two parameters is expressed in sigmoidal fashion

(Figure 9.7). It is possible to calculate from this curve the amount of antigen (as $\mu g\ \mu l^{-1}$) required for a 50% reduction in the cytotoxic activity of the allo-antiserum. This parameter is designated inhibition dosage and named ID_{50}. This value arbitrarily is taken to represent one unit of activity, i.e. the number of units in 1 mg of protein can then be calculated, e.g. if the ID_{50} is 0.05 μg μl^{-1}, the ID_{50} units mg^{-1} will be 20 000 (1000/0.05).

ID_{50} values determined in this way were shown to be quite reproducible[112] and indicate (i) presence of any HL-A specificity under study; (ii) potency of the soluble antigen preparation; and (iii) degree of purification of the antigenic extract.

(b) *Avidity coefficient*—The sigmoidal ID_{50} curve can be converted to a linear function using the Reif[115] modification of the van Krogh equation: $\log g = \log G + 1/m$ [$\log (100 - P)/P$] where g is the ratio of total antigen to total antiserum; P is the potency (expressed as % dead cells) of the serum remaining free in the supernatant following incubation with antigen; $G = g$ when $P = 50\%$; $1/m$ is the slope of the curve. When plotted on a logarithmic scale, the slope of g v. [$(100 - P)/P$] equals $1/m$. The ID_{50} can be read off on the ordinate at the intersection with the linear curve. The slope coefficient expresses the avidity of antigen inhibition, i.e. low values of $1/m$ indicate a strong binding of antibody (i.e. a high AC). The ratio between AC and ID_{50} is expressed arbitrarily as avidity units. The AC is a much more sensitive index of antigen purification than the ID_{50} value as shown in Table 9.9. It is,

Table 9.9 **Serological parameters at various stages of the purification of HL-A antigens**

Antigen	ID_{50}units/mg	ID_{50} Purification	Avidity units/mg (10^3)	Avidity purification
Supernatant, 164 000 g	4 000	1.0	70	1
Precipitate (0.5 saturation) $(NH_4)_2SO_4)$	10 000	2.5	3 500	50
Preparative acrylamide Gel electrophoresis	100 000	25.0	450 000	3 200

however, worth while to mention that in order to convert the sigmoidal curve to a linear function, it is necessary to carry out the inhibition assay with arithmetic rather than geometric dilutions of the antigen preparation. Thus, the procedure is quite time consuming and is not performed routinely in our laboratory.

(c) *Specificity ratio*—The immunological specificity of the alloantigen is reflected by the specificity ratio (SR)[163]. This is the ratio between the concentration of antigen necessary to achieve 50% inhibition of the cytotoxic effect of an alloantiserum directed against an HL-A determinant not present in the donor's phenotype (AD)$_I$ and the concentration required to inhibit an allo-antiserum directed against a determinant *present* in the phenotype of the donor (Ag)$_H$ (Figure 9.7). One of the major limitations in applying SR is the difficulty in obtaining sufficiently concentrated antigenic solutions from which to determine 50% inhibition of the indifferent serum. The value of SR depends upon such variables as (i) amount of alloantibody employed, (ii) antigenic affinities of both homologous and indifferent alloantisera, and (iii) target cells (for a review see Ref. 112).

9.4.2 The absorption test

The relative amounts of HL-A specificities can be evaluated readily by quantitative absorption studies. Aside from aiding studies on cell surface expression and distribution of HL-A determinants, data obtained from this technique makes it feasible to determine soluble antigen yields achieved with different extraction and purification procedures.

In order to conserve alloantisera often in short supply, the following microtechnique has been developed[116]: antiserum (5 µl) is incubated in Beckman microfuge tubes with equal volumes of cell suspension for 60 min at room temperature. The antiserum is then cleared by centrifugation in a Beckman microfuge (5 min, full speed) and the supernatant tested for residual cytotoicity against selected target cells. As control, serum is incubated in parallel with an equal volume of BSS. This same technique is particularly useful in establishing the HL-A phenotype of cultured lymphoid cells. The data can then be compared with that obtained upon direct typing, a procedure which is essential to detect any non-specific inhibition of cytotoxic alloantisera, i.e. CYNAP, phenomena[98]. The same sera employed for the blocking test are used for absorption at 0, 1 and 2 cytotoxic units by absorbing them with increasing concentrations of the same cells used for antigen extraction.

9.4.2.1 Absorption parameters

To facilitate the quantitation of a given number of cells necessary to yield a certain amount of soluble antigen, the following parameters were adopted[117, 118]: (i) absorption dosage (AD_{50}) constitutes the number of cells required to halve the cytotoxic potency of a selected alloantiserum; (ii) cell equivalent (CE_{50}) represents the number of cells from which sufficient soluble HL-A antigen is extracted to achieve 50% inhibition of cytotoxic alloantisera; and (iii) the percentage of recovery is equal to the percentage ratio between absorption dosage (AD_{50}) and the cell equivalents (CD_{50}) required for 50% inhibition of alloantisera.

(a) *Absorption dosage*—The following formula is used to calculate the % absorption from data obtained with the quantitative absorption method:

$$\% \text{ absorption} = 100 - \frac{\% \text{ cells killed by absorbed serum}}{\% \text{ cells killed by non-absorbed serum}} \times 100$$

The percentage of absorption of a cytotoxic alloantiserum is plotted on an arithmetic scale against the concentration of cells added to this alloantiserum. From this sigmoidal curve it is possible to calculate the number of cells required for 50% reduction of the cytotoxic activity of the alloantiserum (AD_{50}).

The AD_{50} parameter indicates presence or absence of any HL-A specificity on the surface of the cell studied as well as the relative concentration of HL-A determinants per cell. This parameter thus makes it feasible to compare the relative amount of the same HL-A specificity on different cells as well as amounts of different HL-A specificities on the same cell. Thus, Table 9.10

Table 9.10 AD_{50} Values for cultured lymphoid cells

Cell line	HL-A	Serum	AD_{50}
WI-L2	2+	TO-11-03	400 ± 50
	5+	D-66	$1\,000 \pm 100$
RPMI 1788	2+	TO-11-03	825 ± 75
	7+	Cutten	$1\,800 \pm 150$

shows that the AD_{50} for HL-A 2 and 7 of cell line RPMI 1788 is double that of cell line WI-L2. However, since the respective surface areas of the cells from the two cultured lines are not known, it is difficult to distinguish clearly whether this difference can be attributed to varying concentrations of the two antigenic specificities on the two cell lines or whether it is merely the result of a difference in the surface area. The difference in AD_{50} for HL-A 2 and 7 and HL-A 2 and five specificities, respectively, could represent an expression of varying concentration of these determinants on the cell surface; however, a difference in affinity of the alloantibody cannot be ruled out and could equally well acount for these data.

(b) *Cell equivalents*—This parameter denoting the number of cells from which one unit of antigenic activity can be extracted can be calculated as follows: $CE_{50} = ID_{50}(C/Pr)$, where C is the number of cells used for antigen extraction and Pr indicates the total yield of protein. For example, if the number of cells used for extraction is 1×10^{10}, the total yield of protein 20×10^3 µg and ID_{50} is 0.1 µg µl^{-1}, the CE_{50} will be 50 000 [0.1 $\times$ 10^{10}/ (20 $\times$ 10^3)]. This parameter is quite useful to compare different cell sources used for antigen extraction. For example, in foetal organs the CE_{50} is considerably lower with kidney cells than with those from either liver or spleen[189]. The CE_{50} also makes possible a comparison of antigens with different specificities extracted from the same cell source. Thus, in cell line RPMI 1780 the CE_{50} value is lower ($CE_{50} = 1200$) for the extraction of HL-A 2 than for that of HL-A 7 antigens ($CE_{50} = 2400$). Finally, determination of CE_{50} values allows one to evaluate the efficiency of different methods of extraction.

(c) *Percentage antigen recovery*—This is determined as follows:

$$\% \text{ recovery} = \frac{AD_{50}}{CE_{50}} \times 100$$

For example, if the AD_{50} (HL-A 2) is 825 (as in cell line RPMI 1788) and the CE_{50} value (HL-A 2) is 1200, then the reccovery of HL-A 2 is 68% (825/1200 $\times$ 100). It must be stressed that this is, of course, only a relative value since the percentage recovery is calculated on the basis of 'absorbing capacity' of the cells and not on the total amount of antigens present on/or within these cells.

In conclusion, serological methods have proven most useful in the study of soluble HL-A alloantigens as they offer a simple and rapid approach for biological evaluation utilising only micro-amounts of reagents. The serologic parameters described are helpful for the standardisation of antigenic activity and can be useful for comparison of data from different laboratories. The quantitative absorption technique offers a means to evaluate antigen yield by different extraction procedures and facilitates the study of antigenic expression on the cell surface. However, it is necessary to point out the limitations of the serological assay of soluble HL-A alloantigens, especially since these methods evaluate only *in vitro* reactivity of cytotoxic alloantisera with these antigens. Thus, such assays are not able to distinguish whether the soluble antigens are true transplantation antigens, i.e. substances which specifically effect allograft survival.

9.5 CHEMICAL AND MOLECULAR NATURE OF HL-A ANTIGENS

Until recently there has been relatively slow progress in the elucidation of the chemical and molecular nature of HL-A antigens. This has been due to a number of circumstances including (a) the chemically complex nature of these antigens due to their intimate association with hydrophobic cell-surface moieties, (b) the non-selective nature of the solubilisation procedures; and (c) the limited amounts of genetically-uniform source materials. Substances as diverse as DNA, lipid, carbohydrate and protein all have been, at one time or another, implicated as the antigenic principle (for reviews see Refs 66 and 119).

More recently the availability of relatively large amounts of cultured lymphoid cells and the development of highly-efficient solubilisation procedures such as 3 M KCl extraction and the application of high-resolution preparative acrylamide-gel electrophoresis have provided the tools to obtain some additional information of the molecular and chemical nature of HL-A antigens[109].

9.5.1 Chemical characteristics

Theoretical considerations and experimental evidence both suggest that H-loci code for polypeptide chains rather than carbohydrate moieties. For example, the finite insertions in the ABO system believed to reflect the action of specific enzymes on precursor molecules are not characteristic of HL-A specificities which are often broadly similar to those seen with polymorphic protein systems. The number of variants characterising the HL-A system may be similar to immunoglobulin allotypes where many mutants are distributed along a limited number of closely-linked structural genes corresponding to many antigenic determinants of a few polypeptide chains. This is in contrast to the ABO system where a limited number of antigenic types are controlled by a few enzymes acting on a common substrate[120].

Available chemical data actually strengthen the hypothesis that HL-A determinants are polypeptide in nature. Thus, antigenic activity is irreversibly destroyed by proteolytic enzymes, e.g. prolonged digestion with papain or trypsin, protein denaturants such as urea and guanidine, pH values >10 and <4, temperatures greater than 50 °C or detergents and complex salts in concentrations sufficient to affect protein confirmation[66].

Thus far there has been relative little evidence suggesting that carbohydrate moieties *per se* are essential for H-antigenic activity, although papain-solubilised H-2 and HL-A antigens were reported to contain from 3–8 % of carbohydrate. However, it is noteworthy that digestion of H-2 antigens with glycosidases and with neuraminedase does not affect their antigenic reactivity *in vitro*[121]. It is also relevant that both guinea-pig transplantation antigens and HL-A antigens solubilised by non-covalent bond cleavage were not found to contain carbohydrates at levels >1 %. Guinea-pig antigen (mol. wt. 15 000) and HL-A antigen (mol. wt. 31 000) would thus contain, respectively, at most one–two carbohydrate residues per mole of antigen. As noted above, the striking amino acid differences between phenotypically different guinea-pig transplantation antigens and HL-A antigens, respectively, together with the phenotypically-determinant differences in peptide maps further argues for H-antigenic determinants to be polypeptide in nature.

9.5.2 Molecular expression of HL-A antigens

Any elucidation of the molecular expression of HL-A antigens is considerably complicated by their cell-membrane association, especially since thus far there is very little known about the detailed cytoarchitecture of mammalian cell membranes. To obtain the gene product of the H-loci in a form amenable to physico-chemical analyses, they have to be obtained in soluble form following their disassociation from the complex hydrophobic lipoprotein lattices on the cell-membrane surface. To gain knowledge of their true molecular expression, H-antigens have to be solubilised without drastically altering their molecular arrangement. This represents a difficult problem which is, of course, not restricted to H-antigens; even extensive research efforts on human blood-group substances have made only very slow progress in elucidating the primary structure of their polypeptide backbone.

In an effort to gain insight into the chemical expression of HL-A antigens, attempts were made to apply proteolysis to obtain fragments with alloantigenic activity. Such antigenic moieties were liberated both by autolysis and papain digestion and subsequently purified by gel exclusion chromatography, ion-exchange chromatography and electrophoresis. To define antigenic activity of these fragments, chromatographic fractions defined by elution peaks were correlated with antigenic profiles obtained by *in vitro* inhibition of alloantisera by narrow effluent fractions. At times antigenic activity was not only present in protein peaks but also in fractions apparently devoid of protein. Individual antigenic specificities appeared to be detectable in broad overlapping peaks and often were detectable in more than one chromatographic fraction in a given effluent profile. Some investigators were able to separate fragments bearing determinants of different segregant series by gel filtration on Sephadex G-150. On the other hand, others separated fragments bearing single and multiple antigenic specificities on DEAE-Sephadex and DEAE-cellulose which yet other workers could only separate on acrylamide gel of Bio-gel P2. The data from these experiments illustrate the difficulty in arriving at meaningful conclusions, regarding the molecular nature of HL-A antigenic determinants when using antigen fragments obtained by the action of proteolytic enzymes. Thus far these various fragments have not been purified and characterised chemically to the point which would permit an evaluation of their significance as far as the molecular nature of H-antigens is concerned (for a review see Ref. 66).

Available data obtained largely from the chemical analysis of H-antigens solubilised by either low-frequency sound or 3 M KCl extraction do permit some conclusions as well as hypotheses concerning the molecular nature of allotype of H-antigens. Thus, there are obvious analogies of H-antigens to immunoglobulin allotypes as H-antigens from histoincompatible donors possess allotypic differences related to protein structure as indicated by their distinct differences in amino acid compositions and peptide maps. Analogous to rabbit and human IgG polypeptide chains, H-antigens also may contain extensive and sharply-divided regions of variability and constancy, with the latter containing some amino acid sequence difference expressing H-allotypy. In this case, functional specialisation of the molecule independent of the histocompatibility system would be expressed in the variable region, as seen in the immunoglobulins where the antibody combining site is thought to be in this region. However, it is also possible that single regions of constant amino acid sequence might have only small defined differences attributable to point mutations. The existing data would be most consistent with the absence of any extended variable region in HL-A antigens as there is seemingly limited detectable heterogeneity of isolated, purified allotypic H-proteins by electrophoretic and peptide mapping techniques. It seems reasonable to conclude that amino acid sequence analysis will be necessary to distinguish the chemical nature of H-allotypy between these two possibilities.

9.5.3 Molecular assembly of H-antigens

It seems reasonable to assume that H-antigens are synthesised by the usual biosynthetic mechanisms even though there are as yet no data regarding messenger RNAs, ribosomal synthesis and generation of nascent polypeptide chains possessing H-specificities. Most likely there are at least two levels of molecular organisation of H-antigens, one at the cytoplasmic level, i.e. assembly of nascent polypeptide chains and the other an organisation of the gene products on the cell surface. If indeed the HL-A genetic model of a set of factors expressed within two mutually exclusive segregant series is correct, then the H genes might translate in the synthesis of four polypeptide chains, one for each of the haplotypic segregant series factors of a heterozygous individual. It seems, indeed, most likely that two factors showing a recombination frequence of *ca.* 1 % controlled by two structural genes as such a recombination frequency corresponds to a distance of 15^5–10^6 nucleotides, i.e. a few hundred average cistrons[122]. Since the LA and FOUR antigens are probably simple proteins, factors of the two series are most likely located on different molecules. Factors within the same segregant series may correspond to antigenic determinants on the same molecule or to antigenic markers situated on different molecules. Such molecules would be expected to have much structural similarity, as they are controlled by adjacent cistrons which arose by gene doubling analogous to the β- and α-chains of haemoglobulins[120].

It seems not very likely that nascent molecules contain the antigenic determinants of the haplotype, i.e. a combination of the two factors, one from each segregant series, are jointly transmitted with the same chromosome. For this occurrence one needs to postulate a polycistronic messenger RNA which seems unlikely in view of the 1 % recombination distance between the LA and FOUR loci. Such a possibility cannot, however, be completely ruled out since one can postulate intrachromosomal translocations similar to those proposed to explain the joining of the V and C regions of Ig polypeptide chains.

While it is tempting to speculate about the cytoplasmic assembly of nascent H-antigen polypeptide chains, it is also possible that there is no assembly at all, but that nascent molecules each bearing one of the four possible H-factors of a heterozygous are each expressed on the cell surface. This assumption is, however, difficult to reconcile with data from antibody blocking tests which suggest a preferential expression of antigenic determinants on the cell surface, i.e. either the haplotype or at least antigenic factors of each series in the 'cis' position[123].

In conclusion, it is, of course, possible to invoke several permutations to explain possible cytoplasmic assembly of nascent H-antigen molecules or recombination of polypeptide chain on the cell surface. However, the limitations of the serological assay method and lack of precise and definite chemical information make this at present an exercise in speculation. Judging from on-going work in several laboratories, it seems likely that there will soon be enough chemical data to reconcile the above speculations with experimentally testable hypotheses.

9.6 PERSPECTIVES ON THE ROLE OF HISTOCOMPATIBILITY ANTIGENS

There are several considerations which suggest that the major histocompatibility antigens have an important biological function. First, a complex polymorphism has been maintained in all mammalian species investigated thus far. Secondly, there has been a consistent expression of HL-A and H-2 antigens on cells maintained in tissue culture even for prolonged periods of time. Thus, human fibroblasts maintain HL-A antigens even in senescence although they lose other specialised features and are morphologically altered[124]. Thirdly, the basic genetic design of histocompatibility systems is remarkably similar in various species suggesting a similarity and indeed a universality in function[125].

The existence of the extensive polymorphism of cell-surface histocompatibility antigens is generally believed to aid in preserving the integrity of the individual; the chemical differences are thought to impede the survival of one individual's cells whenever they invade the tissues of another individual.

However, this postulate is not yet proven and whether it is correct or not remains to be established experimentally.

The polymorphism of the HL-A system is generally believed to confer a selective advantage and thus to be important for the survival of man. Data from family studies do not support the concept of selection at the time of conception. There is also no evidence that selection occurs before birth even when maternal isoimmunisation against alloantigens carried by the foetus has been demonstrated. It seems that pressures for maintaining HL-A polymorphism must occur by selection after birth due to the biological advantages accorded to individuals possessing certain allotypic cell surface markers[126].

Biological superiority in resistance to disease has been studied intensively and individuals possessing certain HL-A phenotypes seem to be less frequently affected by certain diseases. On the other hand, certain antigenic factors are found more frequently in phenotypes of affected individuals. For example, Hodgkin's disease seems to be correlated with an increased frequency of HL-A 5, W5, W15, DA 24 and CM 229. Association of histocompatibility loci with RNA virus infection has been shown by Nandi[127] who demonstrated that R-MTV virus infects only those strains which are compatible at the H-2 locus, suggesting that the virion envelope is coated with part of the preceding host's cell membrane.

Histocompatibility genes, due to the close proximity of the immune response locus IR-1 and of the H-2 locus may well influence immune responsiveness: (a) as a closely-linked gene acting specifically on the binding of antigen to the receptor sites of thymus-derived cells, (b) as an effect of H-antigens acting as receptors due to their stereochemical complementarity; or (c) as a non-specific effect on cell surfaces. Histocompatibility genes might thus be linked to a general responsiveness of the host as described by Biozzi et al.[128].

One of the most basic and intriguing roles of H-antigens was proposed by Burnet[129] who envisioned the threat of deviant cells to the individual as serious as that of any exogenous agent. Burnet proposed that H-surface receptors may serve as checkpoints for wandering recognition lymphocytes serving as watchmen of the immune system. New cell-surface receptors are recognised and destroyed by these 'watchmen.' The selective advantage of this system ensures elimination of foreign and potentially neoplastic clones. In early antogeny, H-antogen receptors on cell surface may even prevent malignancy from being contagious and thus preserve the species. The extensive polymorphism of histocompatibility loci may thus actually provide the variation required to protect the individuality of the members of a species.

At the chemical level, a highly complex problem is coming ever closer to resolution. As in the field of immunoglobulin allotypes, the challenge is to convert a system based on immunogenetic serology into one based on structural genes and translate gene products into amino acid sequences. Although the molecular nature and subunit structure of H-antigens remains to be resolved, there is cause for hope as the genetic polymorphism seems to be expressed by changes in polypeptide structure rather than that of carbohydrates. Thus, it seems feasible to follow in principle the same route taken so successfully for the elucidation of the molecular and chemical structure of the antibody molecule and thus to gain eventually an understanding of H-antigens at the molecular level. If one can judge at all from the saga of the antibody molecule, it would seem reasonable to anticipate that the serology, genetics and physiology of H-antigens will become much more simple and clear once their chemical structure is known[130].

As far as the practical clinical implications of H-antigen research is concerned, it seems relatively unlikely that purified, soluble HL-A antigens will solve all the problems of organ transplantation. Although soluble antigens are more likely to induce tolerance in adult animals than are particulate antigens, the induction of *in vivo* tolerance is as yet far from reality especially since the molecular basis of tolerance at the level of the lymphocyte surface is still unknown. As pointed out by Nossal[130], defined H-antigens will more likely play a role in sorting out phenomena such as enhancement and antibody-mediated tolerance and thus contribute to a better understanding of basic immunological processes. Regardless of whether or not the HL-A system does prove to be the major one controlling transplantation compatibility, it seems likely that chemically defined histocompatibility antigens will play a key role as cell surface receptors affecting input into cells in determining interrelationships between cells and in effecting functional and structural aspects of cell membrane systems. Thus, the polymorphic H-antigens are individuality markers which clearly are crucial for maintaining effective immunological defence and recognition systems of the individual.

Acknowledgement

This is publication number 690 from the Department of Experimental Pathology, Scripps Clinic and Research Foundation, La Jolla, California. This work was supported by United States Public Health Service grant AI 10180, grant 70-615 from the American Heart Association, Inc., Veterans Administration Research support grant Northwestern University Transplantation Research Fund and American Cancer Society grant number IC 84.

References

1. Loeb, L. (1930). *Physiol. Rev.*, **10**, 547
2. Gibson, T. and Medawar, P. B. (1943). *J. Anat.*, **77**, 299
3. Medawar, P. B. (1946). *Brit. J. Exp. Path.*, **27**, 15
4. Simonsen, M. (1962). *CIBA Foundation Symposium on Transplantation*, 185 (G. E. W. Wolstenholme and M. P. Cameron, editors) (London: Churchill)
5. Billingham, R. E., Brent, L. and Medawar, P. B. (1956). *Nature (London)*, **178**, 514
6. Medawar, P. B. (1959). *Cellular and Hormone Aspects of Hypersensitivity States*, 504 (H. S. Lawrence, editor) (New York: Harper Row)
7. Terasaki, P. I. (1970). *Histocompatibility Testing 1970*, 325 (P. I. Terasaki, editor) (Copenhagen: Munksgaard)
8. Cavalli-Sforza, L. L. and Bodmer, W. F. (1971). *The Genetics of Human Populations* (San Francisco: Freeman and Co.)
9. Kissmeyer-Nielsen, F. and Thorsby, E. (1970). *Transplant Rev.*, **4**, 11
10. Dausset, J. (1954). *Vox. Sang. (Basel)*, **4**, 190
11. Miescher, P. and Fauconnet, M. (1954). *Schweiz. Med. Wochnschr.*, **84**, 597
12. Engelfriet, C. P. and Britten, A. (1965). *Vox. Sang.*, **10**, 660
13. Terasaki, P. I. and McClelland, J. (1964). *Nature (London)*, **204**, 998
14. Walford, R. L., Gallagher, R. and Sjaarda, J. R. (1964). *Science*, **144**, 868

15. Aster, R. H., Cooper, H. E. and Singer, D. L. (1964). *J. Lab. Clin. Med.*, **63**, 161
16. Shulman, N. R., Marder, V. J., Hiller, M. C. and Collier, E. M. (1964). *Progr. Hemat.*, **4**, 222
17. Colombani, J., Colombani, M., Benajava, A. and Dausset, J. (1967). *Histocompatibility Testing 1967*, 413 (E. S. Curtoni, P. L. Mattiuz and R. M. Tosi, editors) (Copenhagen: Munksgaard)
18. Colombani, J., Colombani, M. and Dausset, J. (1964). *Ann. N. Y. Acad. Sci.*, **120**, 307
19. Milgrom, F., Kano, K., Barron, A. L. and Witebsky, E. (1964). *J. Immunol.*, **92**, 8
20. Melief, C. J. M., Hart, M., Engelfriet, C. P. and van Loghem, J. J. (1967). *Vox. Sang.*, **12**, 374
21. Boyse, E. A., Old, L. J. and Stockert, E. (1962). *Ann. N. Y. Acad. Sci.*, **99**, 574
22. Wigzell, H. (1965). *Transplantation*, **3**, 423
23. Terasaki, P. I., Vredevoe, D. L. and Mickey, M. R. (1967). *Transplantation*, **5**, 1057
24. Bodmer, W., Tripp, M. and Bodmer, J. (1967). *Histocompatibility Testing 1967*, 341 (E. S. Curtoni, P. L. Mattiuz and R. M. Tosi, editors) (Copenhagen: Munksgaard)
25. Celada, F. and Rotman, B. (1967). *Proc. Nat. Acad. Sci. USA*, **57**, 630
26. Sanderson, A. R. and Batchelor, J. R. (1967). *Histocompatibility Testing 1967*, 367 (E. S. Curtoni, P. L. Mattiuz and R. M. Tosi, editors) (Copenhagen: Munksgaard)
27. Ehrlich, P. and Moregenroth, J. (1901). *Berlin Klin. Wochenschr.*, **38**, 569
28. Landsteiner, K. (1945). *The Specificity of Serological Reactions*, (Boston: Harvard University Press)
29. Forssman, J. (1911). *Biochem. Z.*, **37**, 78
30. Buchbinder, L. (1935). *Arch. Pathol.*, **19**, 841
31. Kaplan, M. H. (1963). *J. Immunol.*, **90**, 595
32. Rapaport, F. T. (1972). *Transplantation Antigens*, 181 (B. D. Kahan and R. A. Reisfeld, editors) (New York: Academic Press)
33. Rapaport, F. T. (1968). *Human Transplantation*, 635 (F. T. Rapaport and J. Dausset, editors) (New York: Grune and Stratton)
34. Rapaport, F. T. and Chase, R. M. (1964). *Science*, **145**, 407
35. Rapaport, F. T., Hanaoka, T., Shimada, T., Cannon, F. D. and Ferrebee, J. W. (1970). *J. Exp. Med.*, **131**, 881
36. Simmons, R. L., Weil, R., Tallent, M. B., Kjelstrand, C. M. and Najarian, J. S. (1970). *Transplant. Proc.*, **3**, 419
37. Hume, D. M., Sterling, W. A., Weymouth, R. S., Siebel, H. R., Madge, G. E. and Lee, H. M. (1970). *Transplant. Proc.*, **3**, 361
38. Ferone, S. and Pellegrino, M. A. (1973). *Contemporary Topics in Molecular Immunology*, 185 (R. A. Reisfeld and W. J. Mandy, editors) (New York: Plenum Press)
39. Hirata, A. A. and Terasaki, P. I. (1970). *Science*, **168**, 1095
40. Pellegrino, M. A., Ferrone, S., Safford, J. W., Hirata, A. A., Terasaki, P. I. and Reisfeld, R. A. (1972). *J. Immunol.*, **109**, 97
41. Ferrone, S., Natali, P. G., Hunter, A., Terasaki, P. I. and Reisfeld, R. A. (1972). *J. Immunol.*, **108**, 1718
42. Dausset, J. (1971). *Transplant. Proc.*, **3**, 8
43. Svejgaard, A. and Kissmeyer-Nielsen, F. (1968). *Nature (London)*, **219**, 868
44. Colombani, J., Colombani, M. and Dausset, J. (1970). *Histocompatibility Testing 1970*, 79 (P. I. Terasaki, editor) (Copenhagen: Munksgaard)
45. Mittal, K. K. and Terasaki, P. I. (1972). *Tissue Antigens*, **2**, 94
46. Dausset, J. and Hors, J. (1971). *Transplant. Proc.*, **3**, 1004
47. Abeyounis, C. J. and Milgrom, F. (1969). *Transplantation*, **1**, 556
48. Sachs, O. H., Winn, H. J. and Russell, P. S. (1971). *J. Immunol.*, **107**, 481
49. Balner, H., Gabb, B. W., Dersjant, H., van Vreeswijk, W., van Leevwen, A. and van Rood, J. J. (1971). *Comparative Genetics and Monkeys, Apes and Man*, 97 (B. Chiarelli, editor) (London: Academic Press)
50. Metzgar, R. J. and Znijewski, C. M. (1966). *Transplantation*, **4**, 84
51. Götze, D., Ferrone, S. and Reisfeld, R. A. (1972). *J. Immunol.*, **109**, 439
52. Medawar, P. B. (1963). *Transplantation*, **1**, 21
53. Hunter, M. S. and Commerford, S. L. (1961). 1. *Biochem. Biophys. Acta*, **47**, 580
54. Manson, L. A., Faschi, G. V. and Palm, J. (1963). *J. Cell. Comp. Physiol.*, **61**, 109
55. Manson, L. A. (1972). *Transplantation Antigens*, 227 (B. D. Kahan and R. A. Reisfeld, editors) (New York: Academic Press)

56. Avis, P. S. G. (1969). *Subcellular Components*, 1 (G. D. Bimie and S. M. Fox, editors) (New York: Plenum Press)
57. Davis, D. A. L. (1966). *Immunology*, **11**, 115
58. Nathenson, S. G. and Davies, D. A. L. (1966). *Proc. Nat. Acad. Sci. USA*, **56**, 676
59. Sanderson, A. R. and Batchelor, J. R. (1968). *Nature (London)*, **219**, 184
60. Sanderson, A. R. (1968). *Nature (London)*, **220**, 192
61. Shinda, A. and Nathenson, S. G. (1969). *Biochemistry*, **8**, 4048
62. Mann, D. L., Rogentine, G. N., Fahey, J. L. and Nathenson, S. G. (1969). *Science*, **163**, 1460
63. Davies, D. A. L. (1969). *Transplantation*, **8**, 51
64. Sanderson, A. R. and Welsh, K. I. (1972). *Transplantation Antigens*, 273 (B. D. Kahan and R. A. Reisfeld, editors) (New York: Academic Press)
65. Mann, D. L. (1972). *Transplantation Antigens*, 287 (B. D. Kahan and R. A. Reisfeld, editors) (New York: Academic Press)
66. Reisfeld, R. A. and Kahan, B. D. (1970). *Advances in Immunology*, vol. 12, 117 (F. J. Dixon and H. G. Kunkel, editors) (New York: Academic Press)
67. Metzgar, R. S., Miller, J. I. and Seigler, H. F. (1972). *Transplantation Antigens*, 299, (B. D. Kahan and R. A. Reisfeld, editors) (New York: Academic Press)
68. Kandutsch, A. A. and Stimpfling, J. H. (1963). *Transplantation*, **1**, 201
69. Graff, R. J. and Kandutsch, A. A. (1966). *Transplantation*, **4**, 465
70. Hilgert, I., Kandutsch, A. A., Cherry, M. and Snell, G. D. (1969). *Transplantation*, **8**, 451
71. Metzgar, R. A., Flanayan, J. F. and Mendes, N. F. (1967). *Histocompatibility Testing 1967*, 307 (E. S. Curtoni, P. L. Mattiuz and R. M. Tosi, editors) (Copenhagen: Munksgaard)
72. Seigler, H. F., Mendes, N. F. and Metzgar, R. S. (1970). *Surgery*, **67**, 261
73. Manson, L. A. and Palm, J. (1968). *Advance in Transplantation*, 301 (J. Dausset, J. Hamburger and G. Mathe, editors) (Copenhagen: Munksgaard)
74. Schwartz, B. D. and Nathenson, S. G. (1971). *J. Immunol.*, **107**, 1363
75. Kahan, B. D. and Reisfeld, R. A. (1971). *Bact. Rev.*, **35**, 59
76. Grabar, P. (1963). *Advan. Biol. Med. Phys.*, **3**, 191
77. Hughes, D. E. and Nyborg, W. L. (1962). *Science*, **138**, 108
78. Nishihara, T. and Doty, P. (1958). *Proc. Nat. Acad. Sci. USA*, **44**, 432
79. Wu, H. and Liu, S. E. (1935). *Proc. Soc. Exp. Biol. Med.*, **28**, 782
80. Kanig, K. and Kunkel, H. (1957). *Hoppe-Seyler Z. Physiol. Chem.*, **309**, 166
81. Hess, E. L., Chun, P. L. and Crowley, R. L. (1964). *Science*, **143**, 1176
82. Billingham, R. E., Brent, L. and Medawar, P. B. (1958). *Transplant. Bull.*, **5**, 377
83. Kahan, B. E. (1972). Transplantation Antigens, 237 (B. D. Kahan and R. A. Reisfeld, editors) (New York: Academic Press)
84. Reisfeld, R. A. and Kahan, B. D. (1970). *Fed. Proc. (Fed. Amer. Soc. Exp. Biol.)*, **28**, 2034
85. Mattern, C., Brackett, S. F. and Olson, B. (1957). *J. Appl. Physiol.*, **10**, 56
86. Pellegrino, M. A., Pellegrino, A. and Kahan, B. D. (1970). *Transplantation*, **10**, 425
87. Kahan, B. D. (1964). *Ph.D. Thesis Dissertation*. University of Chicago
88. Zajtchuk, R., Kahan, B. D. and Adams, W. E. (1966). *Dis. Chest*, **50**, 368
89. Kahan, B. D. (1964). *Fed. Proc. (Fed. Amer. Soc. Exp. Biol.)*, **23**, 352 (Abstr.)
90. Zimmerman, C. E. (1971). *Transplant. Proc.*, **3**, 701
91. Kahan, B. D. and Reisfeld, R. A. (1967). *Proc. Nat. Acad. Sci. USA*, **58**, 1430
92. Kahan, B. D. and Reisfeld, R. A. (1969). *Proc. Soc. Exp. Biol. Med.*, **130**, 765
93. Reisfeld, R. A. (1970). Unpublished observations
94. Kahan, B. D. and Reisfeld, R. A. (1969). *Transplant. Proc.*, **1**, 483
95. Kahan, B. D. and Reisfeld, R. A. (1968). *J. Immunol.*, **101**, 237
96. Wilson, R. E. (1972). *Transplantation Antigens*, 391 (B. D. Kahan and R. A. Reisfeld, editors) (New York: Academic Press)
97. Kahan, B. D., Reisfeld, R. A., Pellegrino, M. A., Curtoni, E. S., Mattiuz, P. L. and Ceppellini, R. (1968). *Proc. Nat. Acad. Sci. USA*, **61**, 897
98. Ferrone, S., Tosi, R. M. and Centis, D. (1967). *Histocompatibility Testing 1967*, 357 (E. S. Curtoni, P. L. Mattiuz and R. M. Tosi, editors) (Copenhagen: Munksgaard)
99. Mann, D. L. and Levy, R. (1971). *Fed. Proc. (Fed. Amer. Soc. Exp. Biol.)*, **30**, 2767
100. Reisfeld, R. A., Pellegrino, M. A. and Kahan, B. D. (1971). *Science*, **172**, 1134

101. Etheredge, E. E. and Najarian, J. J. (1971). *Transplant. Proc.*, **3**, 224
102. Uhlenbruck, G., Voigtmann, R., Salfner, B., Bube, F. W. and Seibel, E. (1973). *Proc. Int. Symp. Standard HL-A Reagents*, in the press
103. Götze, D. and Reisfeld, R. A. (1972). *Fed. Proc. (Fed. Amer. Soc. Exp. Biol.)*, **32**, 643
104. Meltzer, M. S., Leonard, E. J., Rapp, H. J. and Borsos, T. (1971). *J. Nat. Cancer Inst.*, **47**, 703
105. Hofmeister, F. (1888). *Arch. Exp. Pathol. Pharmakol.*, **24**, 247
106. Hamaguchi, K. and Geiduschek, E. P. (1962). *J. Amer. Chem. Soc.*, **84**, 1329
107. Dandliker, W. B. and de Saussure, V. A. (1971). *The Chemistry of Biosurfaces*, 1 (M. L. Hair, editor) (New York: Marrell Dekker, Inc.)
108. Reisfeld, R. A., Ferrone, S. and Pellegrino, M. A. (1973). *Methods of Membrane Biology*, vol. 1 (E. D. Korn, editor) (New York: Plenum Press) in the press
109. Reisfeld, R. A. and Kahan, B. D. (1971). *Transplant. Rev.*, **6**, 81
110. Rodbard, D. and Chrambach, A. (1971). *Anal. Biochem.*, **40**, 95
111. Oh, S., Pellegrino, M. A. and Reisfeld, R. A. (1973). *Fed. Proc. (Fed. Amer. Soc. Exp. Biol.)*, in the press
112. Pellegrino, M. A., Ferrone, S. and Pellegrino, A. (1972). *Transplantation Antigens*, 433 (B. D. Kahan and R. A. Reisfeld, editors) (New York: Academic Press)
113. Walford, R. L., Shanbrom, E., Troup, G. M., Zeller, E. and Ackerman, B. (1967). *Histocompatibility Testing 1967*, 221 (E. S. Curtoni, P. L. Mattiuz and R. M. Tosi, editors) (Copenhagen: Munksgaard)
114. Kahan, B. D., Pellegrino, M. A., Papermaster, B. W. and Reisfeld, R. A. (1971). *Transplant. Proc.*, **3**, 227
115. Reif, A. E. (1966). *Immunochemistry*, **3**, 267
116. Pellegrino, M. A., Ferrone, S. and Pellegrino, A. (1972). *Proc. Soc. Exp. Biol. Med.*, **139**, 484
117. Reisfeld, R. A., Pellegrino, M. A., Papermaster, B. W. and Kahan, B. D. (1970). *J. Immunol.*, **104**, 560
118. Reisfeld, R. A., Pellegrino, M. A., Papermaster, B. W. and Kahan, B. D. (1971). *Immunopathology*, vol. 6, 139 (P. A. Miescher, editor) (New York: Grune and Stratton)
119. Kahan, B. D. and Reisfeld, R. A. (1969). *Science*, **164**, 514
120. Ceppellini, R., Curtoni, E. S., Mattiuz, P. L., Miggiano, V., Scudeller, G. and Serra, A. (1967). *Histocompatibility Testing 1967*, 149 (E. S. Curtoni, P. L. Mattiuz, and R. M. Tosi, editors) (Copenhagen: Munksgaard)
121. Muramatsu, T. and Nathenson, S. G. (1971). *Fed. Proc. (Fed. Amer. Soc. Exp. Biol.)*, **30**, 2768
122. Bodmer, W., Boder, J. G. and Tripp, M. (1970). *Histocompatibility Testing 1970*, 187 (P. I. Terasaki, editor) (Copenhagen: Munksgaard)
123. Dausset, J. and Legrand, L. (1972). *Nature (London)*, **234**, 271
124. Brautbar, C., Pellegrino, M. A., Ferrone, S., Payne, R., Reisfeld, R. A. and Hayflick, L. (1973). *Exp. Cell. Res.*, in the press
125. Klein, J. and Shreffler, D. (1971). *Transplant. Rev.*, **6**, 3
126. Dausset, J. (1973). *Fed. Proc. (Fed. Amer. Soc. Exp. Biol.)*, in the press
127. Nandi, S. (1967). *Proc. Nat. Acad. Sci. USA*, **58**, 485
128. Biozzi, J., Stiffel, C. and Nouton, D. (1968). *Ann. Inst. Pasteur*, **115**, 965
129. Burnet, F. M. (1970). *Nature (London)*, **226**, 123
130. Nossal, G. J. V. (1972). *Transplantation Antigens*, 503 (B. D. Kahan and R. A. Reisfeld, editors) (New York: Academic Press)

Histocompatibility Antigens

Part 2
Genetics of the HL-A and H-2 Major Histocompatibility Systems

W. F. BODMER
University of Oxford

9.7 INTRODUCTION

9.7.1 Blood transfusion and tumour transplantation

Blood transfusion, which is by far the commonest form of transplantation, has a long history which, from the beginning of this century, is intertwined closely with the development of knowledge concerning the transplantation of other tissues. Although the concept of using blood as a therapeutic agent was already familiar in ancient Egypt, blood transfusion as we now know it could not have been practiced until the discovery of the circulation of the blood by Harvey in the seventeenth century. Early enthusiasm for transfusion waned with an inability to obtain satisfactory results. Reaction to transfusion of animal blood into man was explained in the latter part of the nineteenth century by agglutination and haemolysis of the incoming blood by the recipient's serum, but not until Landsteiner's discovery of the ABO blood groups in 1900 was it realised that the same problems attended transfusion of blood from one human into another. Once it was determined that the ABO differences were genetically controlled and that the agglutinins which caused the trouble on transfusion were antibodies such as could be produced by the injection of foreign cells, the combined genetic and immunological basis for 'rejection' of a blood transfusion was established. The recipient is reacting immunologically to genetically determined differences carried by the incoming blood.

The ABO blood group system on its own provided an almost complete answer to the problem of blood transfusion. No such simple answer can be given for the transplantation of other tissues. The pioneer studies with tissues other than blood started with work on transplantation of tumours in the early years of this century. It was found by Jensen[131] in 1902–1903 that live tumours could sometimes be transplanted from one mouse to another and that the success of the transplant of a particular tumour depended on the recipient strain. Following this Loeb found that tumours originating in a particular partially inbred stock of mice, the Japanese Waltzer, mostly grew if transplanted within the stock, but did not grow in unrelated stocks. All the offspring of crosses between Japanese Waltzer and 'common' mice were shown by Tyzzer[132] in 1909 to be susceptible to tumours from Japanese Waltzers, thus establishing that the genetic factors for 'susceptibility' were *dominant*. Further crosses however did not lead to clear-cut Mendelian patterns for the genetic control of susceptibility to the tumours. This was correctly interpreted by Little[133] as showing that many genes must be involved and this led to the development of inbred lines for studies of tumour transplantation by Little, Bittner, Strong, Snell and others, an approach which subsequently dominated the field and made possible many of the most significant advances in transplantation biology.

9.7.2 Inbred strains and the discovery of H-2

Inbred strains are generally produced by continued brother/sister mating over a number of generations, which leads to the production of stocks which are genetically homogeneous. Thus it can be shown that after 12 generations of continued brother/sister mating only 7 % of the loci which were originally heterozygous will still be so, while after 20 generations the proportion of heterozygous loci has dropped to *ca.* 1 %. (The terms *gene* and *locus* tend to be used interchangeably. Strictly speaking the gene is that sequence of nucleotide pairs in the DNA which codes for some basic function, or most simply for a particular polypeptide chain, while locus refers to the position of the gene on the chromosome. Alternative versions of a gene are called *alleles*. An individual who has different alleles in the two homologous chromosomes on which the gene in question is located is called a *heterozygote*. When the two homologous chromosomes carry the same allele, then the individual is a *homozygote*.) Let us first consider the behaviour of a single gene difference controlling tumour transplantation in crosses between two inbred lines and their offspring (see Figure 9.8). P_1 and P_2 are the parent lines, genotypes $A_1 A_1$ and $A_2 A_2$

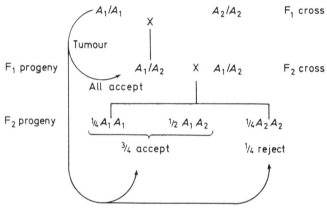

Figure 9.8 Fate of tumour grafts assumed to be controlled by a single gene difference (A_1, A_2) in a cross between two inbred lines and in their offspring

respectively. The cross between the parent lines, called F_1, produces all heterozygous $A_1 A_2$ progeny and the cross between these heterozygotes, called an F_2, produces offspring in the Mendelian proportions $\frac{1}{4} A_1 A_1$, $\frac{1}{2} A_1 A_2$, and $\frac{1}{4} A_2 A_2$. A tumour from P_1 will grow in all F_1 animals since these all have the A_1 allele associated with the P_1 parent. It will, however, only grow in those F_2 animals which have the A_1 gene, namely the $\frac{1}{4} A_1 A_1$ and $\frac{1}{2} A_1 A_2$ genotypes, making $\frac{3}{4}$ in all. The $\frac{1}{4} A_2 A_2$ animals which do not have the A_1 gene will reject the tumour. Suppose now that there are several (say n) such loci at which the parental line carried different alleles affecting tumour transplantation. The F_1 will be heterozygous at all the loci and so all will accept a tumour from P_1. Now, however, only those F_2 individuals which carry the allele derived from P_1 at each of the n loci will accept the P_1 graft. Assuming the loci are all independent (i.e. are not on the same chromosome) this proportion is $(\frac{3}{4})^n$. In such an experiment Little and Tyzzer[134] found that only 3/183 or 1.6 % of the F_2 accepted P_1 grafts suggesting that n was *ca.* 15 $((\frac{3}{4})^{15} = 0.013)$.

As in the case of the blood groups the only satisfactory answer to the further understanding of the transplantation problem was the seemingly hopeless task of identifying the specific loci involved in the rejection of the transplanted tumour. This development was, remarkably, foreshadowed by Landsteiner in his 1930 Nobel lecture[135] who realised the close parallel between the problems of blood transfusion and those of transplantation. While he felt that blood groups other than ABO might have little therapeutic application to blood transfusion, he said that 'they are however, probably related closely to an important field of surgery namely that of the transplantation of tissues'. Comparing the results of early transplantation experiments with his serological studies of blood differences he maintained that 'the agreement between the results of the two independent methods is so striking that one is immediately led to assume that there are differences of substantially the same kind which, on the one hand, determine the individual variations detectable by means of serum reactions and on the other the individually specific behaviour of transplants'. This was the basis on which Gorer in 1936 started the work which led to the discovery of the mouse H-2 system. Gorer[136, 137] described an antigenic difference between two inbred strains of mice which was detected by agglutination of red cells using sera from appropriately immunised rabbits. He first showed that the antigen was inherited as if determined by a single dominant gene. Later data then showed that a tumour which developed in the albino strain, which had the antigen (called II), grew in 35 out of 48 II+ve mice of an F_2 generation with the other strain, whereas none of the 17 F_2 mice that did not have the II antigen would accept the tumour[137]. Gorer thus established a clear relation between this particular blood group antigen and tumour transplantability. He discussed the fact that his data suggested that the growth of the tumour he was working with depended on the action of perhaps just two genes ($35/65 = 0.54$; $(\frac{3}{4})^2 = 9/16 = 0.56$) and pointed out that the more malignant a tumour, the smaller the number of genes controlling its growth. This anticipated the fact that antigen II was relatively 'strong', in the sense that even quite malignant tumours could not grow across a II difference. The II—ve mice in which the tumours from the II+ve strain had grown produced sera which contained anti-II, showing that this antigen was present on the tumour. *Thus the essential law of transplantation is that, for a successful transplant, the donor must not possess antigens which are absent from the recipient.* The relevant antigens are called *histocompatibility antigens* and the dominant genes which determine them, histocompatibility genes[138]. The status of antigen II was firmly established when it was shown by Gorer, Lyman and Snell[139] in 1948 that the corresponding locus, which they now called H-2, was quite closely linked to another well defined gene, called fused, which affected tail development.

Snell[138] realised the importance of developing strains of mice which differed at only one histocompatibility locus and devised a simple breeding system to achieve this, as shown in Figure 9.9. The aim is to produce a stock of strain 1 mice which carries just one strain 2 allele at one of its histocompatibility loci. Generation 0 is a mating between the strains, and generation 1 a mating between their offspring. Out of these offspring mice are selected which are resistant to a strain 1 tumour and these are *back-crossed* to strain 1 mice. The offspring of this mating are intercrossed (generation 3—as in generation 1) and animals resistant to the strain 1 tumour again back-crossed (generation 4—as in generation 2) to a strain 1 mouse. Selection of offspring which are resistant to the strain 1 tumour ensures that these individuals are homozygous for at least 1 histocompatibility allele with respect to which strains 1 and 2 differ (see Figure 9.8). Continued back-crossing, on the other hand, will

Strain 1   Strain 2

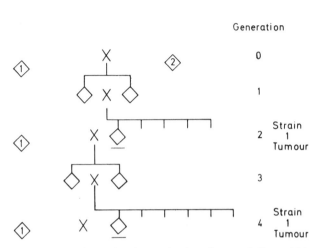

Generation

Figure 9.9   Scheme for the production of *congenic* lines which differ only at a single *histocompitability* locus. Underlined individuals are resistant to the strain 1 tumour

gradually produce offspring which are more and more similar to strain 1 leaving, in the end, only one locus at which the two parents differ. Such strains are called *congenic* and have been the basis for much of the work on H-2 and other histocompatibility systems of the mouse. Using lines developed in this way, Snell and others have defined many different H-2 alleles and also many other histocompatibility (H) loci. Recent estimates have suggested the existence of at least 30 H loci in the mouse[140]. H-2, however, remains by far the strongest as a barrier to transplantation.

9.7.3 Transplantation of normal tissues

Although it was assumed for many years that transplantation of normal tissues should follow the same rules as tumour transplantation this was not firmly established until Medawar's classic experiments on skin transplants in the 1940s. Skin grafting was reported in ancient Egypt more than 3000 years BC, but its systematic and successful practice for the treatment of extensive superficial injury dates to the middle of the nineteenth century. Much of this early work had not distinguished autografts (skin taken from the same individual) from homografts (skin taken from any other individual of the same species). Gradually, however, it became clear that homografts never survived permanently except when carried out between identical twins[141]. This established a genetic basis for graft survival which, however, as in the case of tumour transplantation in the mouse was much more complex than blood transfusion. A single detailed case report by Gibson and Medawar[142], in 1943, of skin grafting carried out on a patient suffering from severe burns established clearly the immunological basis of normal tissue transplantation. Autografts on this patient survived indefinitely and became incorporated as a part of her own skin. The first homograft using skin from a brother of the patient initially was taken and vascularised well. Clear signs of retrogression eventually appeared after the 20th day and the graft was ultimately completely sloughed off, or rejected. Second homografts from the same individual never took properly and started degenerating immediately they were applied. These results established that the rejection of the graft was an immune phenomenon. A period of time was required for the initial graft to sensitise the recipient and initiate rejection. Then once sensitised as in the case of an antibody response, rejection of the second graft was greatly accelerated.

Gibson and Medawar[142] discussed the suggestion that the blood groups discovered by Landsteiner and others may be contributing factors to graft rejection. They rejected this hypothesis, however, because they could find no evidence in their work or in other work reported in the literature that matching for ABO or MN blood groups affected skin graft survival. Apparently in agreement with this, Medawar[143] showed in 1946, using the rabbit, that presensitisation with red cells from a skin donor had no effect on graft survival and that no red cell agglutinins were produced following such a skin homograft. In this same paper, however, Medawar made the all important observation that presensitisation with *leucocytes* did accelerate graft rejection. He thus concluded that, although normal rabbit tissues did not share histocompatibility antigens with red cells, there were such antigens shared with the white cells of the blood. It is a strange accident of history that led to this apparent discrepancy between Gorer's and Medawar's results, due mainly to the fact that one worked with the mouse and the other with the rabbit. H-2 has clearly been shown to be the major histocompatibility antigen system for transplantation of all tissues, so that in the mouse skin and red cells do share major histocompatibility antigens, in contrast to the rabbit.

9.7.4 Studies in man: the discovery of HL-A

There are no inbred human lines and the opportunities for experimental transplantation in man are clearly limited. Thus, as is often the case in human genetics, new strategies were needed to establish the details of histocompatibility genetics for man. Since the early skin graft data had indicated that the known red cell blood groups did not play an important role in transplantation, attention was focused, following Medawar's observations on rabbits, on the possibility of finding blood group-like systems that could be detected on the white cells of the blood. The main initial problem was to find sources of sera for such studies. One obvious source was in sera from individuals who had undergone blood transfusions. These were shown to have antibodies which reacted with the white cells of a high proportion of random donors but proved to be too complex for conventional serological analysis. In 1958, however, Payne[144] and van Rood[145] independently discovered that leucocyte agglutinins could be found in women who had been sensitised by foetal-maternal stimulation as in the case of the Rhesus and, occasionally other, red cell blood groups. Approximately 20–30% of women who have had two or more pregnancies have antibodies that react with their husband's white cells and with those of a significant fraction of the population. This discovery made available sera which, although still largely multispecific, were much less complex than those obtained following multiple transfusion and so were suitable as potential reagents for the establishment of genetic groups. Subsequently, as we shall discuss in the next section, it was shown that the majority of the antibodies present in such sera are directed against the antigens of a genetic system called HL-A which appears to be the human analogue of the mouse H-2 system. Although HL-A antigens are not, in general expressed on red cells and, as already mentioned, early data did not correlate blood group differences with graft survival, more recent results[146,147] demonstrate unequivocally that ABO differences do affect graft survival. No kidney transplants, for example, are now performed in man across an ABO incompatibility. Nevertheless a number of lines of evidence, including correspondence with graft survival, clearly establish the HL-A system as the major histocompatibility antigen system in man.

Although the development of the HL-A system was conceptually closely related to that of H-2 the actual approach used in studying the two systems has been quite different. As already indicated the understanding of the serology and genetics of H-2 came from detailed studies of a relatively small number of inbred mouse lines. The unravelling of the HL-A system, on the other hand, has depended much more on population studies, and so on the statistical methodology which was widely used in the development of the red blood cell groups. The end results, as we shall see, are strikingly similar and emphasise the probable evolutionary homology of the two systems. More emphasis in this review will be placed on the HL-A system solely because that is the area with which I am most familiar.

9.8 GENETICS AND SEROLOGY OF THE HL-A SYSTEM

9.8.1 Serological and statistical techniques

Most of the early work on white cell systems in man made use of a simple agglutination assay using partially purified leukocytes prepared by differential sedimentation of the red cells with high molecular weight polymers, such as Dextran, that induce rouleaux formation. Platelets are removed either by defibrination or differential centrifugation. In the latter case the test is often done in the presence of EDTA which is used as an anticoagulant. A microlymphocytotoxicity assay based on Gorer and O'Gorman's[148] cytotoxicity assay was developed by Terasaki and McLelland[149] and this has become the basis for most of the subsequent studies on the HL-A system. This assay, which uses µl amounts of all reagents and only a few thousand target cells, depends on the killing of partially-purified lymphocytes by specific antibody in the presence of an appropriate source of complement. The lymphocytes are prepared from peripheral blood either by passing mixed white cell suspensions through nylon or cotton fibres or over glass bead columns to remove granulocytes, or more recently by Ficoll–Triosil sedimentation[150] which separates lymphocytes from red cells and granulocytes by a combination of density differences and rouleaux formation. Rabbits provide the only satisfactory source of complement for the human assay. Cell death can be monitored, for example, by direct observation under phase, by uptake of dyes such as Eosin and Trypan blue, as used by Gorer and O'Gorman, by release of absorbed ^{51}Cr or by release of fluorescein following labelling in the presence of fluorescein diacetate[151, 152]. There are a number of papers on these and other techniques in the final section of *Histocompatibility Testing* 1970[153].

Following Shulman and co-workers[154, 155] a complement fixation assay, mainly with platelets, has also been used fairly extensively for HL-A typing. This test became useful in practice after the development of a micro-version comparable in scale to that used for lymphocytotoxicity (see D'Amaro *et al.*[156] and the following papers). Serum, platelets, complement and sensitised red cells are incubated together in appropriate µl amounts and the reactions read by qualitative assessment of the amount of haemolysis. The test has, unfortunately, two major drawbacks. First, comparatively few sera give good reactions with the assay. Secondly, as reactions are run at limiting complement levels, minor anticomplementary effects, which are quite common, give rise to variable results. However, with good sera under appropriate conditions the test gives quite clear cut and reproducible reactions (see *Histocompatibility Testing* 1972[157]—the joint report).

Statistical techniques rather than conventional serological analysis provided the initial basis for the definition of a number of the HL-A antigens, and are still very useful in the initial characterisation of sera. The main reasons for this use of statistics were the multiplicity of available sera, their generally low titres and the difficulty of obtaining adequate amounts of material for large scale absorption. The main statistical tool has been the analysis of 2×2 comparisons of reactions of a set of sera with a random panel of cell donors. As shown in Table 9.11, two sera containing one or more antibodies may

Table 9.11 2×2 **Table for the analysis of the association between a pair of sera tested on a random panel of cell donors: a, b, c, d represent the number of observations of the four possible types of reactions $++$, $-+$, $+-$, and $--$**

		First serum $+$	First serum $-$		1st	2nd
	$+$	$++$ / a	$-+$ / b	a	$+$	$+$
Second serum				b	$-$	$+$
	$-$	$+-$ / c	$--$ / d	or c	$+$	$-$
				d	$-$	$-$

If $b = c = 0$, the sera are identical.
If $b = 0$, serum 2 is 'contained' or 'included' in serum 1, and vice versa if $c = 0$.
The sera may show a significant association. The sign of the association is that of $ad - bc$. The significance of
the association is measured by
$$\chi^2 = \frac{n(ad - bc)^2}{(a + b)(c + d)(a + c)(b + d)}$$
and its magnitude by $(\chi^2/n)^{1/2}$, where $n = a + b + c + d$.
The sera may be independent (χ^2 not significant).

be identical, may be contained one within the other, may be significantly associated or, finally, may be completely independent. There are two main reasons for an association between the reactions of a pair of sera with a random population sample. Either (a) one or both of the sera contain more than one antibody and at least one of the antibodies is common to both sera, or (b) the sera contain antibodies directed against antigens that are associated in the population.

Associations between sera due to shared antibodies can be used as a basis for the definition of antigens using multispecific sera, without recourse to an absorption analysis. The main principle involved is the recognition of a group of associated sera all, or most of which show significant 2 × 2 associations, and which are therefore assumed to share an antibody that defines the corresponding antigen. This statistical approach to the definition of HL-A antigens was pioneered by van Rood[158] in 1962 and led to his original description of the antigens 4a and 4b. The method was further developed by Bodmer, Payne and co-workers in their definition of the antigens HL-A1 and HL-A2[159], (see also Cavalli-Sforza and Bodmer[160], Chapter 5 for a brief review of this approach). An illustration of the way in which a set of multispecific sera can be used to define an antigen is shown in Figure 9.10. The figure is a histogram

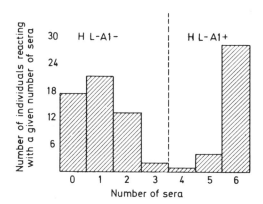

Figure 9.10 Definition of an antigen using a group of multispecific sera

of the number of people who reacted with a given number of six sera, all pairs of which gave significant 2 × 2 associations. These six sera share an antibody which defines the antigen HL-A1. The distribution is clearly bimodal with a minimum at 3–4 sera out of 6. Individuals reacting to four, five or six of the sera are HL-A1+ the remainder HL-A1−. Technical errors account for the fact that some HL-A1+ individuals may not react with all the sera of the group. People reacting to one, two or three sera are, presumably, reacting to antibodies in these sera other than anti-HL-A1. The upper limit to the level of misclassification is set approximately by the three out of 86 individuals who reacted to three or four sera. The definition of the antigen HL-A1 is unambiguous and was later confirmed by absorption studies and the identification of monospecific sera.

A population association between antigens, which is the second reason mentioned above for association between serum reactions may be caused by a number of factors. The antigens may, for example, be the products of interacting genes (as in the case of the red cell antigen Lewis b). There may be departures from random mating with respect to the antigens, or there may be effects of natural selection which tend to favour certain antigenic combinations over others. However, in the case of complex antigenic systems the most likely and most important cause of association is close linkage between the genetic determinants of the corresponding antigens. One example of this is the negative association expected between antigens determined by alleles. Thus, in the ABO system for example the frequency of the type AB in Caucasians, 0.03, is substantially less than the expected product (0.052) of the frequencies of A (0.47) and B (0.11), on the assumption that antigens A and B are determined by genes of two different, unlinked and so independent loci. This was, in fact, the way that the allelism of the genetic determinants for A and B was first established by the mathematician Bernstein in 1924. Family data had previously yielded equivocal results because of appreciable misclassification of the ABO types. In an analogous way, in the early days of HL-A typing, the allelism between two of the first antigens to be described, HL-A1 and HL-A2, was at first established mainly on the basis of their negative population association[159].

9.8.2   The LA and 4 antigen series and their genetic control

The first genetic polymorphism for leukocyte antigens, called Group 4, was described by van Rood[150,161] in 1962. A genetic polymorphism is most simply defined operationally by the existence in one population of two or more alleles at a given locus each of which occurs with an appreciable frequency—say more than 1%. Histocompatibility systems are thus, by their definition, genetic polymorphisms. Initially Group 4 was described as a simple two allele system involving the antigens 4a and 4b and three phenotypes: 4a, 4a4b and 4b. However, as has been the case with so many of the red blood cell groups, it turned out to be a very complex system. What was initially thought to be a second major independent polymorphism, LA, was described soon after by Payne, Bodmer and co-workers[159]. Subsequently, Dausset, Ceppellini, and others presented both family and population association data which showed that the genes for all the antigens were very closely linked, and so that they all belonged to one system, the HL-A polymorphism (see *Histocompatibility Testing* 1967[162], 1970[153] and 1972[157]). It now appears that this system of antigens can be described in terms of two closely linked loci with multiple alleles, corresponding respectively to the LA and 4 series of antigens.

To illustrate this representation we shall first trace the history of the LA antigen series. The two antigens HL-A1 and HL-A2 were first described together by Payne *et al.*[159], though an antigen, Mac described in a preliminary way by Dausset[163] in 1958 later turned out to be essentially the same as HL-A2. Family data and a negative population association between the two antigens indicated, as already mentioned, that they were determined by a pair of alleles. The existence of HL-A1(−)HL-A2(−) individuals indicated the presence of a 'blank' (silent) allele, analogous to O in the ABO system. Subsequently two more antigens, HL-A3 and HL-A9 were described that behaved as if they were determined by two other alleles of this system, still leaving room for a 'blank' allele. The simplest operational criterion for allelism in this contest is that no individual exists who carries on one chromosome, and so transmits together to his offspring, the genetic determinants for two or more of the antigens. Thus, an individual who has two of the allelic set of antigens, say HL-A1 and HL-A2, must be heterozygous for the corresponding genetic determinants, $HL-A1/HL-A2$. No individual should therefore have more than two of the antigens. Data on the expected and observed phenotypic frequencies of a sample of Caucasians with respect to the antigens HL-A1, HL-A2, HL-A3 and HL-A9 are shown in Table 9.12. The expected

Table 9.12 Expected and observed phenotype frequencies for the LA series of HL-A antigens

HL-A1	HL-A2	HL-A3	HL-A9	Observed	Expected*
−	−	−	−	9	7.2
+	−	−	−	8	9.0
−	+	−	−	25	24.2
−	−	+	−	11	10.6
−	−	−	+	5	9.6
+	+	−	−	7	7.8
+	−	+	−	5	4.1
+	−	−	+	5	3.8
−	+	+	−	6	9.0
−	+	−	+	11	8.3
−	−	+	+	6	4.4
			Total	98	98.0

$\chi^2_6 = 5.97$

* The expected phenotype frequencies are based on fitting gene frequencies for each antigen and a 'blank' assuming random mating and so the Hardy–Weinberg law. This states that if alleles $A_i, i = 1 \ldots k$ occur with frequencies p_i then the frequency of genotype $A_iA_j (i \neq j)$ is $2p_ip_j$ and the frequency of A_iA_i is p_i^2. The corresponding estimated gene frequencies for this data are

HL-A1	HL-A2	HL-A3	HL-A9	Blank
0.135	0.289	0.167	0.136	0.276

(Note: italics are generally used for gene symbols, while ordinary roman type refers to the associated antigen or phenotype).

frequencies are based on fitting gene frequencies assuming random mating and the Hardy–Weinberg law (see e.g. Cavalli-Sforza and Bodmer[160] for a discussion of this, and other aspects, of population genetics). The allelism of the genetic determinants of these antigens which is implied by the good fit of the observed and expected frequencies, has now been amply confirmed by family studies[162] which show that no two antigens of the LA series are ever passed on to offspring together. More recent data[153, 157] has increased the

Table 9.13   HL-A Haplotype determination from family data

| | | LA antigens | | | | 4 antigens | | | Haplotype |
	1	3	2	9	7	8	5	12	
Father	1*	1	0	0	1	1	0	0	A/B
Mother	0	0	1	1	0	0	1	1	C/D
Children 1	1	0	1	0	0	1	0	1	A/C
2	1	0	0	1	0	1	1	0	A/D
3	1	0	1	0	0	1	0	1	B/C
4	0	1	1	0	1	0	0	1	B/C
5	0	1	1	0	1	0	0	1	B/C
6	0	1	0	1	1	0	1	0	B/D
7	1	0	1	0	0	1	0	1	A/C

Parental Haplotypes:
Father   A   *1*   *8*
        B   *3*   *7*
Mother   C   *2*   *12*
        D   *9*   *5*

* 1 = presence of antigen   0 = absence

Table 9.14   Average LA and 4 gene frequencies (percentage) in the three major human racial groups (based on histocompatibility testing[157] 1972—joint report)

HL-A		Caucasoid	Mongoloid	Negroid
LA	*1*	12	2	5
Series	*2*	25	18	19
	3	12	1	8
	9	13	41	13
	10	5	7	8
	11	9	13	1
	W29	2	1	5
	W30	4	2	16
	W31	1	0	2
	W32	4	0	4
	W28	5	2	9
	Blank	8	13	10
4	*5*	10	9	8
Series	*7*	11	2	12
	8	7	1	4
	12	11	3	13
	13	2	4	1
	W5	10	6	6
	W10	5	24	6
	W14	3	0	3
	W15	7	16	4
	W16	3	5	1
	W17	6	3	21
	W18	7	1	3
	W21	3	0	1
	W22	2	13	1
	W27	4	4	0
	Blank	9	9	16

number of LA antigens to at least 14, and so virtually filled in the 'blank', at least in Caucasian populations (see Table 9.14).

The 4 series started, as already mentioned, as a simple two antigen system involving antigens 4a and 4b. A number of other antigens were subsequently described that were clearly closely associated with 4a and 4b. It now appears that 4a and 4b are operationally complex, in the sense that each is the sum of a number of constituent specificities. Thus, for example, the antigens HL-A7 and HL-A8 are 'included' in 4b, which means that all individuals classified as either HL-A7 or HL-A8 are also 4b. There still remain people who are 4b but not HL-A7 or HL-A8, indicating that all the constituent antigens of the 4b complex have not yet been described. An exactly similar situation exists with respect to 4a. This complexity may be due to the fact that cross-reacting antibodies, namely those which have affinity for more than one specificity, are relatively common for antigens within each of these complexes, as will be discussed later. A number of antigens, such as HL-A7 and HL-A8, belonging to the 4 series were seen, when they were first described, to behave as if they were determined by a set of alleles analogous to the LA series[164-167]. Subsequently it was recognised that, apart from 4a and 4b, all the major antigens of the 4 series could be represented by a multiple allelic set just like LA[168, 169] (—see also Allen *et al.*[170]). The number of antigens now known in the 4 series is even larger than that at the LA series, being at least 17. (See Table 9.14, and *Histocompatibility Testing* 1972[157]—the joint report).

An example of family data indicating the expected patterns of inheritance of HL-A antigens is shown in Table 9.13. The pattern of reaction to family members is given for each antigen present in at least one member of the family. Allelic antigens present in one parent, for example HL-A1 and HL-A3 in the father, show complementary patterns of inheritance; each child has received from the father the gene for either HL-A1 or HL-A3 and no child receives both these genes or neither of them. The 4 locus antigens of the father HL-A7 and HL-A8, show exactly the same complementary patterns as the LA antigens, with HL-A8 corresponding to HL-A1 and HL-A7 to HL-A3. In other words the pairwise combinations HL-A1,8 and HL-A3,7 are transmitted together to the offspring, exactly as expected if the locus for HL-A1 and 3, LA, is closely linked to that for HL-A8 and 7, 4, and there is no observed recombination. Combinations such as *HL-A1, 8* and *HL-A3,7*, which are controlled by linked genes on the same chromosome and so passed together to the offspring, are called *haplotypes*. An analysis of the inheritance patterns of the maternal antigens shows that her two haplotypes are *HL-A2, 12* and *HL-A9, 5*. The last column in the table shows the inheritance of the four haplotypes using the shorthand labels A (for *HL-A1, 8*), B (for *HL-A3, 7*), C (for *HL-A2, 12*) and D (for *HL-A9, 5*). The only way that an individual's complete HL-A genotype can be firmly established is by studying patterns of inheritance in families such as this, or by using genetic techniques with cells in culture. In the family used as an example each parent had four different HL-A antigens. Somewhat different patterns will be observed if a parent is homozygous at one or other locus, or has an allele which does not correspond to a detectable antigen, namely a 'blank'. The more antigens that are discovered at each locus the lower the incidence of blanks becomes. (See Tables 9.12 and 9.14). It can be shown[41] that, allowing for blanks, with $l-1$

antigens at the first locus and $k-1$ at the second the number of haplotypes is lk, the number of genotypes lk $(lk + 1)/2$ and the number of distinguishable phenotypes

$$(l + \tfrac{1}{2}(l - 1)\,(l - 2))\,(k + \tfrac{1}{2}\,(k - 1)\,(k - 2)).$$

Taking $l - 1$ as 14 and $k - 1$ as 17 these numbers are 270 haplotypes, 36 585 genotypes and 16 324 phenotypes, emphasising the extraordinary variability of the HL-A system.

Recombination between the LA and 4 loci is recognised by exceptions to the rule that pairs of antigens determined by the same haplotype should be inherited together. Since the recombination fraction between the loci is low, great care has to be taken in establishing the validity of any putative recombinants, for example, by ruling out illegitimacy or serological difficulties with the typing. At least 50 well established cases of recombination between the loci have however been described so far[172]. The overall data indicate a recombination fraction of between 0.5 and 1 % with a mean of 0.8 %[173]. Based on certain simplifying assumptions, it is possible to calculate the approximate number of genes encompassed by a recombination fraction of 0.8 %[174, 175].

The calculations give a maximum number which could be as many as 2000 and a minimum estimate of at least 100 or 200, so that there are, most probably, a considerable number of genes between the LA and 4 loci. The possible functions of these genes will be discussed in the final section of this chapter.

Recent data have suggested that the HL-A region is linked to the PGM_3 (Phosphoglucomutase$_3$) locus[176] with an estimated recombination fraction of 21 %. Two other loci have been provisionally associated with this linkage group. Studies with human/mouse hybrids[177] suggested a linkage between HL-A and red cell blood group P, while further family studies have shown evidence for linkage between ADA (red cell adenosine deaminase) and both P and HL-A[178]. The combined data suggests the following very provisional representation of the HL-A linkage group:

HL-A
LA - 4 ———————PGM_3———————ADA———————P
0.8   27   14   35

where the numbers are recombination distances in centimorgans (effectively recombination fractions in per cent).

9.8.3 Cross-reaction between HL-A antigens

Serological cross-reaction is a major feature of the HL-A system. It was first indicated by the existence of cells which could absorb an antibody out of a serum although they did not react with the serum[164, 179]. Furthermore, at the time that the inclusion of 4 locus antigens such as HL-A 5 (then called 4c) in 4a, and others such as HL-A7 in 4b, was first described the possibility that this sort of association between antigens could be due to cross reaction was raised[180]. However, the first clear cut example of cross-reaction involved the two closely related antigens HL-A2 and W28[168, 181]. Thus W28 was first defined by sera which reacted with all HL-A2 positive individuals and also with some individuals who were HL-A2 negative. These sera could not be split by absorption, namely all positive cells, whether HL-A2 positive or not, removed all reactivity from the sera. The HL-A2 negative individuals who reacted to such sera have the W28 antigen, which thus appears to cross-react with HL-A2 as far as these original antibodies were concerned. Subsequently, sera were found which reacted specifically with W28, though the majority of HL-A2 and W28 sera do cross react at least to some extent. Many examples of cross-reaction are now known and it has become apparent that many of the difficulties encountered in characterising sera are due to cross-reaction. In fact, only a small proportion of sera with HL-A antibodies give clean reactions with single well-defined specificities. Further evidence for cross-reaction comes from the production in sera of antibodies against specificities which are not present in the immunising donor[182]. For example, a donor who is HL-A2$^+$ W28$^-$ used with an HLA2$^-$ W28$^-$ recipient will nearly always produce cross-reacting antibodies to W28. This means that sera often contain mixtures of cross-reacting antibodies directed against related antigens.

Several systematic studies on patterns of cross-reaction have recently been published[183-187]. A major feature of these patterns is that, with one possible exception, all the cross-reactions observed so far occur either within the 4 or within the LA series. The only indication of a possible cross-reaction between LA and 4 antigens is the fact pointed out by Bodmer (*Histocompatibility Testing 1970*[153] p. 104) that many, if not most, anti-4a sera also contain antibodies to HL-A9. A diagrammatic representation of the major patterns of cross-reaction between most of the presently known antigens is shown in Figure 9.11. There are several pairs of closely related antigens in addition to HL-A2 and W28. There are also 4 clusters of related antigens with slightly weaker cross-reactions: 1, 10, 11 and 3; W29, W30, W31, W32—the "W19" set; 5, W5, W15, W18 (? W17)—the 4c or Da6 set; and 7, W10, W22 and W27. It is worth noting that the LA antigens seem basically to fall into two groups, namely those connected with HL-A2 (including HL-A9) and those connected with HL-A1. In view of the possible relation between HL-A9 and 4a, this suggests that the LA set of antigens associated with HL-A2 may, in some sense, be analogous to 4a while the remaining LA antigens, associated with HL-A1, are analogous to 4b.

It has been suggested that the partitioning of the 4 series of antigens into those associated with 4a and those associated with 4b is best explained by cross-reaction[168]. However, as indicated in Figure 9.11 the observed major patterns of cross-reaction among the 4 series antigens do not seem to fit into a simple 4a–4b sub-division (in contrast to the LA antigens). There are several quite strong cross-reactions between 4a and 4b associated antigens. This fact, among others, as emphasised by van Rood *et al.*[188] suggests that 4a and 4b are in some way different from the other HL-A antigens which form the two series.

There are two alternative explanations for serological cross-reaction. The first is that an antibody of a single specificity is able to combine with several related chemical structures. The second is that the antigens are complex and that cross-reacting antigens have overlapping chemical similarities. A cross-reacting antibody is then one directed against such an overlapping or common chemical structure. Recent studies using blocking tests have clearly indicated that cross-reacting antibodies combine with different specificities than do non cross-reacting antibodies, clearly favouring the second explanation for cross-reaction in the case of the HL-A system[189, 190]. Thus, Legrand and Dausset[189] showed that adsorption onto a cell of a cross-reacting antibody did not block subsequent absorption of non cross-reacting antibodies by these cells. Richardi *et al.*[190] showed that absorption of F ab fragments from one type of antibody did not block the cytotoxic activity of the other type of antibody. A series of antibodies to such postulated overlapping specificities has been described by Svejgaard *et al.*[191].

The original explanation for the association of 4 series antigens with 4a and 4b was that 4a and 4 b were determined by a gene which was very closely

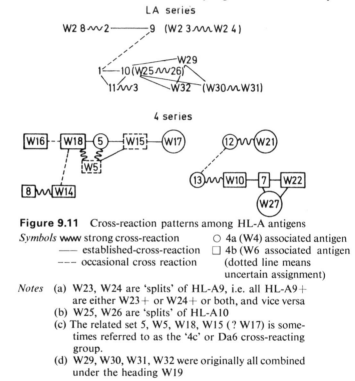

Figure 9.11   Cross-reaction patterns among HL-A antigens

Symbols www strong cross-reaction   ○ 4a (W4) associated antigen
          —— established-cross-reaction   □ 4b (W6 associated antigen
          – – – occasional cross reaction   (dotted line means
                    uncertain assignment)

Notes   (a) W23, W24 are 'splits' of HL-A9, i.e. all HL-A9+
                    are either W23+ or W24+ or both, and vice versa
          (b) W25, W26 are 'splits' of HL-A10
          (c) The related set 5, W5, W18, W15 (? W17) is some-
                    times referred to as the '4c' or Da6 cross-reacting
                    group.
          (d) W29, W30, W31, W32 were originally all combined
                    under the heading W19

linked to those for the other antigens, and that only certain combinations, or haplotypes, were found in a population[166, 180]. Thus HL-A5, a 4a antigen, would only be found on a chromosome which carried the *4a* allele and not on one carrying the *4b* allele. As we shall discuss later, very close linkage can result in such extreme associations. The possibility that 4a and 4b are determined by alleles at a different locus than the other 4 series antigens has, as already mentioned, been repeatedly emphasised by van Rood and his colleagues[188]. As the two locus multiple allele hypothesis developed, emphasis was placed on the definition of apparently monovalent specificities, and associations between antigens of the same locus were explained by cross-reaction.

However, given that cross-reaction is due to overlapping chemical similarities between different antigens the distinction between these two hypothesis for explaining cross-reaction breaks down. Thus, even if the LA and 4 antigens are single polypeptide chains, cross-reacting specificities would most probably be determined by different parts of the polypeptide from non cross-reacting specificities and so, in principle their genetic determinants could be separated by recombination. It has in fact been suggested by Bodmer[175], that alleles which determine pairs of highly cross-reacting antigens, such as HL-A2 and W28, might be evolutionarily related to each other by a single recombination event. Cross-reacting groups, such as the set HL-A5, W5, W18 and W15, might be fitted into a somewhat similar though more complicated evolutionary scheme[142]. It must however be borne in mind[174, 175] that the apparent allelism of the genetic determinants for the LA and 4 antigens does not imply that these antigens are necessarily the products of a single structural gene. Models involving very close linkage between genes with related functions could easily be compatible with the available data. Clearly, the ultimate answer to these questions can only come from a detailed chemical understanding of the nature of the antigens.

9.8.4   Population genetics of the HL-A system

The HL-A system is undoubtedly the most polymorphic system yet known in man. One measure of this, which has already been discussed, is the very large number of HL-A genotypes and phenotypes. The frequency of heterozygotes in a population provides another measure of the extent of polymorphism. Thus in Caucasian populations, for example, at least 75% of individuals are heterozygous at both the LA and 4 loci (and so have four different antigens), and only 1.6% are homozygous at both loci. By way of comparison, the proportion of homozygotes for the Rhesus blood group system, which is the most polymorphic of the red cell blood groups, is 36% while that for the ABO system is *ca.* 56%.

As is the case with most genetic polymorphisms, the frequencies of the different genotypes vary substantially from one population to another. Clearly, the more distantly related are the populations the greater the expected genetic differences between them. Average gene frequencies for the alleles of *LA* and *4* loci in the three major racial groups of man (Caucasian, African, Oriental) are given in Table 9.14. This data was extracted from the results of the Fifth International Histocompatibility Testing Workshop[157] which had population studies as its major theme. The existence of genetic variation between populations means that antigenic combinations found readily in one population may not be so easily available in another, so that such studies can be of great help in the serological definition of antigens. Population genetic studies on HL-A have also contributed to the understanding of the relationships between populations, and to evidence for the existence of natural selection in relation to the HL-A system.

The high level of heterozygosity for the HL-A system reflects the fact that many alleles occur with frequencies of a few per cent. Some antigens, however, clearly show a substantial differential distribution in the major racial groups.

Thus, the antigen HL-A1 occurs predominantly in Caucasoids, its presence in Negroids being accounted for largely by Caucasoid mixture. The antigens HL-A11 and W27 are also absent from Negroids, while W17 and W30 have a much higher frequency in Negroids than in other populations. The antigen HL-A9 occurs with highest frequency in Mongoloids. However, when the split of HL-A9 into W23 and W24 is taken into account (see Figure 9.11), it is almost only W24 which occurs in Mongoloids, while both W23 and W24 are found in appreciable frequencies in Caucasoids and Negroids. The antigens W10 and W22 are also found with high frequency in Mongoloids.

A comparison of these average frequencies clearly hides variation between populations within the racial groups. Significant differences are found, for for example, between Northern and Southern Europeans. Differential variability among populations, both between alleles of one locus and between alleles of different loci, provides evidence for the action of natural selection. This is because natural selection is virtually the only evolutionary factor which can, on average, have different effects on different polymorphic genes[160, 193]. Thus the fact that some HL-A alleles have frequencies which vary much less between populations than others, provides some evidence that the HL-A system is subject to the action of natural selection. One of the most striking features of HL-A gene frequency data is the relative homogeneity of certain populations, notably American Indians and Oceanians, in comparison with most other populations. Thus, in American Indians for example the overall average frequency of HL-A homozygotes is *ca.* 9.5%, which is about five times the comparable frequency in Europeans. Other genetic polymorphisms do not show such a difference in homozygosity[193]. Once again, only the action of natural selection could lead to such differences between genetic systems.

So far our discussion of HL-A variation has been restricted to a separate consideration of alleles at the *LA* and *4* loci. It is of some interest, however, to consider what can be said about the frequencies of the pairwise allele combinations, or haplotypes. If there were statistical independence between the population allele frequencies of the two loci, then one should expect that the frequency of a particular haplotype, say *HL-A1, 8* should be the product of the separate frequencies of the alleles *HL-A1* and *HL-A8*. The extent to which there is an association between the alleles *HL-A1* and *HL-A8* on haplotypes is measured by the difference between the haplotype frequency and the product of the constituent allele frequencies namely:

$$\Delta = p(HL\text{-}A1, 8) - p(HL\text{-}A1)p(HL\text{-}A8) \tag{9.1}$$

where $p(HL\text{-}A1, 8)$, $p(HL\text{-}A1)$ $p(HL\text{-}A8)$ are the respective frequencies of the haplotype and the two alleles. Thus, in typical European populations $p(HL\text{-}A1)$ and $p(HL\text{-}A8)$ are, respectively, *ca.* 0.16 and 0.09, while $p(HL\text{-}A1, 8)$ is *ca.* 0.06. This gives

$$\Delta = 0.06 - 0.16 \times 0.09 = 0.049$$

indicating a substantial positive population association between *HL-A1* and *HL-A8*. Most other Δ values for pairs of alleles for the *LA* and *4* loci are *ca.* 0.01 or less and so generally not significantly different from 0. It is a classical result of population genetics, dating back to Jennings[194] in 1917, that in a random mating population, and in the absence of selection, Δ for two linked loci such a LA and 4 should decrease to 0 at a rate of $(1 - r)$ per generation, where r is the recombination fraction between the loci. Ultimately, therefore, even for very close linkage Δ should be 0, and there should be no association between alleles at the two loci. Clearly, the smaller is r the longer it will take for Δ to approach zero, and so alleles which have not reached equilibrium may be associated, particularly if linkage is very tight. However, given certain types of selection, it is possible for Δ not to be zero even at equilibrium. Fisher[195] in 1930 was the first to realise that selective interaction between pairs of genes could favour closer linkage between them. In terms of a two locus, two allele model, he pointed out that if a and b are the prevailing alleles at the two loci, and A and B new corresponding alleles, then selection in favour of the gametic combination, or haplotype, AB favours closer linkage between the loci. Many theoretical studies have confirmed and extended Fisher's original suggestion[196-198]. and show that such selective interactions can give rise to non zero equilibrium values of Δ, or to *linkage disequilibrium* as it is sometimes called.

As already mentioned, in the absence of selection, Δ decreases at a rate of $(1 - r)$ per generation, or $(1 - 0.008)$ in the case of the HL-A system. Thus, for example, a reduction by a factor of 5 would take n generations, where

$$(1 - 0.008)^n = 1/5$$

giving $n = 200$, corresponding to *ca.* 5000 years in human populations, which even in terms of human evolution is a relatively short time. Statistical considerations suggest that with population samples of just a few hundred, the lower limit for a significant Δ value is *ca.* $0.015-0.02$[192]. Thus it seems likely that Δ values as high as $0.05-0.1$ must be maintained by the type of selective interaction first suggested by Fisher. It can, more generally, be suggested that the fact that interaction between genes with related functions favours closer linkage and relatively high Δ values, indicates that the whole of the HL-A region may consist of a series of genes with interrelated functions. This question will be taken up again in the last section in connection with a discussion of the function of the other genes in the HL-A and H-2 regions.

9.9 GENETICS AND SEROLOGY OF THE H-2 SYSTEM

9.9.1 Serology of H-2 and its interpretation in terms of two regions, D and K

The early studies by Gorer and Snell which established the existence of the mouse H-2 system and its linkage with the fused gene had already suggested that there might be a large number of H-2 alleles with many antigenic specificities. Although the first clear demonstration of a series of alleles was based on Snell's tumour transplantation studies using inbred lines[199, 200], most of the subsequent work has been based on serological analyses using sera raised by immunisation among the inbred lines and their F_1s. The assays used are either Gorer's haemagglutination assay modified in various ways to increase sensitivity, or the lymphocytotoxic assay introduced by Gorer and O'Gorman[148] and modified and refined as already described for HL-A typing.

The likely complexity of anti-H-2 sera was demonstrated by one of Gorer's earliest serological analyses using the inbred strains called C57BL, A and CBA. A serum made in C57BL against A strain tissue was absorbed with CBA cells. The resulting absorbed serum still reacted with strain A cells, showing that the serum had at least two antibodies against two separable specificities present on A strain cells, only one of which was present on CBA. It was later shown by Snell[199] that F_1 hybrids between the inbred strains BALB/C and CBA were susceptible to an A strain tumour. This suggested that the A strain had two components, at first called D and K but now called 4 and 11[201], one of which, 11 (K) was present in CBA and the other, 4 (D), in BALB/C. The 11 component was presumably that which was absorbed out of Gorer's C57 BL anti-A serum by CBA cells, while later studies showed that Gorer's original anti II was most probably directed against the 4 component. The H-2 alleles present (in homozygous state because of inbreeding) in strains BALB/C, CBA and A have been designated $H\text{-}2^d$, $H\text{-}2^k$ and $H\text{-}2^a$ respectively. The results of Gorer's and Snell's experiments suggested that $H\text{-}2^a$ might actually be derived from a recombinant event involving $H\text{-}2^d$ and $H\text{-}2^k$ which brought the two components together on one allele, or haplotype. As more inbred lines were studied, many more serological specificities were defined and it became apparent that several specificities could be associated with any one allele. For example, a serum made in BALB/C against C57 gave rise to an antibody which reacted with CBA and A, as well as C57BL. This, therefore, defined a specificity 5 (then called E), which was present in CBA, A and C57 BL but absent from BALB/C. Two further specificities 3 and 6 (originally C and F) were defined in a similar way[202] giving rise to the pattern shown in Table 9.15.

From this it is clear that Gorer's original C57BL anti-A serum should have contained at least three antibodies, anti-3, anti-4 and anti-11, but since CBA has both 3 and 11, absorption with CBA cells would leave only anti-4. Much use has been made of F_1 hybrids as recipients for immunisation, since this will in general reduce the number of antibodies produced. Thus, for example the F_1 between BALB/C and C57BL will be 3 4 5 6 and so, when immunised by CBA or A strain cells, should produce only anti-11.

The first established cross-overs in the H2 system were described by Allen[203] and Amos et al.[202]. The latter authors, for example, studied a back cross of (A × C57BL) F_1 animals by C57BL, which can be written symbolically as

$$\frac{3\ 4\ 5\ 6\ 11}{5\ 6} \times \frac{5\ 6}{5\ 6}$$

with respect to the H-2 types. In the absence of recombination, all offspring should be either 4^+ 11^+ or 4^- 11^-. Amos et al.[202] found 1 out of 88 mice tested that was 4^- 11^+ and which, on crossing to C57BL, gave 10 4^- 11^- and 11 4^- 11^+ offspring and so was clearly a recombinant. More than 40 H-2 recombinants have so far been described, as will be discussed later. Though the data, as we have indicated it so far, seems to be consistent with a two component structure of the H-2 system, involving mainly just 4 (D) and 11 (K), later recombinants complicated the picture and suggested that the

H-2 system involved a number of components which were separable by re-combinants[204].

The situation was still further complicated when Shreffler and Owen[205] discovered a serologically detected serum protein variant, called Ss, that was associated with the H-2 system. The Ss mouse serum protein was detected by immunodiffusion using a rabbit anti-serum. When a number of inbred strains were tested for this protein, it was found that they fell into two classes: those with a high level, which were mainly H-2k, and those with a low level of the protein in the serum. The difference in levels was sufficiently clear cut for it to be easily shown that the variation was controlled by two alleles at an auto-somal locus. The association with H-2 was shown not to be due to any sero-logical relationship between the Ss protein and the H-2 specificities, suggesting

Table 9.15   Definition of H-2 components in 4 inbred strains (A, BALB/C, C57BL and CBA)

Mouse strain	H-2 allele	Antigenic specificities Present*				
A	a	3	4	5	6	11
BALB/C	d	3	4		6	
CBA	k	3		5		11
C57/BL	b			5	6	

* The numbering system for these specificities is now universally used (Snell *et al.*[201]). The correspondences with the original nomenclature are 3 = C, 4 = D, 5 = E, 6 = F, and 11 = K.

that it was probably due to close linkage between the H-2 system and the gene controlling the Ss protein variation. Subsequent data using H-2 recombinant strains (Shreffler[206] and later) confirmed this and showed that the Ss locus mapped in the middle of the H-2 region. Though this apparently separated the specificities into two groups, with *D* on one side of *Ss* and *K* on the other, H-2 genetic maps of increasing complexity were needed to accommodate the data on other serological specificities, and some apparently irreconcilable inconsistencies in the maps were soon found (for reviews see Stimpfling[207] and Klein and Shreffler[208]).

These paradoxes of the H-2 system were largely resolved when it was realised independently in 1971 by Snell *et al.*[209], Shreffler *et al.*[210] and Thorsby[211] that the data could be reconciled with the existence of just two regions, D and K, for the serological determinants, as was implied by the earliest data obtained by Gorer and Snell on the *H-2ᵈ*, *H-2ᵏ* and *H-2ᵃ* alleles. Snell *et al.*[209] and Thorsby[211] based their analyses on an analogy with the two locus model of the HL-A system, while Shreffler *et al.*[210], approached the problem from a reinterpretation of theirs and other's recombination data.

It had been realised for some time that H-2 specificities could, in general, be divided into two categories. The first, and most common category, included specificities that were determined by many alleles and which are now called 'public'. The second category involved specificities which are determined mostly by just one allele, and so were called by Amos[212] 'private'. A number of the private antigens can be detected only using the lymphocytotoxic test and not by haemagglutination. Cross-reactions between sera, especially those directed against 'public antigens, are also quite common as in the HL-A system. Snell et al.[209] realised that the private H-2 specificities which were detected primarily by relatively high titred lymphocytotoxic sera could be arranged into two series, D and K, which were closely analogous to the LA and 4 series of the HL-A system. Each H-2 allele, or haplotype, defined one K and one D private specificity. The public specificities could, to a large extent, be explained by cross-reactions among the private specificities both within, and to some extent across, the two series. Thorby's[211] interpretation was along the same lines, but did not properly take account of the known definition of private and public specificities. A current interpretation of some of the better known H-2 haplotypes is given in Table 9.16. This is in fact an expanded version of Table 9.15 showing the specificities determined by each haplotype, and distinguishing clearly between private and public, and D and K specificities. The public specificities show patterns of association which are reminiscent of some of the complex cross-reactions that are seen in the HL-A system, and the associations of the 4 series antigens with 4a and 4b. In Table 9.16, for example, it can be seen that 1, 5 and 11 form an 'inclusion' group in the sense that the only observed patterns are 5, 1 5 and 1 5 11. The difficulty with this sort of analysis in the mouse is that it is based effectively on a very small number of observations, being limited mainly to the better known inbred lines of mice and their derivatives. The statistical significance of any observed pattern is, therefore, hard to assess. This limitation of the mouse work was realised long ago by Amos, Gorer and Mikulska[202], and has only begun to change recently following the initiation of studies with wild mice by Micklova and Ivyani[213] and Klein[214]. These studies show a pattern of results that is very similar to the HL-A system in man. Private H2 specificities react quite rarely, while public specificities are comparatively common. Klein[214] has begun to isolate wild H-2 alleles in congenic strains and has shown, in five cases, that

Table 9.16　A simplified version of the H-2 chart

H-2 allele or haplotype	Private specificities K	D	Public specificities*							
a	23	4	1	3	5	6	7	8	11	13
b	33	2			5	6				
d	31	4		3		6		8		13
f	—	9				6	7	8		
j	15	2			5	6	7			
k	23	32	1	3	5			8	11	
p	16	—	1	3	5	6	7	8		
q	17	30	1	3	5	6			11	13
r	25	18	1	3	5	6		8	11	
s	19	—	1	3	5	6	7			

Data based on Klein and Shreffler[208] and Snell et al.[209].

Presence of a number indicates presence of the corresponding specificity

— No specificity detected.

* Only public specificities up to, and including, 13 are listed in this table.

each wild allele carried at least one new private specificity not found on any of a wide range of inbred lines that were tested. Clearly the H-2 system in mice is just as polymorphic as the HL-A system in man.

Stimpfling and Richardson[215], noted that nine recombinants derived from the heterozygous combination $H-2^a/H-2^b$ all carried the determinant for specificity 3, even though only $H-2^a$ and not $H-2^b$ determined this specificity (see Table 9.16). They suggested that some of the anomalies, such as this, which they observed in recombinant strains could be explained by the existence of gene duplications in the H-2 region. This suggestion has been further elaborated by Shreffler et al.[210] to reconcile a bipartite subdivision of the H-2 specificities with the recombination data. Thus, Shreffler et al.[210] suggested that the D and K genetic regions of H-2 have a common evolutionary origin by gene duplication, so that similar specificities may be found in each region. Specificities such as 3, which behave as though they belong in both the D and K regions, could thus represent cross-reactions between closely related, if not identical segments of gene products made by two related genetic sequences one in each region.

As presently interpreted the serology and genetics of the H-2 and HL-A systems are quite similar. The main serological difference seems to be that in the H-2 system there are cross-reactions between D and K specificities, while in HL-A, apart from the possible association between 4a and HL-A9, all cross-reaction occurs within the LA or 4 series. Another difference is, of course, the fact that H-2 can generally be detected on red cells while HL-A cannot. On the other hand, as already mentioned, some of the private H-2 specificities can in some cases only be detected by lymphocytotoxicity, while HL-A specificities can be detected on red cells by sensitive agglutination assays[216, 217]. The difference may simply lie in the relative rates of maturation of red cells in the two species.

It is interesting to compare the development of the H-2 and HL-A systems. Gorer's initial studies were based on the human blood groups as a model and early data indicated a bipartite structure for the H-2 system, partly because of the lucky choice of mouse strains. This was, however, obscured by later work which concentrated on a relatively restricted number of inbred lines. The human studies, although they took their initial cue from the early mouse data had to depend on continued use of population studies as in the development of the blood groups (see e.g. Race and Sanger[218]). This use of population data revealed significant patterns of associations between antigens, leading to a bipartite model which was developed without reference to the early work on the H-2 system. The lack of cross-reaction between LA and 4 antigens was certainly a major factor in the development of the HL-A system. As we have discussed already, and will discuss further in the next section, the two systems have now converged to a remarkable extent so that their similarities are much more striking than any of their differences.

9.9.2 Genetic mapping in and around the H-2 region

Since the linkage of *H-2* with the fused gene was established by Gorer and co-workers in 1948 and the first *H-2* recombinants were described in 1955, much further data has accumulated on the linkage relationships of H-2 and its associated genes. The remarkable *T-t* gene complex, investigated especially by Dunn and his co-workers[219, 220] is known to be on the same chromosome as *Fu* and *H-2*. The *T* allele of the T-t system was discovered as a dominant mutation which shortens the tail. The *t* alleles are recessive factors which affect the development of the axial system of the mouse embryo and, in combination with *T* in a *T/t* heterozygote, result in a tailess mouse. A special feature of many of the *t* alleles is that heterozygous $+ t$ individuals (where $+$ is the normal wild type allele) preferentially transmit *t* bearing gametes to their offspring, so that instead of the usual Mendelian 1:1 ratio, between 80 and 99% of offspring may receive the *t* allele. This property of the *t* alleles is a major influence on their evolution, extending most probably to the relatively closely linked markers such as H-2, and accounts for the high frequency of *t* alleles found in wild populations. Recently Bennet *et al.*[221] have detected a cell surface antigen on sperm that seems to be associated with the *T* allele, emphasising a possible relationship with the functions of the H-2 region. The possible significance of linkage of H-2 with the *T–t* alleles and the fused gene, whose effect is also on skeletal development, were already commented on by Gorer *et al.*[139].

There is another locus, called *Tla*, on the H-2 chromosome which may have a related function, and which is closely linked to H-2, separated from it by a recombination fraction of *ca.* 1.5%. The *Tla* locus controls a series of antigens present only on either thymus or thymic leukaemia cells[222, 223]. In some normal mice these antigens are expressed only on cells from the thymus. However, thymic leukaemia cells always express the antigens and may sometimes express antigens not found in the normal host.

There are two further genetic differences which, like the Ss variation already mentioned, are very closely linked to the H-2 region Following the discovery of the Ss protein, polymorphic variants were sought by immunisation of mice of one strain with partially purified Ss protein from another. Alloimmune sera were found which, by immunodiffusion, detected an antigen called Slp^a that was only expressed in males (Sex limited protein) and whose presence was contolled by a dominant gene[224]. Males castrated before birth do not develop Slp^a, while females treated with testosterone do express Slp^a. Preliminary biochemical studies indicate that Ss and Slp^a are closely related proteins, while genetic studies with recombinants in the H-2 region have not so far separated the genetic control of Ss from Slp^a. Only three of the four possible combinations of high and low levels of Ss and presence or absence of Slp^a have so far been found namely: $Ss^h Slp^a$, $Ss^h Slp^o$ and $SS^1 Slp^o$ (Ss^h = high Ss, Ss^1 = low Ss, Slp^o = absence of Slp^a, from Shreffler and Passmore[224].)

The second genetic difference closely associated with H-2 is that controlling certain types of immune response as also discussed in other chapters. Thus it has been shown by McDevitt and co-workers that the ability of mice to respond to certain branched multi-chain synthetic polypeptides, as well as a number of other antigens, is under the control of one or more closely linked dominant genes which are themselves closely linked to H-2[225, 226]. This immune response controlling genetic region has been called *Ir-1*. Studies by Lilly[227] have shown that there is a recessive gene which controls susceptibility to the Gross virus induced form of murine leukaemia that is also very closely

Location of $Ss-Slp$ inside the H-2 region

Antigens

(a) Heterozygote genotype K region D region Ss phenotype[1]

k	23	32	1
d	31	4	h

(b)

H2 cross-overs		Postulated gene sequence		
		$K-D-Ss$	$Ss-K-D$	$K-Ss-D$
23	4	all h	all l	l or h
31	32	all l	all h	l or h

[1] l = low   h = high

Figure 9.12 (a) shows the genotype and phenotype of the heterozygote being studied
(b) shows the expected Ss phenotypes of H-2 recombinants according to the three possible sequences of the three genes. Observations support the sequence K—Ss—D.

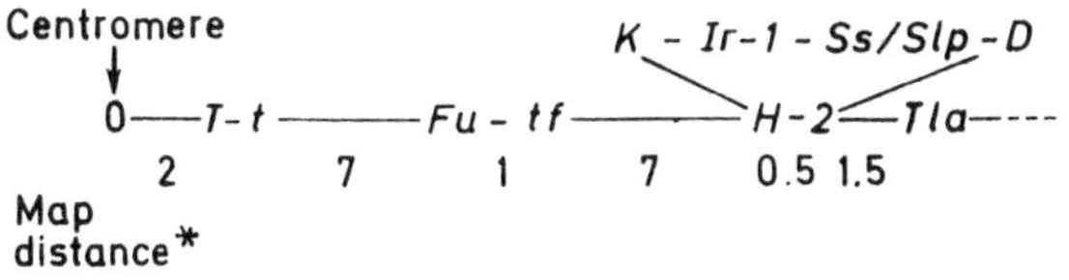

Centromere $K - Ir-1 - Ss/Slp - D$

0——T-t ———————Fu - tf ———————H-2———Tla————

| 2 | 7 | 1 | 7 | 0.5 | 1.5 |

Map distance*

Figure 9.13 A simplified map of mouse linkage group IX

Genes	Phenotypic effects
T-t:	Short tail; axial system defects, segregation distortion, sperm antigen
Fu:	Fused,—short or kinky tails
Tf:	Tufted—waves of hair loss
$H2 K, D$:	Serologically detected determinants
Ss/Slp:	Serum protein/sex limited protein
Ir-1:	Immune response
Tla:	Thymus leukaemia antigen

*Approximate map distances are given in centimorgans.

linked to H-2. Lilly has suggested that the mechanism of this control is via the immune response, which raises the possibility that the relevant gene is in fact Ir-1 (see e.g. McDevitt and Bodmer[228]). The relative genetic position of the Ir-1 and Slp^a genes in the H-2 region have been established by studying H-2 recombinants. An example of this analysis is given in Figure 9.12, which shows how the Ss phenotypes of H-2 recombinants from an H-2^k/H-2^d $\left(\dfrac{23Ss^1\ 32}{31\ Ss^h4}\right)$ heterozygote establish that the Ss gene is located between the K and

D genes. Only this sequence can account for either class of H-2 recombinants, 23 4 or 31 32, being either 1 or h. The Ir-1 locus has, by a similar type of analysis, been placed between K and Ss. Thus, in terms of the order K—Ss—D recombinants between Ss and D place Ir-1 to the left of these two markers, while some (but not all) recombinants between K and Ss place Ir-1 in this region giving the overall sequence K—Ir-1—Ss—D.

A combined map of linkage group IX which includes H-2 and the other markers discussed above is shown in Figure 9.13 The position of the centromere to the left of the T–t and H-2 regions was established by Lyon et al.[229] The average recombination frequency between H-$2D$ and H-$2K$ is ca. 0.5% though there is evidence that this varies to some extent as a function of the H-2 heterozygote genotype. The distance between D and K loci is not significantly different from that between LA and 4, and so presumably encompasses a comparable number of genes some of which have been identified as Ir-1 and Ss/Slp. More discussion of the functions of genes in this region will be given in the next section. Though more than 40 H-2 recombinants have been described (none of which separates Ss from Slp), this number is still probably quite small relative to the size of the region. Thus, while separation of two H-2 associated traits by recombination indicates they are determined by different genes, a lack of separation clearly does not prove the opposite. Thus, as already discussed for the HL-A system, it cannot even be assumed that the serologically detected determinants themselves are controlled by only two genes, D and K rather than two clusters of genes. Selective techniques for the production of recombinants using transplantable tumours[230] should help to alleviate this problem.

9.10 FUNCTION AND EVOLUTION OF MAJOR HISTOCOMPATIBILITY SYSTEMS

9.10.1 Effects of the HL-A and H-2 systems on immune response functions

In addition to their association with graft rejection the H-2 and HL-A histocompatibility systems are associated with other parameters of immunity such as the graft versus host reaction (GVH, usually measured by spleen enlargement following injection of lymphocytes) and the mixed lymphocyte culture response or MLR (sometimes also called MLC). When lymphocytes from different individuals are cultured together they stimulate each other to enlarge and divide and this reaction can be readily quantified by the uptake and incorporation of radioactive thymidine. If one of the sources of cells is inactivated, for example by Mitomycin, then the response of the uninactivated to the inactivated cell population can be assessed in a one-way test. Almost all pairs of individuals stimulate each other in such a test. It was however, shown by Bach and Amos[231], and confirmed by Shellekens et al.[232] and others, that sibs who are identical with respect to their HL-A types do not stimulate each other in an MLR test. This suggested that the MLR response was under the genetic control of the HL-A region. HL-A identical unrelated individuals, however, mostly *do* show mutual MLR reactions[233, 234]. Although some of these reactions could be due to technical errors in typing, giving rise to spurious HL-A identity, this cannot account for all such reactions between HL-A identical unrelated individuals. These results suggest that the MLR reaction can be dissociated genetically from the HL-A antigenic determinants, and this has been confirmed in family studies. Rare combinations (*ca.* 1 %) of HL-A identical sibs have been found which do give rise to an MLR response[235, 236]. This is interpreted as indicating that MLR is controlled by a locus closely linked to *LA* and *4*, but outside the region between these two loci. A schematic example illustrating the rationale behind this interpretation is shown in Figure 9.14. Recombination between *4* and the *MLR* locus separates the

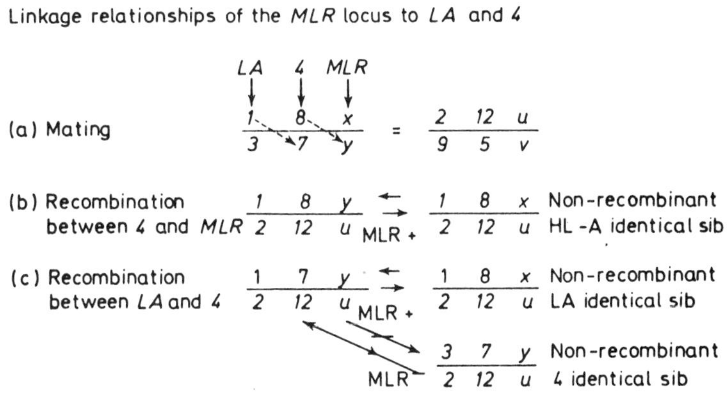

Linkage relationships of the *MLR* locus to *LA* and *4*

Figure 9.14 Linkage relationships of the MLR locus of LA and 4
In (b) HL-A identical sibs stimulate because of MLR locus differences
In (c) *4* locus identical sibs which are different at *LA* do not stimulate, but *LA* locus identical sibs differing at *4* do stimulate

MLR response from HL-A identity. As indicated in Figure 9.14c, the association of MLR response with the *4* rather than the *LA* locus in HL-A recombinants places the *MLR* locus on the *4* side of the HL-A region[237, 238]. A family including two recombinants sibs, one between *LA* and *4* and the other between *4* and *MLR* has been described by Eijsvogel et al.[239]. This gives rise to a situation in which two sibs who differ for at least three HL-A antigens do not stimulate each other in MLR.

Similar, although somewhat less clear, cut, data to those on MLR reactions has been obtained from studies on skin graft survival. HL-A identical sibs show a very significantly prolonged skin graft survival time of *ca.* 20 days, as compared to *ca.* 12 or 13 days for unrelated individuals[231, 241].

This effect is not, however, in general seem among HL-A identical unrelated individuals even if they show no MLR response. Thus it would appear that graft survival may be controlled by one or more genes closely linked to the HL-A region but separable from the LA, 4 and MLR loci[234]. Although recombination between these loci occurs in families with a frequency of only 0.5–1%, all possible combinations of alleles exist in the population at large, as is the case for the LA and 4 antigens themselves. This accounts for the lack of correlation of MLR response and skin graft survival among HL-A identical unrelated individuals.

Recent studies in the mouse have given closely analogous results to those observed in man. Thus Rychlikova *et al.*[242] suggested from a study of H-2 recombinants that the *K* locus of the H-2 system was predominantly associated with the MLR response. Subsequent studies by Demant, Ivanyi, Sorenson, Bach, Miggiano, Nabholz and others, making use of a variety of H-2 recombinants, have provided extensive data on the mapping of MLR, GVH and graft rejection genes in the H-2 region. (see Bach *et al.*[243] and Demant, Festenstein and others personal communication of results of a workshop on Cellular Immunity in Mice held in London in February 1973. (*Transplant Proc.* (in the press)). A schematic summary of these results is shown in Figure 9.15. This includes data on the recently described cell mediated lympholysis

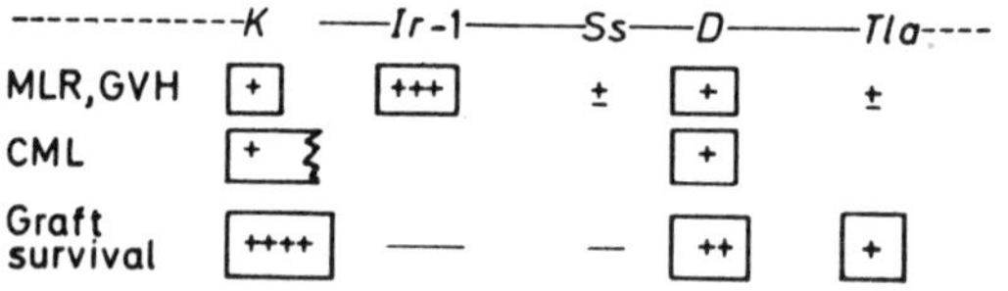

Figure 9.15 Schematic map of the position of genes for the MLR, GVH, graft survival and CML responses in the mouse H-2 region

MLR: Mixed lymphocyte response
GVH: Graft *v.* host reaction
CML: Cell-mediated lympholysis

(CML) reaction[244, 245] which is measured by killing, as indicated by release of ^{51}Cr from labelled target cells, by lymphocytes that have been stimulated *in vitro* by an MLR response. As already emphasised, association of a phenotype with the D and K antigens in recombinants does not by any means imply that the genetic determinants of the phenotype, such as graft survival or CML, are the same as those for the serologically detectable antigens. In particular, there is suggestive evidence for a genetic separation of the *MLR* and *Ir-1* genes. So far the data in the mouse indicate a major MLR gene complex *between* K and D in the mouse, whereas in man the major effect seems to be *outside* the LA to 4 region. This difference between the species may, however, be explained by the fact that the mouse data is based on backcrosses, whereas the human data is necessarily based on combined information from many intercrosses[192]. There is also evidence in the mouse for the existence of a locus not linked to H-2 that has a strong effect on MLR[245].

Further indications of the homology of the H-2 and HL-A regions come from data showing an association between HL-A and susceptibility to a variety of diseases including Hodgkin's disease and systemic lupus erythematosus which are thought to be correlated with immune response differences[228, 246, 247]. These associations have been interpreted in terms of the effects of an immune response type locus separate from, but closely linked to, the *LA* and *4* loci of the HL-A system[228, 248]. Recent data has also provided direct evidence for linkage between HL-A and IgE antibody response to the ragweed allergen E pollen antigen[249, 250]. Preliminary data, furthermore, shows an association between antibody response to the synthetic branched chain polypeptide ((TG)—A—L) originally used in mouse studies and the rhesus monkey major histocompatibility system, which is the homologue of HL-A and H-2 (Balner and McDevitt, personal communication), emphasising the probable existence of an Ir-1 gene complex in the HL-A region.

9.10.2 Functional integration and evolution of the HL-A and H-2 regions

The overall genetic data on the HL-A and H-2 systems clearly suggests that these are genetic regions which contain a large number of closely linked genes with interrelated functions. Such linked gene complexes are predicted by Fisher's theory of the interaction between natural selection and linkage, and data on linkage disequilibrium in the HL-A system provides some evidence for the existence of the required types of selective interaction. Although a number of the genes other than those for the serologically determined antigens have been described, undoubtedly a great many more remain to be discovered. A striking feature of all these genes is that their functions are connected, either directly or implicitly, with the cell surface. This is most clearly the case for the serologically detectable antigens themselves, as well as for the MLR, CML, GVH and graft survival genes. McDevitt's suggestion[226, 251] that the *Ir-1* gene or genes control the synthesis of non immunoglobulin T-cell antigen receptors gives these genes also a clear role on the cell surface. Most recently, the demonstration by Demant et al.[252] that the Ss–Slp protein may control complement levels in the mouse gives even this apparently anomalous gene a cell surface associated function.

It has often been suggested that cell-cell recognition during tissue differentiation and morphogenesis may be mediated by cell surface structures (differentiation antigens), and that the recognition between cells may be controlled by antibody like molecules (recognisers) (see e.g. Refs. [175, 223, 253-256]). I have made the further suggestion that the biological role of many, if not most, of the genes in the major histocompatibility system genetic region lies in the control of the synthesis of a class of differentiation antigens and their recognisers, of which genes such as *Ir-1* and *MLR* are special cases[175]. Following Jerne's[255] suggestion, it seems possible that these genes are evolutionarily quite closely related to the immunoglobulin genes. This would imply that there was a set of genes which were the common evolutionary precursors to both the histocompatibility and immunoglobulin gene complexes, and which were duplicated and separated some time before the evolution of the immune system. As already indicated the multiplicity of genes within the histocompatibility regions probably also arose by a series of duplications, as has been postulated for the immunoglobulins and haemoglobins.

The striking homology between the H-2 and HL-A systems has been emphasised repeatedly. Major histocompatibility systems analogous to H-2 and HL-A have been found in all mammalian species studied so far (man, mouse, rat, rabbit, dog, cow, guinea-pig, pig, Rhesus monkey and chimpanzee) as well as in the chicken (the B blood group system see, e.g. Ivanyi[263]) and even in the toad, *Xenopus laevis*[257]. A two locus structure has also been established in rhesus monkeys, chimpanzees and the dog, and immune response genes linked to the major histocompatibility systems have been found, so far, in the mouse, guinea-pig, rat and probably also in man and Rhesus monkey. Perhaps most surprising of all, direct cross-reactions between the serologically detectable histocompatibility antigens of species as distantly related as man and cow, man and rabbit, man and mouse and mouse and rabbit have been demonstrated[258-262]. This suggests that the polymorphic differences now found within these various species actually predate the separation of the species themselves. A possible way out of this dilemma is to assume that the serologically detectable antigens are actually the products of different genes, and that the genetic polymorphism is for the *control*, of which of the genes is expressed.

Many of the questions raised by the genetic studies of HL-A and H-2 should eventually be answered by studies of the chemistry of the gene products of these regions, and a promising start has already been made as described in the accompanying chapter. If the view of the major histocompatibility systems that I have presented here is essentially correct, then there is much more that remains to be discovered in these regions and in the course of this discovery may lie major clues to the further understanding of the functioning of the immune system and the processes of cell–cell recognition during development and differentiation.

References

131. Jensen, C. O. (1903). *Zbl. Bakt., I. Abt. Ref.*, **34**, 28
132. Tyzzer, E. E. (1909). *J. Med. Res.*, **21**, 519
133. Little, C. C. (1914). *Science*, **40**, 904
134. Little, C. C. and Tyzzer, E. E. (1916). *J. Med. Res.*, **33**, 393
135. Landsteiner, K. (1931). *Science*, **73**, 403
136. Gorer, P. A. (1936). *Brit. J. Exp. Path.*, **17**, 42
137. Gorer, P. A. (1937). *Brit. J. Exp. Path.*, **18**, 31
138. Snell, G. D. (1948). *J. Genet.*, **49**, 87
139. Gorer, P. A., Lyman, S. and Snell, G. D. (1948). *Proc. Roy. Soc. B.*, **135**, 499
140. Bailey, D. W. and Mobraaten, L. E. (1969). *Transplantation*, **7**, 394
141. Bauer, K. H. (1927). *Beitr. Klin. Chir.*, **141**, 442
142. Gibson, T. and Medawar, P. B. (1943). *J. Anat. (London)*, **77**, 299
143. Medawar, P. B. (1946). *Brit. J. Exp. Path.*, **27**, 15
144. Payne, R. and Rolfs, M. R. (1958). *J. Clin. Invest.*, **37**, 1756
145. van Rood, J. J., Eernisse, J. G., and van Leeuwen, A. (1958). *Nature (London)*, **181**, 1735
146. Dausset, J. and Rapaport, F. T. (1966). *Ann. N.Y. Acad. Sci.*, **129**, 408
147. Ceppellini, R., Curtoni, E. S., Mattiuz, P. L., Leigheb, G., Visetti, M. and Colombi, A. (1966). *Ann. N.Y. Acad. Sci.*, **129**, 421

148. Gorer, P. A. and O'Gorman, P. (1956). *Transplant. Bull.*, **3**, 142
149. Terasaki, P. I. and McClelland, J. D. (1964). *Nature (London)*, **204**, 998
150. Böyum, A. (1968). *Scand. J. Clin. Lab. Invest.* **21**, Suppl. 97
151. Rotman, B. and Papermaster, B. W. (1966). *Proc. Nat. Acad. Sci. USA*, **55**/1, 134
152. Bodmer, W. F., Tripp, M. and Bodmer, J. (1967). *Histocompatibility Testing, 1967*, 341. (Copenhagen: Munksgaard)
153. Terasaki, P. I. Ed. (1970). *Histocompatibility Testing 1970*, (Copenhagen: Munksgaard)
154. Shulman, N. R., Aster, R. H., Pearson, H. A. and Hiller, M. C. (1962). *J. Clin. Invest.*, **41**, 1059
155. Shulman, N. W., Marder, V. J., Hiller, M. C., and Collier, E. M. (1964). *Progr. in Hematol.* **4**, 222 (New York: Grune and Stratton)
156. D'Amaro, J., van Leeuwen, A., Svejgaard, A. and van Rood, J. J. (1970). *Histocompatibility Testing, 1970*, 539 (Copenhagen: Munksgaard)
157. Dausset, J. Ed. (1973). *Histocompatibility Testing, 1972* (Copenhagen: Munksgaard)
158. van Rood, J. J. (1962). *Thesis*, Leiden
159. Payne, R., Tripp, M., Weigle, J., Bodmer, W. and Bodmer, J. (1964). *Cold Spring Harbor Sympos. Quant. Biol.*, **29**, 285
160. Cavalli-Sforza, L. L. and Bodmer, W. F. (1971). *The Genetics of Human Populations.* (San Francisco: Freeman and Co.)
161. van Rood, J. J. and van Leeuwen, A. (1963). *J. Clin. Invest.*, **42**, 1382
162. Curtoni, E. S., Mattiuz, P. L. and Mtosi, R. editors (1967). *Histocompatibility Testing 1967* (Copenhagen: Munksgaard)
163. Dausset, J. (1958). *Acta Haematol. (Basel)*, **20**, 156
164. van Rood, J. J., van Leeuwen, A., Schippers, A. M. H., Vouys, W., Frederiks, E., Balner, H. and Eernisse, J. G. (1965). *Histocompatibility Testing, 1965*, 37 (Copenhagen Munksgaard)
165. Dausset, J., Rapaport, F. T., Iványi, P. and Colombani, J. (1965). *Histocompatibility Testing, 1965*, 65 (Copenhagen: Munksgaard)
166. Bodmer, W., Bodmer, J., Adler, S., Payne, R. and Bialek, J. (1966). *Ann. N.Y. Acad. Sci. U.SA*, **129**, 473
167. Ceppellini, R., Curtoni, E. S., Mattiuz, P. L., Miggiano, V., Scudeller, G. and Serra, A. (1967). *Histocompatibility Testing, 1967*, 149 (Copenhagen: Munksgaard)
168. Kissmeyer-Nielsen, F., Svejgaard, A. and Hauge, M. (1968). *Nature (London)* **219**, 1116
169. Dausset, J., Colombani, J., Legrand, L. and Feingold, N. (1968b). *Nouv. Rev. Franç. Hémat.* **8**, 861
170. Allen, A., Amos, D. B., Batchelor, R., Bodmer, W. F., Ceppellini, R., Dausset, J., Engelfriet, C., Jeannet, M., Kissmeyer-Nielsen, F., Morris, P., Payne, R., Terasaki, P., van Rood, J. J., Walford, R., Zmijewski, C., Mattiuz, A. E., Mickey, R. R. and Piazza, A. (1970). *Histocompatibility Testing, 1970*, 2 (Copenhagen: Munksgaard)
171. Mattiuz, P. L., Ihde, D. Piazza, A., Ceppellini, R. and Bodmer, W. F. (1970). *Histocompatibility Testing, 1970*, 193 (Copenhagen: Munksgaard)
172. Weitkamp, L. R., van Rood, J. J., Thorsby, E., Bias, W., Allen, F. H. Jr., Lawler, S. D., Dausset, J., Mayr, W. R., Bodmer, J., Ward, F. E., Seignalet, J., Payne, R., Kissmeyer-Nielsen, F., Gatti, R. A., Sachs, J. A. and Lamm, L. U. (1973). *Human Heredity* (in the press)
173. Svejgaard, A, Bratlie, A., Hedin, P. J., Högman, C., Jersild, C., Kissmeyer-Nielsen, F., Lindblohm, B., Lindblohm, A., Löw, B., Messeter, L., Möller, E., Sandberg, L., Staub-Neilsen, L. and Thorsby, E. (1971). *Tissue Antigens*, **1**, 81
174. Bodmer, W. F., Bodmer, J. G. and Tripp, M. (1970). *Histocompatibility Testing, 1970*, 187 (Copenhagen: Munksgaard)
175. Bodmer, W. F. (1972). *Nature (London)*, **237**, 139
176. Lamm, L. U., Svejgaard, A. and Kissmeyer-Nielsen, F. (1971). *Nature New Biol.*, **231**, 109
177. Fellous, M., Billardon C., Dausset, J. and Frézal, J. (1971). *C.R. Acad. Sci. (Paris)*, **272 D**, 3356
178. Edwards, J. H., Allen, F. H., Glenn, K. P., Lamm, L. U. and Robson, E. B. (1973). *Histocompatibility Testing, 1972*, 745, (Copenhagen: Munksgaard)
179. Ferrone, S., Tosi, R. M., and Centis, D. (1967). *Histocompatibility Testing 1967*, 357 (Copenhagen: Munksgaard)

180. Bodmer, W. F. and Payne, R. (1965). *Histocompatibility Testing, 1965, Series Haematologia*, **11**, 141, (Copenhagen: Munksgard)
181. Dausset, J., Colombani, J., Colombani, M., Legrand, L. and Feingold, N. (1968). *Nouv. Rev. Franç. Hémat.*, **8**, 398
182. Bodmer, J. G., Coukell, A., Bodmer, W. F., Payne, R. and Shanbrom, E. (1970). *Histocompatibility Testing, 1970*, 175, (Copenhagen: Munksgaard)
183. Colombani, J., Colombani, M. and Dausset, J. (1970). *Histocompatibility Testing, 1970*, 79, (Copenhagen: Munksgaard)
184. Dausset, J. (1971). *Transplant. Proc.*, **3**, 1139
185. Ceppellini, R. (1971). *Proc. First Intern. Congr. Immunol.*, 973, (New York: Academic Press)
186. Thorsby, E., Kissmeyer-Neilsen, F. and Svejgaard, A. (1970). *Histocompatibility Testing, 1970*, 137, (Copenhagen: Munksgaard)
187. Mittal, K. K. and Terasaki, P. I. (1972). *Tissue Antigens*, **2**, 94
188. van Rood, J. J., van Leeuwen, A., Koch, C. T. and Van Santen, M. C. T. (1970). *Histocompatibility Testing, 1970*, 483, (Copenhagen: Munksgaard)
189. Legrand, L. and Dausset, J. (1973). *Histocompatibility Testing, 1972*, 441 (Copenhagen: Munksgaard)
190. Richiardi, P., Carbonara, A. O., Mattiuz, P. L. and Ceppellini, R. (1973). *Histocompatibility Testing, 1972*, 455, (Copenhagen: Munksgaard)
191. Svejgaard, A., Staub-Nielsen, L., Ryder, L., Kissmeyer-Neilsen, F., Sandberg, L., Lindholm, A. and Thorsby, E. (1973). *Histocompatibility Testing, 1972*, 465, (Copenhagen: Munksgaard)
192. Bodmer, W. F. (1972). *Histocompatibility Testing, 1972*, 611, (Copenhagen: Munksgaard)
193. Bodmer, W. F., Cann, H. and Piazza, A. (1973). *Histocompatibility Testing, 1972*, 753, (Copenhagen: Munksgaard)
194. Jennings, H. S. (1917). *Genetics*, **2**, 97
195. Fisher, R. A. (1930). *The Genetical Theory of Natural Selection*. (2nd edn. 1958 New York: Dover)
196. Bodmer, W. F. and Felsenstein, J., *Genetics* (1967), **52**, 237
197. Karlin, S. and Feldman, M. W. (1970). *Theoret. Population Biol.*, **1**, 39
198. Franklin, I. and Lewontin R. C. (1970). *Genetics*, **65**, 77
199. Snell, G. D. (1951). *J. Nat. Cancer Inst.*, **11**, 1299
200. Snell, G. D. Smith P. and Gabrielson F. (1953). *J. Nat. Cancer Inst.*, **14**, 457
201. Snell, G. D., Hoecker, G., Amos, D. B. and Stimpfling, J. H. (1964). *Transplantation*, **2**, 777
202. Amos, D. B., Gorer, P. A. and Mikulska, Z. B. (1955). *Proc. Roy. Soc. B* **144**, 369
203. Allen, S. L. (1955). *Genetics*, **40**, 627
204. Gorer, P. A. and Mikulska, Z. B. (1959). *Proc. Roy. Soc. B*, **151**, 57
205. Shreffler, D. C. and Owen, R. D. (1963). *Genetics*, **48**, 9
206. Shreffler, D. C. (1965). *Wistar. Inst. Sympos. Monogr. No. 3*, 11, (Philadelphia: Wistar Institute Press)
207. Stimpfling, J. H. (1971). *Ann. Rev. Genetics*, **5**, 121
208. Klein, J. and Shreffler, D. C. (1971). *Transplant. Rev.*, **6**, 3
209. Snell, G. D., Cherry, M. and Démant, P. (1971). *Transplant. Rev.*, **3**, 183
210. Shreffler, D. C., David, C. S., Passmore, H. C. and Klein, J. (1971). *Transplant. Proc.*, **3**, 176
211. Thorsby, E. (1971). *Europ. J. Immunol.*, **1**, 57
212. Amos, D. B. (1962). *Ann. N.Y. Acad. Sci. USA*, **97**, 69
213. Micklová, M. and Iványi, P. (1971). *Immunogenetics of the H-2 System*, (Basel: Karger)
214. Klein, J. (1972). *Transplantation*, **13**, 291
215. Stimpfling, J. H. and Richardson, A. (1965). *Genetics*, **51**, 831
216. Morton, J. A., Pickles, M. M. and Sutton, L. (1969). *Vox. Sang.*, **17**, 536
217. Morton, J. A., Pickles, M. M., Sutton, L. and Skov F. (1971). *Vox. Sang.*, **21**, 141
218. Race, R. R. and Sanger, R. (1968). *Blood Groups in Man*, (Oxford: Blackwells)
219. Dunn, L. C. (1964). *Science*, **144**, 260
220. Bennett, D. and Dunn, L. C. (1971). *Proc. Sympos. Immunogenetics of the H-2 System*, 90, (Basel: Karger)

221. Bennett, D., Goldberg, E., Dunn, L. C. and Boyse, E. A. (1972). *Proc. Nat. Acad. Sci. USA*, **69**, 2076
222. Boyse, E. A., Old, L. J. and Stockert, E. (1966). *IVth Imternat. Symp.*, 23, (Basel: Schwabe and Co. Publ.)
223. Boyse, E. A. and Old, L. J. (1969). *Ann. Rev. Genet.*, **3**, 269
224. Shreffler, D. C. and Passmore, H. C. (1971). *Proceedings of Symposium on Immunogenetics of the H-2 System Prague*, 58 (Basel: Karger)
225. McDevitt, H. O. and Benacerraf, B. (1969). *Advan. Immunol.*, **11**, 31
226. Benacerraf, B. and McDevitt, H. O. (1972). *Science*, **175**, 273
227. Lilly, F. (1970). *Comparative Leukemia Research 1969*, 213, (Basel/New York: S. Karger)
228. McDevitt, H. O. and Bodmer, W. F. (1972). *Amer. J. Med.*, **52**, 1
229. Lyon, M. F., Butler, J. M. and Kemp, R. (1968). *Genet. Res.*, **11**, 193
230. Shreffler, D. C. (1971). *Proc. of the Symp. on Immunogenetics of the H-2 System. Prague*, 138 (Basel: Karger)
231. Bach, F. and Amos, D. B. (1967). *Science*, **156**, 1506
232. Shellekens, P. Th. A., Vriesendorp, B., Eijsvogel, V. P., van Leeuwen, A., van Rood, J. J., Miggiano, V. and Ceppellini, R. (1970). *Clin. Exp. Immunol.*, **6**, 241
233. Eijsvogel, V. P., Shellekens, P. Th. A., Vriesendorp. B., van Leeuwen, A., Koch, C. and van Rood, J. J. (1970). *Histocompetibility Testing, 1970*, 523, (Copenhagen: Munksgaard)
234. Koch, C. T., Eijsvogel, V. P., Frederiks, E. and van Rood, J. J. (1971). *Lancet*, **2**, 1334
235. Plate, J. M., Ward, F. E. and Amos, D. B. (1970). *Histocompatibility Testing, 1970*, 531, (Copenhagen: Munksgaard)
236. Yunis, E. J. and Amos, D. B. (1971). *Proc. Nat. Acad. Sci. USA*, **68**, 3031
237. Dupont, B., Nielsen, L. S. and Svejgaard, A. (1971). *Lancet*, **2**, 1336
238. Lebrun, A., Sasportes, M., Lebrun, D. and Dausset, J. (1971). *C.R. Acad. Sci. (Paris)*, **273**, 2130
239. Eijsvogel, V. P., du Bois, M. J. G. J., Melief, C. J. M., de Groot-Kooy, M. L., Koning, C., van Rood, J. J., van Leeuwen, A., du Toit, E. and Shellekens, P. Th. A. (1973.) *Histocompatibility Testing, 1972*, 501, (Copenhagen: Munksgaard)
240. Ceppellini, R. (1968). *Human Transplantation*, 21 (J. Daussel and F. Rapaport, editors). (New York: Grune and Stratton)
241. Dausset, J., Rapaport, F. T., Legrand, L., Colombani, J. and Marcelli-Barge, A. (1970). *Histocompatibility Testing, 1970*, 381, (Copenhagen: Munksgaard)
242. Rychlikova, M., Démant, P. and Iványi, P. (1971). *Nature (London)*, **230**, 271
243. Bach, F. H., Bach, M. L., Sondel, P. M. and Gnanasigamoni Sundharadas (1972). *Transplant. Rev.*, **12**, 30
244. Lightbody, J. J., Bernoco, D., Miggiano, V. C. and Ceppellini, R. (1971). *G. Batt. Virol.*, **64**, 243
245. Festenstein, H., Sachs, J. A. and Oliver, R. T. (1970). *Proceedings of Symp. Immunogenetics of the H-2 System. Prague*, 170, (Basel: Karger)
246. Dausset, J. (1972). *Progress in Clinical Immunology*, 116, (New York: Grune and Stratton)
247. Walford, R. L., (1972). *Transpl. Rev.*, **8**, 1
248. Bodmer, W. F. (1973). *International Symposium on Hodgkin's Disease, Stanford University, Calif., 1972*, (in the press)
249. Marsh, D. G., Bias, W. B., and Hsu, S. H. (1973). *Science*, **179**, 691
250. Levine, B. B. and Stember, R. H. (1972). *Science*, **178**, 1201
251. McDevitt, H. O., Bechtol, K., Grumet, F. C., Mitchell, G. F. and Wegmann, T. G. (1971). *Proc. First Intern. Cong. Immunol.* 495, (New York: Academic Press)
252. Démant, P., Capková, J., Hinzová, E. and Vorácová, B. (1973). *Proc. Nat. Acad. Sci. USA*, **70**, 863
253. Moscona A. (1957). *Proc. Nat. Acad. Sci. USA*, **43**, 184
254. Boyse, E. A. and Old, L. J. (1970). *Immune Surveillance*, 5, (New York: Academic Press)
255. Jerne, N. K. (1971). *Europ. J. Immunol.*, **1**, 1
256. Burnet, F. M. (1971). *Nature (London)*, **232**, 230
257. Du Pasquier, L. and Miggiano, V. C. (1973). *Transplant. Proc.* (in the press)

258. Iha, T. H., Gerbrandt, G., Bodmer, W. F., McGary, D. and Stone, W. H. (1969)· *Abstr. Amer. Soc. Hum. Genet.*
259. Iha, T. H., Gerbrandt, G., Bodmer, W. F., McGarry, D. and Stone, W. H. (1973). *Tissue Antigens* (in the press)
260. Albert, E., Kano, K., Abeyounis, C. J. and Milgrom, F. (1969). *Transplantation*, **8,** 466
261. Ivašková, E., Dausset, J. and Iványi, P. (1972). *Folia Biologica (Praha)*, **18,** 194
262. Abeyounis, C. J. and Milgrom, F. (1969). *Transplant. Proc.*, **1,** 556
263. Ivanyi, P. (1970). *Current Topics in Microbiology and Immunology*, **53,** 1 (Berlin: Springer Verlag)

10
Antigen Recognition and Cell-receptor Sites

W. E. PAUL

National Institute of Allergy and Infectious Diseases, Bethesda, Maryland

10.1 INTRODUCTION

The activation of immunocompetent cells to proliferate and differentiate into antibody-secreting cells or into cells mediating the various cellular immune functions depends upon a specific interaction between antigen and responsive cell, that is, cellular activation is dependent upon a mechanism by which the cell recognises antigen.

The concept of a cellular recognition mechanism in immune responses was initially proposed by Ehrlich[1]. Although Ehlrich's terminology was quite different from that used today, many of the main elements of modern selective theories of the immune response were present in Ehrlich's hypothesis. He envisioned that antigen interacted with a recognition structure on the cell surface, that this interaction led to a response of the cell, and as part of the response, molecules identical to the recognition structure were produced in large quantities and were secreted by the cell.

In one key respect, however, the 'side-chain' theory of Ehrlich differs from the concept which has dominated contemporary immunological thinking. Thus, a key postulate of the clonal selection theory of Burnet[2] is that individual cells functioning as precursors of antibody-secreting cells or as precursors of cells mediating cellular immune responses have antigen recognition units of a single specificity. The wide repertoire of the organism derives from the existence of a large number of cells, or clones of cells, each with antigen-recognition units of distinct specificity.

A considerable portion of modern immunological research is concerned with the analysis of the nature and specificity of the antigen recognition units, or receptors, of immunocompetent cells and substantial progress has been made in this area. In many respects, the results obtained provide confirmation for the key tenets of the clonal selection theory. None the less, the direct study of receptors of immunocompetent cells is still in a relatively early stage. In this chapter, I will review several aspects of the antigen-recognition mechanisms important in the immune response.

10.2 MACROPHAGES

One important complexity of the immune response is the participation of three cell types in many immunological phenomena. Antigen recognition appears to occur to some extent in each cell type.

As has been already discussed in previous chapters of this volume, the cells which are specifically activated by antigen are lymphocytes, of which two major classes exist, the thymus dependent (T) and the thymus independent (B). These cell types have distinct immunological functions and, it also appears, major differences in their antigen-recognition mechanisms. Before discussing the receptors of B and T lymphocytes, which form the major topic of this chapter, some consideration of the role of the macrophage in antigen recognition is required.

The precise role of the macrophage in the initiation of immune responses is still a subject of some controversy. Thus, it has been proposed that the macrophage functions as:

(a) An antigen trapping cell which displays antigen on its surface, perhaps in a particularly favourable array for lymphocyte activation.

(b) A cell which digests large molecules or particles into smaller substances which might be more capable of initiating immune responses.

(c) A cell which processes antigen by complexing it to RNA or other substances thereby producing an exceedingly potent antigen (super-antigen).

(d) A cell which has a nutritional or trephocytic role in the maintenance of lymphocyte function.

(e) A cell in which the main antigen-recognition events occur and which dictates subsequent immune responses of lymphocytes through the transfer of informational RNA.

For each of these potential roles for macrophages a degree of experimental support has been provided and mechanisms (a)–(d) are not mutually exclusive. The information-transfer thesis, (e) which is radically different from each of the others, is clearly the most controversial and the one for which experimental evidence must be regarded as the least secure.

The thesis which currently has the widest support is that the prime function of the macrophage is as an antigen-concentrating cell which displays antigen on its surface (a). In many respects, the macrophage is ideally suited for this role. Its anatomical location is such that it encounters antigen rapidly after introduction into the animal and in an environment through which lymphocytes pass with high frequency. Many agents bind to its surface 'non-specifically'[3]. The word non-specifically is placed in quotation marks as it principally reflects the limited state of our knowledge concerning this surface phenomenon rather than a precise characterisation of the mechanism of interaction between antigen and cell surface. The macrophage also bears surface receptors for certain forms of immunoglobulin G[4, 5], particularly aggregated IgG, and for the third component of complement (C3)[6]. Thus, it can bind free circulating antigen either by virtue of its 'non-specific' sites or through cytophilic antibody already present on its surface, bound by the receptor for IgG. Furthermore, antigen–antibody complexes or antigen–antibody–complement complexes may bind to macrophages through the receptors for aggregated IgG and for C3, respectively.

In vitro studies indicate that macrophage function is of particular importance in the initiation of thymus-dependent immune responses while the stimulation of antibody production by thymus-independent antigens either does not require macrophages at all or requires many fewer such cells[7, 8]. Definitive *in vivo* studies on this issue are not yet available as experimental models of animals with a *specific* deletion of macrophage function have been difficult to achieve.

10.3 LYMPHOCYTES

The lymphocytes, as the *specific* cells of the immunological system, must occupy the centre of the stage in any consideration of antigen-recognition mechanisms. Certain postulates of the nature of their receptors are implicit in clonal-selection theories and in attempts to adhere to a unitary theory of antigen recognition. I initially state these concepts here so that in consideration of results of current research one can have a clear view of the potential implications of any given outcome.

(a) Cells which are differentiated precursors of antibody-secreting cells or of cells specifically involved in cellular immune responses are committed in regard to the specific antigens by which they may be stimulated.

(b) This commitment is reflected in the specificity of the surface receptor which they bear. For precursors of antibody-secreting cells, the antigen-binding receptor is equivalent in its binding characteristics to the antibody which will be secreted by the descendent of the precursor.

(c) The chemical nature of the receptor on the precursor of an antibody-secreting cell is immunoglobulin as the product of the descendent cell is immunoglobulin. Cells participating in cellular immune responses do not produce easily detectable amounts of immunoglobulin; thus, it is not *necessary* that the antigen-binding receptor of the precursors of such cells be immunoglobulin. None the less, as the postulation of two independent sets of distinct recognition molecules increases the complexity of the system, immunoglobulin should be regarded as the principal candidate for the receptor of these cells.

10.3.1 B Lymphoctyes

The thymus-independent lymphocytes (in the bird—the Bursa-derived lymphocytes) have, as their principal role, the production of antibody-secreting cells and of specific memory cells. The B lymphocytes may be identified by a series of surface markers which include differentiation antigens for which no biological function is yet known (MBLA)[9], surface receptors which may have a general, rather than specific, role in antigen recognition (receptors for aggregated Ig[10, 11] and receptors for C3[12]) and surface immunoglobulin, which plays the role of antigen-binding receptor[13, 14].

10.3.1.1 *Surface immunoglobulins*

Immunoglobulin on the surface of at least some lymphocytes was first demonstrated by the capacity of anti-immunoglobulin sera to cause rabbit lymphocytes to transform, *in vitro*, into blastoid cells and to synthesise DNA. This key finding was reported by Sell and Gell[15] and for several years was the principal evidence which indicated that immunoglobulin existed on the surface of such cells.

Sell and Gell demonstrated that antibodies specific for immunoglobulin class or for allotypic forms of immunoglobulin were effective in stimulating *in vitro* DNA synthesis by rabbit lymphoid cells. Moreover, through the study of lymphocytes of neonatal rabbits heterozygous at an allotype locus, they showed that the surface immunoglobulin responsible for this effect does not derive from circulating immunoglobulin[16]. The serum immunoglobulin of neonatal rabbits is almost completely maternal in origin; these animals have themselves secreted very little, if any, immunoglobulin. Thus, heterozy-gous neonatal rabbits have no detectable serum immunoglobulin of paternal allotype. Nevertheless, peripheral lymphocytes obtained from such rabbits are stimulated fully as effectively by antisera directed at allotypic determin-ants of the paternal type as by antisera specific for maternal allotypic deter-minants. Thus, the surface immunoglobulin must derive, in large measure, from the responsive lymphocytes.

This *in vitro* demonstration, albeit indirect, was paralleled by an *in vivo* phenomenon—allotype suppression—which led to the same conclusion[17, 18]. Infusion of antisera directed at paternal allotypic determinants into a hetero-zygous neonatal rabbit results in profound and prolonged suppression in the production of serum immunoglobulin of that allotype. These two findings constituted the main experimental evidence for the existence of immuno-globulin on lymphocyte surfaces until more recent, direct studies.

In the last several years a variety of procedures to demonstrate directly immunoglobulin on lymphocyte surfaces have been introduced. One principal method has been to utilise anti-immunoglobulin antibodies bearing an easily-detectable marker and to search for the marker on lymphocyte surfaces.

The first such procedure used for this purpose was the mixed antiglobulin technique of Coombs and his colleagues[19]. This procedure involves the use of lymphocytes, anti-immunoglobulin antibody and erythrocytes coated with immunoglobulin. If immunoglobulin exists on the lymphocyte, then anti-immunoglobulin should bind it to the immunoglobulin-bearing erythro-cyte leading to a mixed agglutinate or rosette, in which lymphocytes and erythrocytes are present. This approach provided a direct demonstration of surface immunoglobulin on certain lymphocytes and has also been used to investigate the class and allotype of immunoglobulin on lymphocyte surfaces. Nevertheless, the mixed antiglobulin test is difficult to perform and requires numerous controls. Although useful in the hands of highly skilled and experienced investigators, this procedure has largely been superseded by the use of fluorescent, radioactive and enzymatic markers.

Lymphocyte populations from a variety of sources contain variable num-bers of cells which bind fluorescent or radioactive anti-immunoglobulin anti-body to their surface[14]. These cells must be distinguished from cells containing cytoplasmic immunoglobulin. The latter are plasma cells and lymphocytes which are in the process of synthesising immunoglobulin for secretion. Such cells may or may not have surface immunoglobulin[20]. In general, if live cells are treated with anti-immunoglobulin at reduced temperatures, only surface immunoglobulin is detected as appreciable amounts of the reagents do not enter the cell under such conditions. Figure 10.1a is an electron micrograph illustrating surface immunoglobulin on a lymphocyte. In this case, the anti-immunoglobulin antibody had been covalently labelled with horse radish peroxidase. An electron-dense reaction product indicates the localisation of immunoglobulin on the cell surface.

Although the fraction of lymphocytes which may be identified as immu-noglobulin bearing varies depending on tissues and species of origin, appre-ciable numbers of immunoglobulin-bearing cells are found in all lymphoid tissues except thymus. Moreover, thymus deprivation achieved either by neo-natal thymectomy or adult thymectomy, lethal irradiation and reconstitution

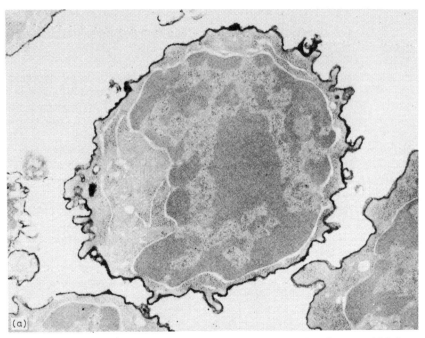

Figure 10.1 Electron micrographs of guinea-pig lymph node lymphocytes which have bound anti-immunoglobulin antibody labelled with horse radish peroxidase. The intense dark areas represent reaction product and indicate the location of surface immunoglobulin. (a) Lymphocyte incubated with anti-immunoglobulin at 4 °C. Note uniform surface distribution of product.

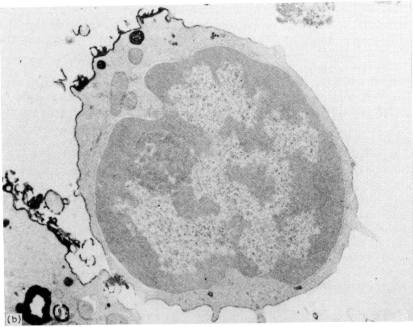

(b) After initial exposure to anti-immunoglobulin at 4 °C, the cell was maintained at 37 °C for 30 min. Label is now concentrated over one pole of cell indicating migration of surface immunoglobulin

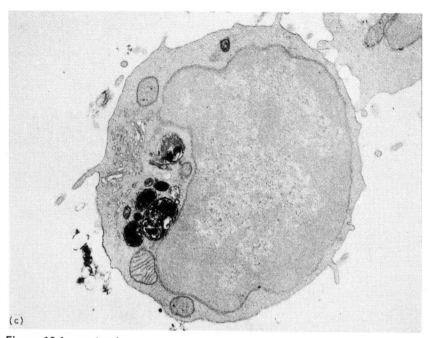

Figure 10.1—*continued*
(c) This cell was maintained at 37 °C for 1 h after initial labelling. All reaction product is now within cytoplasmic vesicles indicating endocytosis of surface complexes
I am indebted to Dr. Alan Rosenthal for permission to show these micrographs.

with bone marrow cells results in an increase in the fraction of immuno-globulin bearing cells in the spleen of the mouse[21]. Similarly, destruction of T lymphocytes by cytolysis with specific antisera results in a marked increase in the number of cells with easily-detectable surface immunoglobulin[22]. Finally, as discussed below, populations highly enriched in T cells, are lacking cells bearing sufficient immunoglobulin to be detected by conventional autoradiography[23]. Thus, it is clear that easily-detectable surface immunoglobulin is found on many B lymphocytes and few, if any, T lymphocytes. A functional correlate of this morphological finding is that procedures which remove immunoglobulin-bearing cells from a population remove precursors of antibody-forming cells. One demonstration of this is provided by the passage of lymphoid cell populations over columns packed with plastic beads to which anti-immunoglobulin antibody has been adsorbed[24]. The effluent of such columns contain few if any immunoglobulin bearing cells and are similarly depleted of precursors of antibody secreting cells although T lymphocytes are preserved and, indeed, enriched in such populations.

The amount of immunoglobulin on the surface of an immunoglobulin-bearing cell has been estimated in several ways. One method has been to use lymphocyte surface immunoglobulin to compete with iodinated soluble immunoglobulin for binding to anti-immunoglobulin antibody[25]. By determining the number of lymphocytes required for a given degree of inhibition and by comparing this to the amount of soluble unlabelled immunoglobulin required for a similar degree of inhibition, an estimate can be achieved of the amount of immunoglobulin per cell. It is important to recognise that the estimate is in terms of equivalents of soluble immunoglobulin molecules and cannot, with certainty, be translated into the number of molecules on a cell surface. The value obtained by this procedure is of the order of 100 000 molecules per B cell. An alternate approach is to measure the maximum number of anti-immunoglobulin molecules which can bind to a cell surface by plotting binding data according to the approach of Scatchard and determining by extrapolation, the number of anti-immunoglobulin molecules bound at infinite ligand concentration. An estimate of 70 000–80 000 anti-immunoglobulin molecules is achieved in this way[26]. However, since a value for the number of anti-immunoglobulin molecules which bind to a single molecule of surface immunoglobulin is not available, one cannot determine the number of immunoglobulin molecules on the cell membrane with certainty. As a first approximation, a mean value of *ca*. 10^5 immunoglobulin molecules per immunoglobulin-bearing cell may be taken. A final point on this issue however, is that such an estimate gives no indication of the degree of heterogeneity which may exist within the B cell population in regard to the number of surface immunoglobulin molecules per B cell. Observations of immunoglobulin density on human leukaemia cells suggests that considerable heterogeneity may exist[27].

Let us now turn to the problem of the distribution of the immunoglobulin over the surface of the cell. Two major, and conflicting, views exist on this issue. One suggests that immunoglobulin molecules are distributed randomly over the surface of the cell and are capable of diffusing freely in the plane of the membrane, even at relatively low temperatures[28, 29]. This view is based on immunofluorescence studies in which fluorescent-univalent anti-immunoglobulin molecules (Fab pieces) label B lymphocyte surfaces diffusely and on thin-section electron micrographs, such as that shown in Figure 10.1a, in which cells labelled at low temperature with anti-immunoglobulin–horse radish peroxidase conjugate show a diffuse distribution of marker. The other view is that immunoglobulin exists on the surface of the cell in a network; that is, that a degree of organisation of the distribution of surface immunoglobulin exists. Studies which have supported this view were carried out by observing the localisation, at low temperature, of labelled anti-immunoglobulin by the technique of freeze etching[30]. The latter technique allows large areas of the cell surface to be viewed. It is clear that whatever the initial disposition of immunoglobulin, the use of divalent anti-immunoglobulin antibody allows a lattice to form on the surface of the cell. At either room temperature, or at 37 °C, this lattice migrates to one pole of the cell where it has the appearance of a cap (Figure 10.1b). Subsequently, the antigen–antibody complex is internalised and enters lysosomes (Figure 10.1c). Although sufficiently detailed studies have not yet been performed to allow a definitive choice between the two major views, the rapid formation of the antigen–antibody complex on the cell surface suggests considerable freedom in immunoglobulin movement in the plane of the membrane and is more in keeping with a random initial distribution of surface immunoglobulin. If this is correct, then the observation of networks of immunoglobulin on the cell surface may represent early stages of aggregation of surface Ig by anti-Ig occurring even at reduced temperature.

It should be clear that this sequence of events (lattice formation, cap formation, internalisation) on the lymphocytes surface is not unique for immunoglobulin molecules. It has now been reported for a whole series of surface components[31]. Further, the role of redistribution of cell-surface immunoglobulin in stimulation of that cell is very far from clear. A recent, potentially very important, finding is that several hours after endocytosis, induced by anti-immunoglobulin, immunoglobulin reappears on the cell surface, apparently in quantities greater than were initially present[29]. It has been suggested that cell stimulation may result from repeated contacts between stimulants and receptors leading to several rounds of such increased expression of surface immunoglobulin.

An alternative to the use of anti-immunoglobulin antibody for the demonstration and analysis of cell-surface immunoglobulin is to label membrane components covalently and to purify labelled immunoglobulin from extracted surface protein. This strategy has been used in the radioiodination of membrane proteins and demonstration of iodinated immunoglobulin. The labelling is achieved by the use of lactoperoxidase and H_2O_2 to generate iodine from iodide. As the lactoperoxidase appears to be excluded from the cell, labelling with radioiodine is largely restricted to surface proteins. The second step in this procedure is to extract as much of the labelled material as possible, usually through the use of a non-ionic detergent or urea and acetic acid. The extracted material is then initially purified by precipitation with anti-immunoglobulin antisera in the presence of added non-radioactive immunoglobulin as carrier and the precipitate is reduced, alkylated and analysed by electrophoresis with sodium dodecyl sulphate–acrylamide gel.

Studies of immunoglobulin on the surface of mouse B lymphocytes indicate that the vast majority of extractable immunoprecipitable immunoglobulin is IgM in class with a mol. wt. of ca. 180 000 Dalton[32, 33]. This suggests that, in this instance at least, the bulk of the surface immunoglobulin is monomeric IgM. Uhr and his colleagues[34] have shown that the ratio of radioactivity present on heavy and light chains of immunoglobulin is similar for immunoglobulin iodinated on the cell surface and immunoglobulin iodinated in free solution. Similarly, immunoglobulin labelled internally with tritiated amino acids has a similar distribution of radioactivity in heavy and light chains to that of surface-labelled immunoglobulin. This suggests that no major region of the immunoglobulin molecule on the cell surface is inaccessible to the labelling reagents and, therefore, that surface immunoglobulin has a superficial location in the membrane. This would be in keeping with the fluorescence observations which indicate rapid movement of surface Ig on the cell surface.

If cells are surface labelled with[125] I by the lactoperoxidase procedure and are then held, in the living state, at 37 °C, labelled immunoglobulin appears in the culture medium and does so quite quickly[33-36]. The material which appears has the characteristic of a lipoprotein suggesting that, on the surface of the cell, immunoglobulin is associated, non-covalently, with other molecules, including lipids, and that this complex is shed as a single unit.

The shedding procedure depends upon activity of the cell. It requires both energy metabolism and active protein synthesis. Moreover, the shed molecules appear to be replaced by new unlabelled surface IgM molecules. This suggests that 'shedding' may be a normal activity of immunoglobulin-bearing cells and may be part of the general physiology of membrane turnover. It has been suggested that such shed molecules play a role in the immune response; the formation of complexes with antigen in the vicinity of the cell from which the surface immunoglobulin has been shed may serve as an antigen-concentrating mechanism and, indeed, may aid in the binding of antigen to the cell surface. Although this is an interesting possibility, no receptor for aggregated IgM on the B cell surface has been described so that the antigen–antibody complexes formed under these conditions would not be expected to adhere to B lymphocytes.

The introduction of the surface-labelling procedures provides a potential method for the precise evaluation of immunoglobulin molecules and of other surface molecules of lymphocytes. There is no doubt that this powerful tool will be widely used and that improvements in this technique should allow a very detailed analysis of membrane-associated molecules.

10.3.1.2 Are different allotypic forms and classes of immunoglobulin expressed on the surface of a single cell?

The ability to demonstrate immunoglobulin on the surface of B lymphocytes, which include precursors of antibody-secreting cells, allows us to ask some specific questions about the degree of commitment of such cells. Studies of antibody secreting cells have established that an individual cell secretes immunoglobulin of a single class[37], allotype[38], specificity[39] and affinity[40]. It seems virtually certain that the immunoglobulin molecules produced by a single antibody-secreting cell are of one primary structure. In its purest form, the clonal-selection theory holds that the antigen-sensitive precursor of this cell should have precisely the same molecule as its antigen-binding receptor, perhaps with some modification so that the molecule can function properly in the cell membrane.

It is clearly established that immunoglobulin exists on B cell surfaces, and, as will be described in the subsequent section, functions as the antigen-binding receptor of the B cell. We will delay a consideration of the specificity restriction of B cells until the section on antigen binding. In this section, we consider the issues of allotype and class expression.

These problems are in one major respect different from each other. The question of expression of one or both allotypic forms of a polymorphic molecule asks whether one or both alleles at a single genetic locus are activated in an individual cell whereas the expression of more than one immunoglobulin class on a single cell implies the activation of genes at separate loci.

Whether both allotypic forms of immunoglobulins are expressed on a single immunoglobulin-bearing cell was first approached by Sell in his studies of lymphocyte activation by anti-immunoglobulin antibodies[41]. Antisera to the rabbit L-chain immunoglobulin determinants b4 and b5 stimulate transformation by lymphocytes of the appropriate genetic constitution. However, the maximal response of lymphocytes from heterozygous rabbits (b4b5) was considerably less than the maximal response of lymphocytes from b4b4 homozygotes to anti-b4 or of lymphocytes from b5b5 homozygotes to anti-b5. This led Sell to suggest that individual lymphocytes from b4b5 heterozygotes could be stimulated either by anti-b4 or anti-b5 but not by both and that allelic exclusion for immunoglobulin genes existed in B cells.

Wolf et al. have used the mixed antiglobulin procedure to measure the frequency of rabbit peripheral blood lymphocytes which bear only one or, alternatively, both allotypic forms of immunoglobulin[42]. Their result was that a substantial fraction of the cells possessed immunoglobulin of both allotypes on their surface. Strikingly, however, the fraction of immunoglobulin-bearing cells which appeared to express both allotypes was very low in young rabbits and quite considerable in older animals.

Studies by Pernis et al.[43] and from our laboratory[44] using simultaneous binding of two distinct fluorescent antibodies or of fluorescent and radioactively-labelled antibodies reveal that the vast bulk of immunoglobulin-bearing cells have surfaces of immunoglobulin of only one allotypic form.

The apparent disagreement between results obtained by the mixed antiglobulin test and by immunofluorescence and autoradiography appears to have been resolved by recent studies of Jones et al. using double label immunofluorescence[45]. These authors found that substantial numbers of lymphocytes from heterozygous rabbits bound antibodies directed at both allotypic forms of immunoglobulin. However, they observed that exposure of the cells to pronase removed the surface immunoglobulin. When the immunoglobulin reappeared, presumably through new synthesis, cells bore immunoglobulin of but a single allotype. This strongly suggests that the great majority of immunoglobulin bearing cells express the product of but one allele at an activated immunoglobulin locus. It would appear that small amounts of immunoglobulin can, under certain conditions, adhere to cells and lead to confusing results, particularly when highly sensitive techniques are used.

Attempts to resolve the question of class of immunoglobulin on cell surfaces have met with similar difficulties and lack of agreement among investigators. Indeed, the problem here may be even more difficult to resolve. That is so because it appears very likely that cells which secrete immunoglobulin G are descended from a cell which at some stage of its development possesses surface IgM. Studies by Cooper and his colleagues[46-48] suggest that in the chicken, a cell bearing IgM and found in the Bursa of Fabricius is the progenitor of both IgM and IgG bearing peripheral lymphocytes and that a 'switch' in expression of surface immunoglobulin class appears to be a normal ontogenetic event, occurring independently of antigenic stimulation. In the mouse, studies of the suppression by anti-immunoglobulin antibody of an in vitro primary antibody response also suggest that an IgM bearing cell is the predecessor of an IgG-secreting cell[49]. In these studies, however, the transition in expressed immunoglobulin appears to be an antigen-driven event. Finally, Pernis and his colleagues have demonstrated that some rabbit cells which contain (and secrete) IgG have surface IgM[50].

Analysis of the class of immunoglobulin on the surface of lymphocytes has demonstrated the presence of substantial numbers of cells bearing each of the major immunoglobulin classes. Table 10.1 reviews reported values for numbers of immunoglobulin-bearing cells of each class in the mouse. These results bear comment. Obviously, the agreement between the various laboratories is very poor. Nonetheless, the bulk of the data suggest that μ-bearing cells, although relatively numerous, hardly predominate in the population of immunoglobulin-bearing cells to a sufficient degree to explain the finding that surface immunoglobulin labelled by iodination procedures is almost exclusively μ. Whether this latter finding may reflect a greater density of

Table 10.1 **Mouse splenic lymphocytes bearing surface immunoglobulin of various classes**

	Positive lymphocytes (%)			
Antiserum	Rabellino et al.[25]	Jones et al.[51]	Nossal et al.[23]	Takahashi et al.[20]
anti-κ	45	29	46	41
anti-μ	10	18	46	31
anti-a	6	4	29	<10
anti-γ_1	19	0	3	<10
anti-γ_2	12	10	19	<10

The study of Rabellino et al. used fluorescent-labelled antibody; Jones et al. and Nossal et al. used [125I]-labelled antibody. Takahashi et al. determined the frequency of immunoglobulin bearing cells by lysis with antibody and complement.

immunoglobulin on μ-bearing cells than on γ-bearing cells is uncertain. Whether more than one class of immunoglobulin is simultaneously expressed on the surface of an individual B cell is also unresolved. The data reported by Rabellino et al.[25], Jones et al.[51] and Takahashi et al.[20] suggest that the sum of the percentage of cells bearing each of the major H-chain classes is similar to the percentage of cells bearing light chains. This would imply that few, if any, cells bear detectable immunoglobulin of more than a single class. On the other hand, the study of Nossal and his colleagues[23] certainly points to the opposite conclusion.

Recently, Fröland and Natvig[52] have reported results of simultaneous binding studies with labelled antisera against human IgM and IgG subclasses. They did not observe any doubly-staining human lymphocytes. Thus, the balance of reports thus far favours the concept that, in most instances, an individual immunoglobulin-bearing cell has a predominance of a single class of immunoglobulin on its surface, but the disagreement between several highly competent groups of workers leaves this issue in doubt.

10.3.1.3 Antigen-binding B cells

The nature and specificity of antigen-binding receptors had been a subject of major interest long before surface-binding procedures were introduced. Evidence gained from the analysis of changes in antibody affinity during the course of the immune response and from the specificity of the antibody produced in anamnestic responses to antigens cross-reactive with the initial immunogen suggested strongly that the specificity of the receptor on the precursor of the antibody-secreting cell was equivalent to that of the antibody[53].

It had long been known that the avidity of antibody in the serum of animals recently immunised was relatively low whereas the avidity of antibody present at a longer interval after immunisation was quite high. By studying the antibody response to hapten–protein conjugates, Eisen and Siskind[54] demonstrated that such avidity increases could be explained by an increase in the average intrinsic association constant for the reaction between antibody and hapten. Subsequent work demonstrated that secreted antibody was also of higher affinity long after immunisation[55,56]. Thus, the affinity increase could not be ascribed to a preferential neutralisation of high-affinity antibody by antigen. The simplest explanation for this phenomenon was that, in the population of precursor cells, individual lymphocytes had surface receptors of distinct affinity and the receptors of different cells differed from each other in their affinity. Initially, sufficient antigen was present so that cells possessing receptors of high, intermediate and perhaps even low affinity could bind and be stimulated by antigen. However, as antigen concentration fell, only cells with receptors of relatively high affinity could bind sufficient antigen to continue to be stimulated. The key postulate for this explanation was that the affinity (and specificity) of the receptor of the precursor cell resembled that of the antibody secreted by the descendent. Indeed, it would seem very difficult to explain this phenomenon if this postulate were not correct.

The other line of evidence, strongly suggesting that the receptor on the precursor cell must closely resemble the product, came from the analysis of stimulation of secondary responses by cross-reactive antigens. The key elements of these experiments had been foreshadowed by the investigation of the phenomenon of 'original antigenic sin' in the response of humans and experimental animals to influenza vaccine[57,58]. However, the experiments performed in hapten–carrier systems are somewhat clearer.

If mice are primed with the hapten–carrier conjugate 4-hydroxy-3,5-diiodophenylacetyl (DIP)–chicken gamma globulin (CGG), transfer of spleen cells from these mice to irradiated syngeneic recipients prepares the recipient for secondary responses to DIP–CGG[59]. Indeed, if spleen cells from the primed donors are incubated with DIP–CGG *in vitro*, washed and then infused into the recipients, a substantial secondary anti-DIP response develops without the need for subsequent antigen challenge. This suggests that antigen became associated with cellular receptors during the *in vitro* incubation period. If the cells are incubated with DIP–aminocaproic acid (DIP–EACA), a univalent ligand capable of binding to anti-DIP antibody but without the capacity to initiate anti-DIP antibody responses, the response to DIP–CGG is diminished markedly. If a cross-reactive ligand, 4-hydroxy-3-iodo-5-nitrophenylacetyl (NIP)–EACA, is used as an inhibitor, the anti-DIP response is only partially diminished. What is striking, however, is that the cross reactivity pattern of the anti-DIP antibody molecules produced under these conditions is different from that of 'normal' anti-DIP molecules. Thus, in the normal secondary response to DIP–CGG, there is a substantial fraction of molecules which bind NIP–EACA quite well whereas in the secondary response, obtained when the cells have been incubated with NIP–EACA, the degree of cross reaction with NIP–EACA is diminished markedly. This indicates that cells bearing receptors which react with either DIP or NIP–EACA are blocked by NIP–EACA whereas cells bearing receptors for DIP which do not bind NIP are not blocked by NIP–EACA. The descendents of the latter cells produce anti-DIP antibody which does not bind NIP–EACA. Again, this explanation is only tenable if the specificity (cross-reaction pattern) of the receptor and the antibody are very similar.

Many other experiments of this type have given important but indirect evidence on the nature and specificity of antigen recognition units on immunocompetent cells. The virtue of these studies is that they deal with immune responses and thus are clearly germane to the binding characteristics of a receptor involved in cell activation. The defect of these experiments is that the cell on which the receptor is located cannot always be identified with certainty and the evaluation of the binding characteristics requires an immune response in which amplification factors may exaggerate or diminish differences between different compounds in their interaction with cellular receptors.

A more direct method to analyse the antigen-binding character of B lymphocytes involves their specific removal from a population by adherence to an immunoadsorbent. For example, incubation of lymphoid cells with antigen bound to solid particles, such as beads of glass[60], plastic[60], agarose[61] or polyacrylamide[62] or to nylon fibres[63], results in removal of antigen-binding cells (see later) and diminishes the capacity of the cell population to transfer primary or secondary responsiveness to an irradiated recipient. In some instances, cells which had bound to the adsorbent have been recovered either by mechanical methods[60, 63] (shaking beads or plucking nylon fibres) or by specific elution with free ligand[62]. The recovered cell population is somewhat enriched in its capacity to transfer responses, although generally a source of T cells must be added if the recovered cells are to express their function. This reinforces the concept that it is the specific B cells, in most instances, which are preferentially bound to antigen–adsorbent complexes.

These procedures, which may be considered as affinity chromatography of lymphocytes, hold great promise for obtaining specific sub-populations of cells. However, the available techniques still have several problems. Often there is considerable non-specific binding of lymphocytes to the adsorbent. This obviously precludes substantial subsequent purification. Procedures which diminish non-specific binding (e.g. very rapid flow rate when columns are used) also tend to diminish the fraction of specific cells which bind. Another major problem is that individual antigen-binding cells form many bonds with an individual antigen–particle complex, so that dissociation of the cells is very difficult. If the cell is eluted from the adsorbent with free ligands, major membrane rearrangements may result from this interaction with antigen. Similarly, mechanical dissociation of cells from the adsorbent carries with it a risk of damage to the cell. None the less, procedures of this type, particularly the polyacrylamide-bead method, provide a base upon which efficient and specific separation procedures may be built subsequently.

Another approach to the specific fractionation of cells on the basis of the specificity of their antigen–binding receptors utilises an electronic fluorescence-activated cell sorter[64]. In this technique, a subpopulation of cells is labelled with a fluorescent ligand and then fluorescent cells are separated from non-fluorescent cells. For example, keyhole limpet haemocyanin (KLH), labelled with fluorescein, is incubated with lymphocytes and a small fraction of the cells bind the fluorescent molecules to their surface. The cells are then placed into a device in which a narrow stream of cells is exposed to a laser with a frequency which will excite fluorescein. Cells which fluoresce are detected by a photomultiplier tube. The stream is then broken up into a series of very small droplets and an electrical charge is placed onto droplets which contain fluorescent cells. The droplets pass through an electrical field in which charged droplets are deflected and are collected separately from non-charged droplets. Cell populations depleted of, and markedly enriched in, antigen-binding cells and in precursors of antibody-secreting cells may be obtained in this way[65]. Thus far, this procedure has been used mainly to study cells from immunised animals. This approach appears capable of achieving highly-purified cell populations and may be very useful in the future.

As mentioned above, it is now possible to detect and to study directly antigen-binding by receptors on B lymphocytes. Incubation of normal lymphocytes with antigens labelled with radioactive iodine, certain enzymes, fluorescein or large particles, results in the binding of these antigens by small numbers of lymphocytes. The cells which have bound antigen can be identified by virtue of the marker associated with the antigen. In general, best results are obtained when populations of lymphocytes depleted of macrophages are used and when incubation is carried out at reduced temperature and in the presence of sodium azide. Radiolabelled antigens have been used quite widely for the detection of antigen binding cells[61, 66-68]. I describe here studies performed by Davie and I on the antigen-binding cells of guinea-pigs. In most respects, our results are similar to those obtained with lymphocytes from other species.

Among the lymph-node lymphocytes of non-immunised guinea-pigs, we find routinely that *ca.* 0.04% of the cells bind ^{125}I-labelled-2,4-dinitrophenyl-guinea-pig albumin ($[^{125}$I]DNP–GPA) when a concentration of 0.2 µg of DNP–GPA ml^{-1} is used[61]. It must be emphasised that the number of antigen-binding lymphocytes detected depends to some extent upon the concentration of ligand. Thus, increasing the concentration of $[^{125}$I]DNP–GPA increases the number of lymphocytes which bind the antigen; similarly, diminishing the concentration of $[^{125}$I]DNP–GPA decreases the number of lymphocytes which bind sufficient antigen to be detected as positive. Obviously, this reflects the fact that there is a heterogeneity of antigen-binding cells in respect to the affinity of their receptors. When very low ligand concentrations are used, only cells with high-affinity receptors bind sufficient ligand to be detected as positive. When high ligand concentrations are used, cells with low-affinity receptors also are able to bind antigen. This concentration-dependent variability in the number of antigen-binding lymphocytes emphasises a principal difficulty in the use of the direct antigen-binding procedures, that is, the problem of relating the capacity of a cell to bind antigen to its ability to be activated by that antigen. At the present time, it is not known with certainty what concentration of ligand will distinguish cells with receptors of sufficiently high affinity to be activated from cells with receptors of such low affinity that they can rarely, if ever, be activated by antigen. Consequently, conditions which are used in antigen-binding assays have, to some extent, an arbitrary quality.

One very satisfactory demonstration that at least some of the cells which bind radioactive antigens to their surface are important in the immune response is the so-called 'antigen-suicide' experiment[69]. Incubation of lymphocytes with [^{125}I]antigens of very high specific activity diminishes or abolishes the capacity of these cells to transfer responsiveness to those antigens to irradiated recipients. This appears to be due to destruction of the cell due to radiation originating from the labelled antigen on its surface. Such a technique should allow a determination of the affinity distribution of the receptors of 'true precursors' through the correlation of the concentration of radioactive ligands and the degree of depression of subsequent responsiveness.

The frequency of DNP–GPA binding lymphocytes is relatively similar in cell populations obtained from each of the peripheral lymphoid organs of non-immunised guinea-pigs. Strikingly, however, antigen-binding cells are absent from the thymus. This suggests that immature T cells fail to bind sufficient antigen to be detected as positive by short-term radioautography with ligands of intermediate specific activity (*ca.* 10–50 µCi µg^{-1}). Furthermore, virtually all the DNP–GPA binding lymphocytes of normal guinea-pigs have large amounts of surface immunoglobulin. This finding, which strongly suggests that the vast bulk of the antigen-binding cells are B lymphocytes, was obtained by sequential incubation of cells with [^{125}I]DNP–GPA and fluorescent anti-Ig. After development of radioautographs, antigen-binding cells were identified under dark field illumination with a tungsten light source; by switching to an ultraviolet light source, with appropriate excitation and nosepiece filters, it was shown that essentially all the cells which had bound antigen had also bound anti-immunoglobulin[61].

Although it appears that antigen-binding cells detected by short-term autoradiography with antigens of intermediate specific activity are largely B cells, it has been reported that antigen-binding thymus cells and T lymphocytes can also be identified particularly when longer exposure periods and higher specific activity antigens are used[70]. We will consider this issue in the section on T cell receptors.

10.3.1.4 *Surface immunoglobulin on antigen-binding cells*

The demonstration that most antigen-binding cells have large amounts of sufrace immunoglobulin not only indicates that they are B cells but also suggests that the antigen-binding receptors of B cells are immunoglobulin. Indeed, preincubation of lymphoid cells with anti-immunoglobulin antibody prevents antigen from binding to the surface of B lymphocytes. This is strong evidence that immunoglobulin is the receptor, although final proof awaits the isolation of immunoglobulin from the surface of a cell which can bind a given antigen and the demonstration that this immunoglobulin binds that antigen. Recently, Cone *et al.* have reported initial steps to the achievement of this end[71].

The class of immunoglobulin acting as receptor for antigen appears to vary to some extent from species to species. Thus, reports concerning lymphocytes from non-immune mice, capable of binding either flagellin or haemocyanin, demonstate that anti-μ antibodies block binding to a very large extent whereas anti-γ antibodies block little or not at all[72]. On the other hand, antigen-binding cells in non-immunised guinea-pigs may have either γ_1, γ_2 or μ on their surface[73].

As was mentioned in the section on immunoglobulins on B lymphocytes, there is suggestive evidence that a 'switch' in the class of immunoglobulin expressed on the surface of the mouse lymphocyte appears to occur. The 'switch' appears to be from IgM to IgG and seems to be an antigen-driven event. This is consistent with the observed predominance of surface μ on antigen-binding cells in non-immunised mice. In support of the antigen-driven 'switch', Greaves and Hogg[74] have reported that many cells, obtained from *immune* mice, which form rosettes with sheep erythrocytes appear to have surface γ while rosette-forming B lymphocytes from non-immune mice bear surface μ determinants. On the other hand, Cooper and his colleagues (see earlier) studying the ontogeny of immunoglobulin bearing cells in the chicken have reported that the appearance of cells bearing IgG does not depend upon antigenic stimulation. The observation that many antigen-binding cells in non-immune guinea-pigs have receptors of the IgG class suggests that an antigen independent pathway for the generation of γ-bearing cells may also exist in mammals.

10.3.1.5 Specificity of antigen-binding cells

The antigen-binding cells of non-immune animals are highly specific. Thus, guinea-pig lymphocytes capable of binding [^{125}I]DNP–GPA are blocked from doing so by prior incubation with non-radioactive DNP-proteins, such as DNP–GPA, DNP–bovine serum albumin, DNP–bovine fibrinogen and DNP–haemocyanin. In addition, the univalent hapten ε-DNP-L-lysine also blocks binding although relatively high concentrations (*ca.* 10^{-3}M) are required. These ligands do not block the binding of human serum albumin to lymphocytes nor do proteins without DNP groups block the binding of [^{125}I]DNP–GPA to lymphocytes.

In addition to demonstrating the specificity of antigen-binding lymphocytes these blocking studies indicate that the antigen-binding receptors of the DNP–GPA binding cells are highly hapten (DNP) specific and in that regard these receptors resemble the serum antibody which develops as a result of immunisation with DNP–GPA.

Whether antigen-binding cells possess only a single set of specific receptors or, alternatively, antigen-binding receptors or more than one specificity has not yet been established unequivocally. Both the relatively small number of lymphocytes capable of binding any individual antigen and the existence of allelic exclusion in the expression of B lymphocyte immunoglobulin strongly suggests that individual B lymphocytes cannot possess very large numbers of receptors of different specificities. Similarly, the capacity to impair specifically an immune response to one antigen but not another by treatment of cells with highly radioactive antigens or by passing cells over immunoadsorbents support this specialisation of B cells. These considerations rule out the possibility that B cells have a very large number of different types of receptors but they do not exclude the possibility that B cells possess a *limited* number of different receptors. Indeed, Sercarz and his colleagues[75] have reported that individual B lymphocytes may occasionally bind more than a single antigen. Their observations do not *establish* that more than a single receptor is expressed on any cell because of the likely possibility that a single receptor may be capable of binding several different 'cross-reactive' antigens. Studies of myeloma proteins with antigen-binding character establish that very unexpected cross reactivities may exist (e.g. DNP and menadione[76, 77]) and thus the fact that an individual cell may bind two apparently unrelated antigens does not constitute proof that that cell has two distinct sets of receptors. To establish the number of different types of receptors on an individual cell will require the isolation of immunoglobulin from a normal or malignant B cell and an examination of its degree of homogeneity. At the current time, it appears most likely that individual B cells express only one set of receptors.

10.3.1.6 Antigen-binding cells in immunity and tolerance

Upon immunisation, the number of cells capable of binding the antigen used for immunisation increases markedly. The increase usually precedes the increase in the number of antibody-producing cells and, in some cases at least, the increased number of antigen-binding cells is preserved after the number of antibody-secreting cells has diminished[78]. At least some of these antigen-binding cells must be 'memory cells' as removing them from a population by passage over specific immunoadsorbents removes the capacity of that population to transfer a secondary response to an irradiated recipient[79].

Examination of the apparent affinity of the receptors of antigen-binding cells demonstrates that with increasing time after immunisation the average affinity of receptors in the cell population rises[80, 81]. This supports the concept, described above, that increases in antibody affinity result from a selection by antigen among precursor cells with receptors of varying affinity, so that when antigen has become very limiting, only cells with high-affinity receptors continue to be stimulated and so predominate in the population.

The number of antigen-binding cells present in tolerant animals has been the subject of considerable attention recently. Unfortunately, in many experiments the form of tolerance induced has not been established as affecting B lymphocytes, so that an evaluation of the number of antigen-binding cells in such animals may not be germane. There are some experiments, however, in which clear B-cell tolerance exists and in which the number of antigen-binding cells has been evaluated. Even in such cases, no uniformity has yet been achieved. The number of specific rosette-forming cells in mice tolerant to bacterial lipopolysaccharide[82] or to pneumococcal polysaccharide[83] have been reported to be normal or even slightly elevated. On the other hand, guinea-pigs in whom DNP-specific tolerance has been induced by a DNP conjugate of a non-immunogenic amino acid copolymer have markedly diminished numbers of cells capable of binding [^{125}I]DNP–GPA[84].

Considerably more study of this area is required, particularly since the evaluation of antigen-binding receptors offers a new approach to the study of the mechanism of tolerance induction.

10.3.1.7 Requirements for B-cell activation

In most instances, the activation of B cells by antigen either requires, or is markedly augmented by the function of T lymphocytes. There are several antigens, however, for which B-cell activation appears not to require participation of T cells. It has been suggested that the structure of such 'thymus-independent' antigens may give important clues to the requirements for antigen activation of B cells.

Among the antigens which have been reported to activate B cells directly are type-specific pneumococcal polysaccharide, bacterial lipopolysaccharide, polymerised flagellin and certain hapten conjugates of this substance and polyvinylpyrollidine. All of these molecules are of very high molecular weight and are characterised by the possession of repeating units with a regular spacing between them. It is a distinct possibility that the activation of B cells can be accomplished when single molecules of immunogen each bind to several receptors on the cell surface. As the receptors are normally spaced quite widely, many molecules bearing repeating units (hapten conjugates of albumins or γ-globulins) may be too small to bind more than a single, divalent receptor. This would, presumably, be an insufficient stimulus for direct activation. It must be noted, however, that this model of the type of binding required for B cell activation probably explains only one aspect of cell stimulation. Thus, antibody responses to thymus-independent antigens are generally restricted to the production of IgM molecules. It appears that stimulation of IgG production is much more dependent on T cell function and that appropriate presentation of antigen, even in a large array, fails to duplicate this T cell activity.

10.3.2 T Lymphocytes

The nature of the antigen recognition molecules on T lymphocytes has been much more difficult to determine than was the case for those of B lymphocytes. There is a substantial body of experiments strongly suggesting that the antigen binding receptor of a T lymphocyte is an immunoglobulin molecule and these will be discussed in a subsequent section. It is fair to say, however, that for every positive report concerning T-cell immunoglobulin and its role as receptor, a negative experiment may also be cited. Moreover, it has been suggested that the T cell may bear a recognition molecule which is not immunoglobulin in character. The study of mixed lymphocyte reactions and of histocompatibility-linked immune response genes has, indeed, led to the proposal that molecules coded for by genes within the major histocompatibility complex may be the key recognition molecules for some or all T cells.

10.3.2.1 Surface immunoglobulin of T cells

Although the bulk of investigators studying the binding of fluorescent or radioactive anti-immunoglobulin to lymphoid cells report that thymus cells and peripheral T lymphocytes do not bind anti-immunoglobulins, occasional descriptions of such binding have appeared. Hammerling and Rajewsky have reported that a hybrid antibody consisting of anti-immunoglobulin and anti-southern bean mosaic virus binds to essentially all lymph node lymphocytes but not to thymocytes[85]. In their experiments, southern bean mosaic virus was added to the cell suspension and cells which bound the hybrid antibody were detected by electron microscopy. In view of the fact that T lymphocytes constitute a majority of the lymph node lymphocytes, the authors conclude that peripheral T cells possess easily detectable surface immunoglobulin. These findings are distinctly unusual in comparison to the great majority of reports on this topic. It is possible that the observations of Hammerling and Rajewsky may be explained by postulating that immunoglobulin exists on T lymphocytes but that the bulk of the molecule lies deep in the membrane so that determinants against which *most* sera are directed are not available. Another possibility is that T-cell immunoglobulin is of an unusual class and that the antibodies used by Hammerling and Rajewsky could interact with that immunoglobulin although most anti-immunoglobulin antibodies fail to bind to the putative T-cell immunoglobulin. Finally, the possibility must be considered that the hybrid antibody preparations contained some molecules directed at membrane components other than immunoglobulin and are not identifying immunoglobulin on T cells.

Nossal and his colleagues[23] have reported that anti-immunoglobulin antibodies bind to both thymus cells and T lymphocytes. In their studies, however, the binding could only be detected by a very sensitive sandwich autoradiographic technique while more conventional procedures failed to detect binding to such cells. They estimated that an individual T cell possessed fewer than 1000 immunoglobulin molecules. Indeed, erythrocytes appeared to bind the same amount of anti-immunoglobulin antibody as did T cells.

Finally, the use of the lactoperoxidase procedure to label membrane proteins has also led to disparate findings on the part of two laboratories, both studying mouse lymphocytes. Vitetta *et al.*[86] detect immunoglobulin on B cells but fail to find any on T cells. Indeed, they can add B cells to a suspension of thymocytes in a ratio of 1:400 and easily detect the surface immunoglobulin on those added B cells. This indicates that thymocytes must have less than 1/400 as much immunoglobulin as B cells, unless there is some major difference in the capacity to label T-cell proteins or to extract the labelled material from T cells.

On the other hand, Marchalonis and his associates report that iodinated immunoglobulin can be extracted from thymocytes and T lymphocytes which have been labelled by the lactoperoxidase method[87]. Their results suggest that the amount of surface Ig on T cells may be similar to that on B cells. As with so many of the other controversial topics in this area, the reason for the difference between the two groups has not yet been resolved. The Australian group (Marchalonis *et al.*) suggests that T-cell immunoglobulin is not extractable from cell membranes with the non-ionic detergents which Vitetta, Uhr and their colleagues use, although B-cell immunoglobulin may be extracted in this way. On the other hand, they report that their extraction procedure (9 M urea–1.5 M acetic acid) is effective in solubilising immunoglobulin from both B and T cells. However, Vitetta and Uhr have not been able to confirm these findings. Indeed, their results indicate that the acid-urea procedure is less efficient than non-ionic detergents in extraction of immunoglobulin.

Finally, Cone, Sprent and Marchalonis[71] have reported that in tissue culture, lymphocytes from CBA mice which are sensitive to the histocompatibility antigens of C57Bl/6 mice, shed membrane immunoglobulin, which binds to C57Bl/6 lymphocytes but not to CBA lymphocytes. Thus, they imply that they have isolated T-cell immunoglobulin and that it is specific for antigens to which the cells are sensitive.

To summarise, the question of surface immunoglobulin on T cells remains unresolved. Moreover, the simple demonstration of a few immunoglobulin molecules on a T lymphocyte is not necessarily proof that such immunoglobulin is produced by these cells and has not been passively adsorbed by them. Indeed, Grey et al.[88] have recently shown that cultured T lymphocytes may adsorb small amounts of immunoglobulin from the culture medium and retain it on their surface.

10.3.2.2 Blocking of T-lymphocyte activation by anti-immunoglobulin

Several reports that anti-immunoglobulin sera may block the capacity of T lymphocytes to respond to or bind antigen have appeared. Greaves et al.[89] have reported that an Fab fragment of anti-L-chain antibody blocks the in vitro activation of human peripheral blood lymphocytes by antigens. Mason and Warner[90] have described experiments in which the incubation of mouse cells in anti-L or anti-μ sera inhibited the capacity of those cells to transfer delayed hypersensitivity reactions to syngeneic hosts or to initiate graft versus host reactions in semi-allogeneic recipients. Each of these reactions are largely, or exclusively, T-cell functions and thus the experiments suggest that surface immunoglobulin on T cells has an important role in antigen recognition. However, other investigators have failed frequently in their attempts to perform similar experiments. A more detailed consideration of the positive and negative experiments on this subject is found in the review of Crone et al.[91].

Perhaps the most convincing evidence that has yet been presented that surface immunoglobulin is important in T-cell activation is the report of Basten et al.[92] using the radioactive antigen 'suicide' technique described previously. In this study, the capacity to transfer primary antibody responses to chicken γ-globulin (CGG) and to sheep erythrocytes (SRBC) to lethally irradiated syngeneic mice was studied. The transfer of immune responsiveness required a source of T lymphocytes and of B lymphocytes as both CGG and SRBC are 'thymus-dependent' antigens. Incubation of either the B or T cells with [^{125}I]CGG of high specific activity abolished the response of the recipient to CGG although the response to SRBC was unimpaired. Thus, the 'suicide' procedure affected T cells as well as B cells. The crucial finding of

Basten *et al.* was that preincubation of the T cells with anti-mouse immu-globulin blocked the capacity of [^{125}I]CGG to inhibit the anti-CGG response. The interpretation of this finding is that the anti-immunoglobulin sera bound the surface immunoglobulin of the T cell and prevented the binding of [^{125}I]CGG which would have led to T-cell destruction. The one reservation which can be entertained here is the possibility that anti-mouse immuno-globulin might cross-react with CGG and thus block by binding the radio-active antigen rather than the receptor.

10.3.2.3 Antigen-binding by T lymphocytes

Although the binding of radioactive antigens to T lymphocytes and to thymus cells has not been generally observed, some investigators report that such binding may be detected. Dwyer *et al.*[70] find that anti-immunoglobulin sera blocks such binding while Engers[93] reports that it does not.

A system more widely used to study antigen-binding by T cells is the formation of rosettes of sheep erythrocytes (or conjugated sheep erythrocytes) around individual mouse lymphocytes. Rosette forming lymphocytes are relatively rare in non-immunised mice and increase in number after immuni-sation. The identification of rosette-forming lymphocytes as of the T or B lines has generally been accomplished by lysis with antisera specific for surface antigens of the T or B cells and evaluation of the residual cells. Using such techniques, a substantial fraction of rosette-forming cells have been reported to be T lymphocytes by several, but not all, investigators[20, 94-97].

It has been reported that the formation of SRBC rosettes by mouse spleen cells can be inhibited by anti-immunoglobulin sera. Rosette forming T cells from non-immunised mice are blocked from binding erythrocytes by anti-L-chain sera but not by anti-H-chain sera. Rosette forming T cells from mice which have been immunised to sheep erythrocytes can be inhibited by some anti-μ sera as well as anti-L-chain sera. Greaves and Hogg[74] have suggested that the common property of the inhibitory anti-μ-sera is that they are specific for hinge region determinants while non-inhibitory anti-μ-sera lack such specificity. They propose that the surface immunoglobulin of T cells is of the μ-class and that only the Fab ends are exposed in non-sensitised cells. They envisage that, upon activation, a larger segment of the immuno-globulin molecule becomes exposed but that this is still less than the extent of exposure of immunoglobulin on B cells.

One cautionary note in the use of rosette formation to evaluate T-cell receptors may be drawn from the study of the lymphocytes of bursectomised agammaglobulinemic chickens. These birds have a marked, if not complete, deficit of B lymphocytes but possess a normal T-lymphocyte system. Theis and Thorbecke[98] report that no rosette-forming cells can be found among the splenic lymphocytes of such chickens either prior to, or following, immunisation.

10.3.2.4 Apparent specificity of T-cell receptors

Another striking feature of the antigen recognition system of T lymphocytes is the range of specificities which can serve to activate these cells. The T-cell system appears to have specificity characteristics which are very different from those of B-cell receptors or serum antibody molecules[99]. This difference in specificity has been most widely investigated for the responses to hapten–protein conjugates. Animals immunised to various hapten–protein conjugates produce antibodies which can bind to the haptenic group itself, to the protein carrier molecule, and to determinants unique to the conjugate. In the immune response to 2,4-dinitrophenyl (DNP) conjugates, for example, anti-DNP antibody frequently accounts for a majority of the specific antibody produced. Analysis of the fine specificity of this antibody reveals that ε-DNP-L-lysine contributes 70% or more of the interaction energy in the binding of anti-DNP antibody to the immunogen[100, 101].

Cellular immune responses of animals immunised with DNP-proteins rarely can be demonstrated to have a high degree of *independent* hapten specificity. That is, these T cell responses are elicited by the hapten-carrier conjugate used for immunisation and to a lesser extent by DNP-conjugates of closely-related proteins. However, DNP-conjugates of unrelated proteins induce meagre responses and the concentration of antigen required for these responses is markedly in excess (*ca.* $10^4:1$) of the concentration of the immunising antigen required for a similar response[99, 102].

Analysis of specificity of elicitation of cellular immune responses, either *in vivo* (delayed hypersensitivity) or *in vitro* (stimulation of DNA synthesis) indicates a very complex specificity pattern. For example, guinea-pigs immunised with trinitrophenyl (TNP) guinea-pig albumin (GPA) demonstrate vigorous delayed hypersensitivity skin reaction to TNP-GPA but absent or meagre responses to a TNP conjugate of GPA in which an aminocaproate group is interposed between the TNP radical and the protein[103]. Similarly, the magnitude of the response is diminished markedly by changes in the structure of the haptenic group, itself. Thus, lymphocytes from guinea-pigs immunised to DNP–GPA give a vigorous *in vitro* response (DNA synthesis) to DNP–GPA and a more meagre response to TNP–GPA. Moreover, *o*-nitrophenyl–GPA, which differs from DNP–GPA by only a single nitro group, fails to stimulate any response[104]. Many other examples of the precise specificity of this system could be cited, but it suffices to say that the T-cell recognition system distinguishes changes in the structure of the haptenic group, in the nature of the carrier molecule and in the mode of linkage between hapten and carrier.

Further support for the distinctive specificity characteristics of the B- and T-cell recognition systems stems from an analysis of antibody and cell-mediated cytotoxicity in allogeneic mouse systems[105-107]. For example, the immunisation of C3H mice with mastocytoma cells derived from DBA/2 mice leads to the development of a population of T lymphocytes which mediates the *in vitro* destruction of the DBA/2 cells and to the production of antibodies cytotoxic for DBA/2 cells. The DBA/2 and C3H mice are of different H-2 types. That is, the C3H mouse is H-2^k and the DBA/2 is H-2^d. They differ from each other at both of the major histocompatibility loci of the H-2 region. (i.e. the H-2K and H-2D genes). T cells from C3H mice immune to the DBA/2 mastocytoma will lyse target cells from other mouse strains if those strains are identical to the DBA/2 at either the H-2K or H-2D loci but they fail to lyse cells from animals which differ at both these loci, even if these mice share H-2 controlled antigenic determinants with the DBA/2 mouse, such as for example is true of the C57Bl/6 mouse. The C57Bl/6 mouse differs from the DBA/2 at both the H-2K and H-2D loci but C57Bl/6 lymphocytes possess at least six H-2 antigenic determinants present on DBA/2 cells and absent from the C3H cells. Antisera from C3H mice immunised with DBA/2 cells are quite efficient in lysing C57Bl/6 cells but lymphocytes from C3H mice fail to destroy C57Bl/6 cells. Thus, a major difference in specificity of T cells on the one hand and antibody (and presumably B cells) on the other is illustrated in this system.

The fact that B cells and serum antibodies efficiently recognise haptenic structures and histocompatibility *determinants*, whereas T cell responses highly specific for such structural elements are rare, has suggested that T cells may utilise an entirely different recognition system than B cells. One obvious objection to reaching such a conclusion is that the analysis of T-cell recognition systems involves the initiation of an immune response whereas antibody and B-cell receptors have been studied by direct binding procedures. More direct evaluations of T-cell specificity are available from two relatively-recent studies.

Firstly, incubation of lymph node cells, from guinea-pigs immunised with DNP–GPA, with agarose beads to which DNP–GPA has been coupled, removes from the cell population those cells which can be stimulated by DNP–GPA to synthesise DNA. Incubation of DNP–GPA immune lymph node cell populations with DNP–BSA–agarose beads has no effect whatever in diminishing the subsequent response to DNP–GPA[104]. As the *in vitro* DNA synthetic response requires T cells, this suggests that the capacity of T cells to bind to antigen shows the same specificity pattern as that observed by studying the capacity of antigen to initiate a T-cell response.

The other type of direct binding study has involved the use of hapten-coated erythrocytes to form rosettes with cells of immunised and non-immunised animals. Möller, Bullock and Mäkelä[108] have reported that some cells which form rosettes with erythrocytes coated with the 4-hydroxy-3,5-dinitrophenylacetyl (NNP) can be lysed with anti-θ serum. θ is a determinant restricted in the mouse lymphoid system to thymocytes and T lymphocytes. Thus, these rosette-forming cells would appear to be hapten-specific T cells. Their analysis of the capacity of the univalent ligand NNP–aminocaproate to inhibit the formation of such rosettes suggests that the interaction of hapten with receptor is of quite low affinity. It is not yet clear if these cells are functionally hapten specific in the sense that they may be activated by hapten on a carrier different from that used in priming.

In summary, hapten-specific T-cell responses are rare. There is not yet sufficient data to determine whether T lymphocytes with highly hapten-specific receptors do not exist or alternatively whether such cells are not activated by the hapten-carrier conjugates generally used for immunisation. The lack of hapten-specific T cells would constitute major supportive evidence for a qualitative distinction in the nature of B- and T-cell receptors.

10.3.2.5 Is the T-cell receptor immunoglobulin?

The experimental data on this topic is still highly controversial and no reviewer, however critical, can resolve the problem simply by recounting the experiments on both sides of the issue. The solution needs much more study and would certainly benefit from new and imaginative approaches. Indeed, a consideration of the histocompatibility-linked immune response genes and the study of the recognition structure responsible for mixed lymphocyte reactions may provide such a framework for answering these questions. Consequently, I will conclude this chapter on antigen recognition by briefly describing these two areas and their possible relation to antigen recognition by T lymphocytes.

10.4 IMMUNE RESPONSE GENES

In the last several years, many examples of genetic factors controlling the immune response to individual antigens or to related groups of antigens have been described. The analysis of the cellular and molecular basis of specific genetic defects gives us another approach to the understanding of antigen recognition mechanisms.

In view of the great heterogeneity of the antibody molecules produced in response to most individual antigens, it would not be anticipated that the failure to demonstrate a given immune response would be due to an absence of an individual variable (v) region gene. Indeed, until very recently, instances of genetic control of specific immune response operating at the level of the genes for immunoglobulin molecules have not been observed. Blomberg et al.[109] have now reported that the anti-dextran antibody response of mice appears to be under the control of a gene linked to those genes controlling the structure of immunoglobulin heavy-chain constant regions. As the anti-dextran antibody response appears to be quite homogeneous, this suggests that more careful analysis of other antibody responses should yield additional instances of genetic control of the antibody response mediated by structural genes for immunoglobulins.

A large group of immune responses have now been shown to be controlled by autosomal dominant genes which do not appear to be the structural genes for serum-type immunoglobulin molecules. Many of these immune response (Ir) genes, are linked to the gene complex controlling the major histocompatibility antigens in mice, guinea-pigs and rats[110, 111]. A large body of evidence now exists to indicate that these histocompatibility-linked Ir genes function primarily, if not exclusively, in T lymphocytes. Two of the important observations which have led to this conclusion are: (a) Guinea-pigs lacking a given Ir gene fail to make cellular immune responses (T-cell responses) to the antigens the response to which is controlled by that gene[112]; (b) The difference between 'responder' and 'non-responder' mice in one system (the response to the branched-chain polymer of tyrosine, glutamic- acid, D, L-alanine and lysine [(T,G)–A—L]) is lost when both groups are thymus-deprived[113], that is, 'non-responder' mice which have been thymectomised, irradiated and reconstituted only with bone marrow respond to (T,G)–A—L to the same extent as sham thymectomised animals of the same genotype whereas 'responder' mice which have been thymus deprived resemble non-responders in their capacity to produce antibody upon immunisation with (T,G)–A—L.

On the other hand, functional defects in the B-cell pool seem to be less important. Thus, 'non-responder' guine-pigs and mice have been shown to possess normal numbers of B lymphocytes capable of binding the antigens to which their response is absent or impaired[114, 115]. Moreover, if antigens which elicit a poor response are linked to immunogenic molecules, a vigorous antibody response ensues[116]. This indicates that specific B cells are not only present in non-responders but that, under appropriate conditions, these cells can be activated.

The products of Ir genes must contribute in some way to the antigen recognition system of the T lymphocytes as they control responses to individual antigens or to limited sets of related antigens. Indeed, the question can immediately be framed as to whether the product of a histocompatibility linked Ir gene is the antigen-binding receptor of the T cell. This question cannot yet be answered definitively. Two recent studies suggest that it must be considered very seriously.

Firstly, genetic analysis demonstrates that more than a single, and probably many, genetic loci for Ir genes exists within the H-2 region of mice. Lieberman and Humphrey[117, 118] have recently described H-2 linked Ir genes controlling the immune response of inbred mice to BALB/c myeloma proteins of the IgA and IgG (γ_{2a}) classes. By analysing the response of congenic mice whose H-2 regions are derived from recombinations between the H-2^a and the H-2^b chromosomes, Lieberman and her colleagues[119] have shown that the responses to these two sets of proteins are controlled by separate genetic loci in the H-2 complex, both located in the region between the H-2K and the Ss-Slp genes. More recent, and still very preliminary studies, suggest that a gene controlling immune responses to γ_{2b} (IgH) myeloma proteins may be found either in the region between the Ss-Slp genes and the H-2D gene or to the 'right' of the H-2D gene[120]. This would imply that a large number of loci for Ir genes may exist and may be located over a wide area within the gene complex controlling major histocompatibility antigens. Thus the possibility exists that the 'Ir regions' of genome may encompass sufficient genetic material to allow a quite discriminatory antigen-recognition system. Indeed, a very cogent example of the discriminatory power of this system stems from the analysis of the response of inbred guinea-pigs to limiting doses of the DNP conjugates of bovine serum albumin (BSA) and guinea-pig albumin (GPA). The immune response to low doses of DNP–BSA is controlled by an Ir gene linked to strain 2 histocompatibility (H) genes[121] while the immune response to low doses of DNP–GPA is controlled by an Ir gene linked to strain 13 H genes[122] and thus these two very similar compounds can be easily distinguished by Ir gene products.

The second recent finding pointing to the crucial role of Ir gene products in antigen recognition stems from an analysis of the role of alloantisera in blocking *in vitro* T cell responses to antigens under genetic control[123]. The immune response of guinea-pigs to the DNP conjugate of the copolymer of L-glutamic acid and L-lysine (DNP–L-GL) is controlled by an Ir gene linked to strain 2 H gene complex while the response to the copolymer of L-glutamic acid and L-tyrosine (GT) is controlled by a gene linked to strain 13 H gene complex. (Strain 2 × strain 13)F$_1$ hybrid guinea-pigs respond to both antigens. Peritoneal exudate lymphocytes from hybrid guinea-pigs immunised with DNP–L-GL and GT in complete Freund's adjuvant respond vigorously *in vitro* to both DNP–L-GL and GT and to purified protein derivative (PPD) of tuberculin. If an alloantisera directed at strain 2 histocompatibility antigens (13 anti 2 sera) is added to the culture, the response to DNP–L-GL is ablated while the response to GT and to PPD is preserved. Similarly, an anti-13 alloantiserum (2 anti-13) blocks the response of F_1 cells to GT but not to DNP–GL or to PPD (Table 10.2). This demonstrates the importance of Ir

Table 10.2   Inhibition of activation of $(2 \times 13)F_1$ lymphocytes by alloantisera
(From Shevach, Paul and Green[123], by courtesy of Rockefeller Univ. Press)

Stimulant	Normal	Serum 13 anti 2	2 anti 13
0	3499*	1479	1484
DNP–GL	68361	1231	46385
GT	17070	12147	1770
PPD	20049	12086	15159
PHA†	56887	44281	28094

* CPM of tritiated thymidine incorporated into TCA precipitable material by peritoneal exudate lymphocytes from $(2 \times 13)F_1$ guinea-pigs immunised with DNP–GL and GT emulsified in complete Freund's adjuvant. Data adapted from reference 123. DNP–GL responsiveness is linked to strain 2 H genes; GT responsiveness to strain 13 H genes.
† PHA = phytohemagglutinin.

gene products in antigen recognition and suggests that the gene product is expressed on the cell surface.

The crucial questions which remain unanswered are: (a) How do the alloantisera block Ir gene-controlled functions? (b) What is the nature of the product of the Ir gene? (c) How does the product function in the recognition of antigen by T cells? Two major possibilities to explain the capacity of alloantisera to block Ir gene-controlled functions can be envisaged. Either the alloantisera bind to histocompatibility determinants which are very close to Ir gene products on the cell surface and block by 'steric hindrance' or the alloantisera contain antibodies which are specific for the Ir gene products themselves. Attempts to resolve this are now in progress.

The nature and function of the Ir gene products are still matters for speculation. Whether they represent the antigen-binding receptors and whether such receptors are of a molecular class different from immunoglobulin is still unknown.

10.5 MIXED LYMPHOCYTE REACTIONS

One striking example of antigen- recognition which has been discussed in some detail in previous chapters is the mixed lymphocyte response (MLR). This response is largely mediated by T lymphocytes and is exceptional in that the response to lymphocytes differing at the major H locus engages a large fraction of all the T lymphocytes. In the mouse, mapping studies suggest the crucial region of genome controlling MLR is located between the H-2K and Ss-Slp genes[124, 125] while in the human it is located to the 'right' of the second series locus in the HLA region[126]. What is very uncertain now is the molecular basis of the recognition of disparity in this system and the relation between the so-called MLR gene and the Ir genes.

10.6 CONCLUSION

The immune response is remarkable in the wide diversity of foreign substances which can be recognised and against which a prompt and vigorous response can be mounted. The nature of the mechanism allowing this sophisticated appreciation of foreign substances is one of the most fascinating and important biological problems. As I have attempted to show in this chapter, recognition is a multi-step process, involving three cell types and, in all likelihood, more than a single type of recognition structure. Although we have accumulated a great body of information on the antigen-binding character of antibodies and, to a lesser extent, of receptors on B lymphocytes, our understanding of the remaining aspects of this system remain very limited. Indeed, the nature of T-cell recognition structures and of the product and mechanism of function of Ir genes are among the major unsolved problems of contemporary immunology.

References

1. Ehrlich, P. (1900). *Proc. Roy. Soc. (London)*, **66**, 424
2. Burnet, F. M. (1959). The Clonal Selection Theory of Acquired Immunity (Cambridge: Cambridge University Press)
3. Unanue, E. R. (1972). *Advan. Immunol.*, **15**, 95
4. Boyden, S. V. (1963). *Cell-Bound Antibodies*, 7 (B. Amos and H. Koprowski, editors) (Philadelphia: Wistar Institute Press)
5. Berken, A. and Benacerraf, B. (1966). *J. Exp. Med.*, **123**, 119
6. Huber, H., Polley, M. J., Linscott, W. D., Fudenberg, H. H. and Müller–Eberhard, H. J. (1968). *Science*, **162**, 1281
7. Mosier, D. E. (1967). *Science*, **151**, 1573
8. Shortman, K. and Palmer, J. (1971). *Cell Immunol.*, **2**, 399
9. Raff, M. C., Nase, S. and Mitchison, N. A. (1971). *Nature (London)*, **230**, 50
10. Basten, A., Miller, J. F. A. P., Sprent, J. and Pye, J. (1972). *J. Exp. Med.*, **135**, 610
11. Dickler, H. B. and Kunkel, H. G. (1972). *J. Exp. Med.*, **136**, 191
12. Bianco, C., Patrick, R. and Nussenzweig, V. (1970). *J. Exp. Med.*, **132**, 702
13. Coombs, R. R. A., Feinstein, A. and Wilson, A. B. (1969). *Lancet*, **ii**, 1157
14. Raff, M. C., Sternberg, M. and Taylor, R. (1970). *Nature (London)*, **225**, 553
15. Sell, S. and Gell, P. G. H. (1965). *J. Exp. Med.*, **122**, 423
16. Gell, P. G. H. and Sell, S. (1965). *J. Exp. Med.*, **122**, 813
17. Dray, S. (1962). *Nature (London)*, **195**, 677
18. Mage, R. G. (1967). *Cold Spring Harbor Symp. Quant. Biol.*, **32**, 203
19. Coombs, R. R. A., Gurner, B. W., Janeway, C. A. Jr., Wilson, A. B., Gell, P. G. H. and Kelus, A. S. (1970). *Immunology*, **18**, 417
20. Takahashi, T., Old, L. J., McIntire, K. R. and Boyse, E. A. (1971). *J. Exp. Med.*, **134**, 815
21. Unanue, E. R., Grey, H. M., Rabellino, E., Campbell, P. and Schmidtke, J. (1971). *J. Exp. Med.*, **133**, 1188
22. Shevach, E., Green, I., Ellman, L. and Maillard, J. (1972). *Nature New Biol.*, **235**, 19
23. Nossal, G. J. V., Warner, N. L., Lewis, H. and Sprent, J. (1972). *J. Exp. Med.*, **135**, 405
24. Grey, H. M., Colon, S., Campbell, P. and Rabellino, E. (1972). *J. Immunol.*, **109**, 776
25. Rabellino, E., Colon, S., Grey, H. M. and Unanue, E. R. (1971). *J. Exp. Med.*, **133**, 156
26. Stobo, J. D., Talal, N. and Paul, W. E. (1972). *J. Immunol.*, **109**, 701

27. Pernis, B., Terrarini, M., Forni, L. and Amante, L. (1971). *Progress in Immunology*, **1**, 95
28. Taylor, R. B., Duffus, P. H., Raff, M. C. and de Petris, S. (1971). *Nature New Biol.*, **233**, 225
29. Loor, F., Forni, L. and Pernis, B. (1972). *Europ. J. Immunol.*, **2**, 203
30. Karnovsky, M. J., Unanue, E. R. and Leventhal, M. (1972). *J. Exp. Med.*, **136**, 907
31. Unanue, E. R., Perkins, W. D. and Karnovsky, M. J. (1972). *J. Exp. Med.*, **136**, 885
32. Vitetta, E., Bauer, S. and Uhr, J. W. (1971). *J. Exp. Med.*, **134**, 242
33. Cone, R. E., Marchalonis, J. J. and Rolley, R. T. (1971). *J. Exp. Med.*, **134**, 1373
34. Uhr, J. W. Personal communication.
35. Vitetta, E. S. and Uhr, J. W. (1972). *J. Immunol.*, **108**, 577
36. Vitetta, E. S. and Uhr, J. W. (1972). *J. Exp. Med.*, **136**, 676
37. Bernier, G. M., Ballieux, R. E., Tominaga, K. T. and Putnam, F. W. (1967). *J. Exp. Med.*, **125**, 303
38. Pernis, B., Chiappino, G., Kelus, A. and Gell, P. G. H. (1965). *J. Exp. Med.*, **122**, 853
39. Nossal, G. J. V. and Mäkelä, O. (1962). *J. Immunol.*, **88**, 604
40. Klinman, N. R. (1971). *J. Immunol.*, **106**, 1330
41. Sell, S. (1968). *J. Exp. Med.*, **128**, 341
42. Wolf, B., Janeway, C. A., Jr., Coombs, R. R. A., Catty, D., Gell, P. G. H. and Kelus, A. S. (1971). *Immunology*, **20**, 931
43. Pernis, B., Forni, L. and Amante, L. (1970). *J. Exp. Med.*, **132**, 1001
44. Davie, J. M., Paul, W. E., Mage, R. G. and Goldman, M. B. (1971). *Proc. Nat. Acad. Sci.* (*USA*), **68**, 430
45. Jones, P. P., Herzenberg, L. A. and Cebra, J. J. Submitted for publication
46. Kincade, P. W., Lawton, A. R., Bockman, D. E. and Cooper, M. D. (1970). *Proc. Nat. Acad. Sci. USA*, **67**, 1918
47. Cooper, M. D., Cain, W. A., Van Alten, P. J. and Good, R. A. (1969). *Internat. Arch. Allergy*, **35**, 242
48. Cooper, M. D., Lawton, A. R. and Kincade, P. W. (1972). *Contemporary Topics in Immunology*, **1**, 33
49. Pierce, C. W., Solliday, S. M. and Asofsky, R. (1972). *J. Exp. Med.*, **135**, 675
50. Pernis, B., Forni, L. and Amante, L. (1971). *Annal. N.Y. Acad. Sci.*, **190**, 420
51. Jones, G., Torrigiani, G. and Roitt, I. M. (1971). *J. Immunol.*, **106**, 1425
52. Fröland, S. S. and Natvig, J. B. (1972). *J. Exp. Med.*, **136**, 409
53. Siskind, G. W. and Benacerraf, B. (1969). *Advan. Immunol.*, **10**, 1
54. Eisen, H. N. and Siskind, G. W. (1964). *Biochemistry*, **3**, 996
55. Andersson, B. (1970). *J. Exp. Med.*, **132**, 77
56. Davie, J. M. and Paul, W. E. (1972). *J. Exp. Med.*, **135**, 660
57. Fazekas de St. Groth, S. and Webster, R. G. (1966). *J. Exp. Med.*, **124**, 341
58. Fazekas de St. Groth, S. and Webster, R. G. (1966). *J. Exp. Med.*, **124**, 347
59. Mitchison, N. A. (1967). *Cold Spring Harbor Symp. Quant. Biol.*, **32**, 431
60. Wigzell, H. and Andersson, B. (1969). *J. Exp. Med.*, **129**, 23
61. Davie, J. M. and Paul, W. E. (1971). *J. Exp. Med.*, **134**, 495
62. Truffa-Bachi, P. and Wofsy, L. (1970). *Proc. Nat. Acad. Sci. USA*, **66**, 685
63. Edelman, G. M., Rutishauser, U. and Millette, C. F. (1971). *Proc. Nat. Acad. Sci. USA* **68**, 2153
64. Bonner, W. A., Hulett, H. R., Sweet, R. G. and Herzenberg, L. A. (1972). *Rev. Sci. Instrum.*, **43**, 404
65. Julius, M. H., Masuda, T. and Herzenberg, L. A. (1972). *Proc. Nat. Acad. Sci. USA*, **69**, 1934
66. Naor, D. and Sulitzeanu, D. (1967). *Nature (London)*, **214**, 687
67. Byrt, P. and Ada, G. L. (1969). *Immunology*, **17**, 503
68. Humphrey, J. H. and Keller, H. U. (1970). Developmental Aspects of Antibody Formation and Structure Vol. 2, 485. (J. Sterzl and I. Riha, editors) (Prague: Academia Publishing House of the Czechoslovak Academy of Sciences)
69. Ada, G. L. and Byrt, P. (1969). *Nature (London)*, **222**, 1291
70. Dwyer, J. M., Warner, N. L. and Mackag, I. R. (1972). *J. Immunol.*, **108**, 1439
71. Cone, R. E., Sprent, J. and Marchalonis, J. J. (1972). *Proc. Nat. Acad. Sci. USA*, **69**, 2556
72. Warner, N. L., Byrt, P. and Ada, G. L. (1979). *Nature (London)*, **226**, 942

73. Davie, J. M., Paul, W. E. and Asofsky, R. A. (1972). *Fed. Proc. (Fed. Amer. Soc. Exp. Biol.)* **31**, 735
74. Greaves, M. F. and Hogg, N. M. (1971). *Progress in Immunology*, **1**, 111
75. Miller, A., DeLuca, D., Decker, J., Ezzell, R. and Sercarz, E. E. (1971). *Amer. J. Path.*, **65**, 451
76. Jaffe, B. M., Simms, E. S. and Eisen, H. N. (1971). *Biochemistry*, **10**, 1693
77. Rosenstien, R. W., Musson, R. A., Armstrong, M. Y. K., Konigsberg, W. H. and Richards, F. F. (1972). *Proc. Nat. Acad. Sci. USA*, **69**, 877
78. Davie, J. M., Rosenthal, A. S. and Paul, W. E. (1971). *J. Exp. Med.*, **134**, 517
79. Wigzell, H. and Mäkelä, O. (1970). *J. Exp. Med.*, **132**, 110
80. Davie, J. M. and Paul, W. E. (1972). *J. Exp. Med.*, **135**, 643
81. Davie, J. M. and Paul, W. E. (1972). *J. Exp. Med.*, **135**, 660
82. Sjöberg, O. and Möller, E. (1970). *Nature (London)*, **228**, 780
83. Howard, J. G., Elsen, J., Christie, G. H. and Kinsky, R. G. (1969). *Clin. Exp. Immunol*, **16**, 513
84. Katz, D. H., Davie, J. M., Paul, W. E. and Benacerraf, B. (1971). *J. Exp. Med.*, **134**, 201
85. Hämmerling, U. and Rajewsky, K. (1971). *Europ. J. Immunol.*, **1**, 447
86. Vitetta, E., Bianco, C., Nussenzweig, V. and Uhr, J. (1972). *J. Exp. Med.*, **136**, 81
87. Marchalonis, J. J., Cone, R. E. and Atwell, J. L. (1972). *J. Exp. Med.*, **135**, 956
88. Grey, H. M., Kubo, R. T. and Cerottini, J. C. (1972). *J. Exp. Med.*, **136**, 1323
89. Greaves, M. F., Torrigiani, G. and Roitt, I. M. (1969). *Nature (London)*, **222**, 885
90. Mason, S. and Warner, N. L. (1970). *J. Immunol.*, **104**, 762
91. Crone, M., Koch, C. and Simonsen, M. (1972). *Transplant Rev.*, **10**, 35
92. Basten, A., Miller, J. F. A. P., Warner, N. L. and Pye, J. (1971). *Nature New Biol.*, **231**, 105
93. Engers, H. D. (1972). *Fed. Proc. (Fed. Amer. Soc. Exp. Biol.)*, **31**, 735
94. Greaves, M. F. and Möller, E. (1971). *Cellular Immunol.*, **1**, 372
95. Haskill, J. S., Eliot, B. E., Kerbel, R., Axelrad, M. A. and Eidinger, D. (1972). *J. Exp. Med.*, **135**, 1410
96. Bach, J. F. and Dardenne, M. (1972). *Cell. Immunol.*, **3**, 11
97. Lamelin, J.-P., Lisowska-Bernstein, B., Matter, A., Reyser, J. E. and Vassalli, P. (1972). *J. Exp. Med.*, **136**, 984
98. Theis, G. A. and Thorbecke, G. J. (1972). *Fed. Proc. (Fed. Amer. Soc. Exp. Biol.)*, **31**, 775
99. Paul, W. E. (1970). *Transplant Rev.*, **6**, 130
100. Paul, W. E., Siskind, G. W. and Benacerraf, B. (1966). *J. Exp. Med.*, **123**, 689
101. Levin, H. A., Levine, H. and Schlossman, S. F. (1971). *J. Exp. Med.*, **133**, 1199
102. Paul, W. E., Siskind, G. W. and Benacerraf, B. (1968). *J. Exp. Med.*, **127**, 25
103. Benacerraf, B. and Levine, B. B. (1962). *J. Exp. Med.*, **115**, 1023
104. Davie, J. M. and Paul, W. E. (1970). *Cellular Immunol.*, **1**, 404
105. Mauel, J., Rudolf, H., Chapuis, B. and Brunner, K. T. (1970). *Immunology*, **18**, 517
106. Brondz, B. D. (1968). *Folia Biologica*, **14**, 115
107. Brondz, B. D. and Goldberg, N. E. *Folia Biologica*, **16**, 20
108. Möller, E., Bullock, W. and Mäkelä, O. Personal communication
109. Blomberg, B., Geckeler, W. R. and Weigert, M. (1972). *Science*, **177**, 178
110. McDevitt, H. O. and Benacerraf, B. (1969). *Advan. Immunol.*, **11**, 31
111. Benacerraf, B. and McDevitt, H. O. (1972). *Science*, **175**, 273
112. Benacerraf, B., Green, I. and Paul, W. E. (1967). *Cold Spring Harbor Symp. Quant. Biol.*, **32**, 567
113. Mitchell, G. F., Grumet, F. C. and McDevitt, H. O. (1972). *J. Exp. Med.*, **135**, 126
114. Davie, J. M., Paul, W. E. and Green, I. (1972). *J. Immunol.*, **109**, 193
115. Dunham, E. K., Unanue, E. R. and Benacerraf, B. (1972). *J. Exp. Med.*, **136**, 403
116. Green, I., Paul, W. E. and Benacerraf, B. (1966). *J. Exp. Med.*, **123**, 859
117. Lieberman, R. and Humphrey, W., Jr. (1971). *Proc. Nat. Acad. Sci. USA*, **68**, 251
118. Lieberman, R. and Humphrey, W., Jr. (1972). *J. Exp. Med.*, **136**, 1222
119. Lieberman, R., Paul, W. E., Humphrey, W., Jr. and Stimpfling, J. H. (1972). *J. Exp. Med.*, **136**, 1231
120. Lieberman, R. Personal communication
121. Green, I. and Benacerraf, B. (1971). *J. Immunol.*, **107**, 374

122. Green, I., Paul, W. E. and Benacerraf, B. (1972). *J. Immunol.*, **109,** 457
123. Shevach, E. M., Paul, W. E. and Green I. (1972). *J. Exp. Med.*, **136,** 1207
124. Bach, F. H., Widmer, M. B., Segall, M., Bach, M. L. and Klein, J. (1972). *Science*, **176,** 1024
125. Klein, J., Widmer, M. B., Segall, M. and Bach, F. H. (1972). *Cellular Immunol.*, **4, 442**
126. Yunis, E. J. and Amos, D. B. (1971). *Proc. Nat. Acad. Sci. USA*, **68,** 303

11
Complement

P. J. LACHMANN

Royal Postgraduate Medical School, London

11.1 INTRODUCTION

The term 'complement' is applied to a system of factors occurring in normal serum that are activated characteristically by antigen–antibody interaction and subsequently mediate a number of biologically significant consequences[1].

It is the principal effector mechanism for antibody mediated allergic reactions. Complement may also be looked upon as one of the enzyme-cascade systems described by McFarlane[2] as the 'triggered enzyme systems of blood plasma'. These include, besides complement, the blood clotting and fibrinolytic mechanisms, and the renin-angiotensin and kinin systems. All are effector mechanisms which in response to trigger stimuli can produce a rapid and amplified effect. All consist of multiple components which circulate in plasma generally in inactive form and undergo sequential activation. Typically, the product of one reaction is the catalyst of the next, producing a characteristic cascade effect. Homeostatic mechanisms for limiting activation are another common feature and are particularly well seen in the case of complement.

As a heat-labile serum co-factor in immune haemolysis and bactericidal reactions, complement has been recognised since the end of the nineteenth century[3-5]. It was soon recognised to be multifactorial and to show a complicated reaction pattern[6], but detailed immunochemical studies became possible only in the 1960s with the development of improved techniques for the isolation of minor components from serum. Since the original identification of C3 as βlc-globulin[7] the great majority of the complement factors have been substantially isolated and characterised.

Even compared with the other triggered enzyme systems complement has turned out to be surprisingly complex and current work is revealing yet more factors and interactions.

If the intricacy of the checks and balances that are built into an enzyme cascade indeed reflect its biological importance, then complement studies should at least not prove trivial.

11.2 GLOSSARY

Erythrocyte = E
Antibody = A
Complement components. The factors involved in the lysis of antibody coated erythrocytes (EA) by the so-called 'classical pathway' are called the complement *components* and have been given numbers. They are designated C1–C9. In general, the numerical sequence follows the order of their reaction but for historical reasons the first four components in order of activation are still called: C1, C4, C2 and C3.
Intermediate complexes. These are designated EAC followed by the components that have reacted, e.g. EAC142 or EAC1$\sim$7 for complexes with the first three or first seven components respectively.
Activation of components. Where components acquire an enzymic or other demonstrable biological activity this is designated by a bar over the components, e.g. C$\overline{1}$ is the enzymatically active form of C1 and C$\overline{56}$ is the activated complex of C5 and C6 that takes part in reactive lysis.

Where a site capable of binding to cell membranes or other molecules is activated this is sometimes denoted by a suffix*, e.g. $C\overline{567}*$ is the nascent form of $C\overline{567}$ that can bind to erythrocytes.

The alternate pathway factors. No generally agreed terminology for the factors yet exists. The factors involved are given names (e.g. 'C3-proactivator convertase') based on their postulated functions or (e.g. glycine rich β-glycoprotein) on immunoelectrophoretic and chemical data, or (e.g. Properdin) are traditional.

The terminology of other factors involved with the complement system are explained in the relevant sections.

11.3 THE IMMUNOCHEMISTRY OF COMPLEMENT

The lysis of sheep erythrocytes coated with rabbit antibody by guinea-pig or human complement was for many years the model of complement activity to which the greatest attention was given and on which most of our knowledge of complement is based. The reaction can usefully be considered in five stages (see Figure 11.1).

11.3.1 Stage 1: The initiation of complement fixation

$$EA + C1 \xrightarrow{\text{Ca}^{2+}} EAC1$$

The first component of complement (C1) occurs in plasma as a macromolecular complex with a sedimentation coefficient of around 18 S[8]. Calcium ions are needed to hold this complex together and if these are chelated by EDTA the complex breaks into three proteins called, C1q, C1r and C1s[9].

11.3.1.1 C1q

C1q is the component that carries the binding site for fixed antibody, and for this reason has attracted particular interest from protein chemists. It was

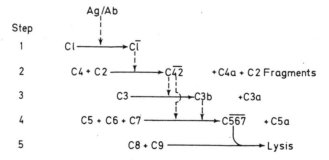

Figure 11.1 The reaction sequence in immune haemolysis. The five main steps of the pathway are shown. Details are given in the text

originally isolated by the usual combinations of ion exchange chromatography, preparative electrophoresis and Sephadex gel filtration[15] but more recently, ingenious techniques for its isolation have been described based on its extreme insolubility[10]; its extremely basic nature allowing it to precipitate with acidic polymers like DNA[11]; or upon its physiological property of binding to aggregated gamma globulin[12]. Clq has a mol. wt. of *ca.* 400 000 and occurs in serum at a concentration of 100–200 µg ml^{-1}. It has been reported by Reid, Lowe and Porter[13] that there are three different types of polypeptide chain, part of each of which resembles collagen in sequence and in sensitivity to collagenase. Furthermore, the molecule is made up of probably six sub-units each containing one of each type of polypeptide chain. Electron-microscopic studies of Clq have shown a molecule with some resemblance to a bunch of flowers. There is a central sub-unit joined by connecting strands to six terminal sub-units[14].

Although it is not known with certainty which part of the molecule binds to antibody, the polyvalence of Clq in this respect (one Clq molecule binding to *ca.* five IgG molecules[15]) would suggest that the reaction site is in the 'flower heads'.

It has been known since 1961[16] that in the presence of EDTA, Clq can precipitate aggregated gammaglobulin. The same is true for soluble immune complexes and the demonstration of precipitin lines in gel between Clq and biological fluids is now widely used as a test for detecting immune complexes[11]. Although the precipitin reaction of Clq can be brought about only by aggregated or complexed gamma globulin, it is possible to show by ultracentrifugation studies that Clq will bind monomeric IgG[17]. This capacity to associate with Clq mirrored the capacity of different immunoglobulins to activate the classical complement pathway. Thus it was shown[18] that binding of CĪ was strong with human IgG 1 and 3 subclasses; weaker with IgG 2; and was not shown by IgG 4, IgA, IgD, IgE or F(ab')$_2$. Most, but apparently not all, IgM is strongly complement binding. In some other species, notably in the guinea-pig and in ruminants such as cows and sheep it is possible to separate the subclasses of IgG by electrophoresis. Thus in the guinea-pig the IgG 1 (fast) subclass is unreactive with Cl, the IgG 2 (or slow) subclass is reactive[19]. In the ruminant[20] the situation is reversed and it is the slow IgG 2 subclass that is non-reactive with Cl.

Besides aggregated immunoglobulins certain other materials will precipitate Clq. These include polyanions like DNA as has already been mentioned. Certain bacterial endotoxins also precipitate Clq[21] (see later).

11.3.1.2 Clr

Clr has a sedimentation coefficient of *ca.* 7 S, a mol. wt. of *ca.* 170 000, is very heat labile and is an essential component for Cl activity[22, 23]. It has been shown[24] that Clr may act proteolytically upon Cls to activate it. This can be inhibited by the CĪ inhibitor (see later). It has been suggested that the action of Clr upon Cls is normally inhibited by calcium ions and that the fixation of Clq in some way abolishes this inhibition[25].

11.3.1.3 C1s

C1s is the sub-unit of C1 that carries the proenzyme site which on activation is converted to $C\bar{1}$, the enzyme which subsequently acts on C4 and C2. C1s has recently been purified by affinity chromatography on a column of benzamidine linked to Sepharose[26], benzamidine being a competitive inhibitor of $C\bar{1}$. C1s has a sedimentation coefficient of 4 S and a mol. wt. of 79 000. Its serum concentration is 22 µg ml^{-1}. C1 can be measured enzymatically by its hydrolysis of acetyltyrosine ethyl ester[27] and is the predominant esterase with a preferential activity on this substrate generated in blood plasma. Its physiological activity is presumably proteolytic and its only known substrates are the two succeeding complement components C4 and C2.

The nature of the reaction between C1 and immunoglobulins is still under study (see Chapter 00). It appears that some site in the third domain of the heavy chain is involved[28]. To obtain C1 activation, reaction is needed either with two closely adjacent IgG molecules or with a single IgM molecule[29]; but in the latter case it may be necessary that at least two of its valencies have reacted with antigen.

In the haemolytic reaction C1 reacts rapidly with EA and the C1 binds to the antibody molecule. The complex $EAC\bar{1}$ is stable at low ionic strength but under physiological conditions the binding is relatively loose and activated C1 can move from site to site on the erythrocytes. At low temperature and normal ionic strength C1 dissociates rapidly from EA[30]. This behaviour of C1 has been utilised by Borsos and Rapp[31] as the basis of an ingenious and highly-sensitive test for complement fixation—the 'C1 fixation and transfer test'.

11.3.2 Stage 2: The generation of C3 convertase

$$EAC1 + C4 + C2 \xrightarrow{\quad Mg^{2+} \quad} EAC142$$

Two further complement components are required in this reaction: C4 and C2.

11.3.2.1 C4

C4 or β1E-globulin was purified from human serum by Müller-Eberhard and Biro[32]. Its great susceptibility to $C\bar{1}$ (and possibly to other plasma proteases) makes C4 more difficult to isolate in active form than might be expected. It is a glycoprotein with a sedimentation coefficient of 10 S, a mol. wt. of 240 000 and a serum concentration of 400–500 µg ml^{-1}. It was the originally described hydrazine or ammonia-sensitive component of complement[33] and is also destroyed by high concentrations of salts like KCNS[34]. C4 is the primary substrate of $C\bar{1}$. A fragment, C4a, is split off[35, 36] and the remaining major fragment, C4b, while in the nascent state has an activated binding site which is capable of combining with receptors on the cell membrane or on IgG molecules or on other C4 molecules. The duration of this nascent state is immeasurably short and binding occurs only in the immediate vicinity of the activation.

Thus the addition of C$\bar{1}$ to a stirred mixture of E and C4 (i.e. where C4 activation occurs in free solution) achieves little or no fixation of C4 to the cell membrane. Even in the ongoing haemolytic reaction the uptake of C4 on EAC1 (i.e. where C4 is activated on the cell surface) is usually less than 10% of that offered[37]. The attachment of the C4 (and of C3) to the cell membrane is believed to be by hydrophobic bonding[38] on the basis of its resistance to elution by strong salt, weak acid or alkali and thiol reagents. Nascent C4 (and nascent C3) will bind to a wide variety of substances: for example, cell membranes, antibody molecules, the predominantly polysaccharide yeast cell walls, the pure protein bacterial flagella and pure phospholipid artificial membranes.

11.3.2.2 C2

C2 was originally defined as a heat-labile pseudoglobulin complement component. The component has been purified[39] and is a basic β-pseudoglobulin with a sedimentation coefficient of 5.5 S, a mol. wt. of ca. 120 000 and occurring at a serum concentration of 20 and 40 μg ml^{-1}. Human C2 has 2–3 free SH groups[40] and its activity can be greatly enhanced by oxidation at critical concentrations of iodine[41].

In the presence of magnesium ions C2 will bind to EAC4 in the absence of C$\bar{1}$. This binding is reversible and shows paradoxical temperature dependence (i.e. binding occurs to a greater extent in the warm). It is not associated with any splitting of C2 and has been used as the basis of a method of purifying C2[42]. However, if C$\bar{1}$ is present C2 is split, the larger fragment, remaining attached to the C4, and the complex forming the second complement enzyme, 'C3 convertase' or C$\overline{42}$. Of the other C2 fragments formed one is of substantial mol. wt. ca. 60 000[39] but a further small C2 fragment has been described by Donaldson et al.[43]. This fragment has biological activity resembling that of kinins and is discussed again in the section on hereditary angio-oedema. Although C$\bar{1}$ will act upon C2 on its own, this reaction is much less effective than C$\bar{1}$ action on C2 in the presence of C4[44].

11.3.2.3 C42

C$\overline{42}$ is unstable having a half-life under physiological conditions of ca. 7 min. The C2 moiety elutes in inactive form into solution leaving C4 bound at the complement fixation site where it can react with further C2 to generate further C$\overline{42}$.

The generation of C$\overline{42}$ does not need to take place on a surface. If purified preparations of C$\bar{1}$, C4, and C2 are incubated together in solution, active C$\overline{42}$ is formed. This reaction is not inhibited if the C$\bar{1}$ and C4 are first incubated together showing that the inactivation of C4 brought about in this way affects its membrane binding site and not its receptor site for C2[45].

Once C3-convertase is generated at the complement fixation site, there is no further requirement for C1 which can now be inactivated by di-isopropyl-fluorophosphate or eluted with EDTA without affecting the course of the subsequent reactions. That C3-convertase activity is found in EDTA shows that either magnesium ions are required only in the formation of the complex and not in its activity or that the magnesium is so firmly bound that EDTA cannot chelate it.

11.3.3 Stage 3: The fixation of C3

$$\text{EAC142} + \text{C3} \xrightarrow{\hspace{6cm}} \text{EAC1423}$$

C3 is the 'bulk' component of the complement system. Its serum concentration is *ca.* 1.2 mg ml^{-1} in man. It is a glycoprotein with a sedimentation coefficient of 9.5 S and a mol. wt. in the region of 200 000. The native molecule contains two free SH groups and two disulphide bonds reducible by 10^{-3}M. dithiothreotol[40].

C3 was originally described as the complement component that could be removed by absorption with yeast[46] a phenomenon related to the 'alternate pathway' of complement fixation to be discussed below. C3 shares with C4 a capacity to be inactivated by ammonia, hydrazine or KCNS although the inactivation of C3 is less complete. C3 is extremely sensitive to proteolysis[143] and the initial products appear to be substantially the same whether this is brought about by C3-convertase or by trypsin, plasmin, thrombin or merely by standing in serum.

C$\overline{42}$ action splits off a small fragment, C3a, with a mol. wt. of *ca.* 7000. This shows biological activity as a chemotactic agent and as an anaphylatoxin (see later). It is the large fragment, C3b, which when nascent has a binding site analogous to that already described for C4 and, becomes attached to the cell membrane. The fixation of C3b at the complement-fixation site brings about several biologically-important consequences, principally the C3 adherence reactions and the feed-back into the alternate pathway. These reactions as well as the homeostatic mechanisms acting upon C3 fixation and the subsequent fate of the bound C3 are discussed in greater detail in later sections. Up to *ca.* 20% of the C3 offered to an EAC142 cell may be bound around the complement fixation site. This is a substantial amount of C3 and it can be shown that C3-coating of say a virus particle or bacterial flagellum in a complement fixation reaction completely covers the structures[47, 48]. The split C3 that is not bound at the complement fixation site is liberated into solution as C3b (β1G-globulin) but is rapidly further broken down in serum to C3c (β1A-globulin) and more slowly a further breakdown product, C3d (a2D-globulin) is also formed.

The antigenicity of C3c and C3d are distinct[50] and are called the A and D determinants of C3 respectively. A further antigenic specificity, the B antigen, is found only in native C3 and occurs neither in C3c nor in C3d. Native C3 contains this B antigen and the A antigen but the D antigen is hardly, if at all, detectable in native C3[51]. In man, C3c has a faster mobility than native C3 and on immunoelectrophoresis the characteristic double arc of C3–C3c (β1C–β1A) globulin is seen when there is any C3 breakdown. In the mouse, on the other hand, C3c is of a lower mobility than C3 and in the rabbit the two mobilities are almost identical.

11.3.4 Stage 4: The generation of the heat-stable intermediate

$$EAC1423 + C5 + C6 + C7 \longrightarrow EAC1423567$$

For the generation of the so-called heat-stable intermediate both $C\overline{42}$ and C3b are required at the complement-fixation site and three further complement components C5, C6 and C7 are involved.

11.3.4.1 C5

C5 is a well-characterised protein–β1F globulin. It was isolated by Nilsson and Müller-Eberhard[52] and completely purified by Nilsson, Tomar and Taylor[53]. C5 has a sedimentation coefficient of 8.7 S and a serum concentration of *ca.* 75 µg ml^{-1}. It bears some resemblance to C3 and to C4 in showing some sensitivity to hydrazine and to salts such as KCNS but it is the most difficult of these components to inactivate.

11.3.4.2 C6

C6 is a β-globulin with a sedimentation coefficient of 5.8 S and a molecular weight in the region of 150 000. It has been most completely purified by Arroyave and Müller-Eberhard[54], although the final product showed a much lower specific activity than that of C6 in serum. Serum concentrations of *ca.* 60 µg ml^{-1} [54] and 11 µg ml^{-1} [55] have been quoted for human serum and 35 µg ml^{-1} [55] for rabbit serum. C6 in human serum is very heat labile at 56 °C and both haemolytic activity and antigenicity are reduced considerably after even 5 min and can no longer be detected after 1 h. By contrast, rabbit C6 shows no significant fall in haemolytic or antigenic activity after 1 h at 56 °C. Most of the work on C6 was made possible by the existence of strains of rabbit that are genetically deficient in this component (see a later section).

11.3.4.3 C7

C7 was isolated by Thompson and Lachmann[56]. It is a β-globulin with a sedimentation coefficient of 5.7 and a mol. wt. of *ca.* 140 000. It is stable in serum at 56 °C.

Monospecific antisera had been prepared to all three components from human serum and they are antigenically non-cross-reacting.

During the immune haemolytic reaction $C\overline{42}$ and C3b are both required for the activation of C5 and C6. The final product after the interaction of C7, is a complex, $C\overline{567}$, which when nascent has a hydrophobic binding site comparable to that already discussed for C3 and C4 and is capable of binding to membranes. It is significantly different, however, in that its half-life is (relatively speaking) long, *ca.* 30 s, and this allows the complement reaction to be to some extent 'contagious' at this point, i.e. $C\overline{567}$ can be fixed at sites distant from the complement fixation site[37].

Although in physiological conditions intermediates between EACl~3 and EACl~7 may not occur, it is possible at low ionic strength to show that the components react sequentially[58,59] C5 is the first component to interact. A small fragment, C5a, with a mol. wt. of 15 000 is split off. This has biological activity as an anaphylatoxin and a chemotactic factor. The large fragment, C5b, binds to the complement fixation site. The binding, however, is not stable. C6 is the next component to be bound. No split product of C6 has yet been identified and the nature of the reaction is not known. However, a stable activated complex of C5 and C6 ($C\overline{56}$) can in some circumstances be released from the complement fixation site (see below) and is presumably a normal, albeit evanescent, reaction intermediate.

C7 is the last of the three to react. The binding of $C\overline{56}$ with C7 requires no other factors. The trimolecular complex $C\overline{567}$ leads to the formation of the heat-stable intermediate. The name 'heat-stable' implies that the intermediate survives several hours at 37°C implying that $C\overline{42}$ is now no longer required, neither indeed is C3. As far as is known, the $C\overline{567}$ complex fixed on a membrane is all that is needed to prepare it for lysis by C8 and C9. Only a minority of the $C\overline{567}$ found is normally bound to membrane. The remainder escapes into solution where it shows biological activity as a chemotactic factor.

11.3.4.4 Reactive lysis

Much of what is known of this fourth step of the complement reaction sequence is based on studies of a phenomenon known as 'Reactive lysis'[56,57,60]. It was observed that the activation of the 'alternative pathway' (q.v.) in a minority of human sera led to the generation of an activated complex of the fifth and sixth components of complement $C\overline{56}$. The features in human sera that allow $C\overline{56}$ to be generated is a relative excess of C5 and C6 over C7 and this occurs in the 'acute phase of inflammation'. $C\overline{56}$ was isolated from the activated 'acute phase' sera[57] and shown to be a complex of one molecule of C5 with one molecule of C6. $C\overline{56}$ associates spontaneously with one molecule C7. The nascent $C\overline{567}$ formed in solution will bind to any suitable surface present and convert it to the functional state of the heat stable intermediate. Thus mixing $C\overline{56}$, E and C7 allows the intermediate $EC\overline{567}$ to be made, i.e. a cell having neither antibody nor any of the complement components acting before C5. These cells are lysed by C8 and C9 in a way wholly comparable to conventional immune haemolysis. Similarly it is possible to bring artificial phospholipid dispersions (Liposomes) to the $LC\overline{567}$ stage and then to lyse them with C8 and C9[61]. This is the most simplified system available for the study of membrane damage by complement.

11.3.5 Stage 5: The terminal stages of complement lysis

EAC1423567 (or EC567) + C8 + C9 ⟶ Lysis

Two further components are required to bring about lysis: C8 and C9.

11.3.5.1   C8

C8 is a basic protein and migrates in the fast γ-region. It was isolated by Manni and Müller-Eberhard[62] and has a sedimentation coefficient of 8.0 and a mol. wt. of 150 000.

11.3.5.2   C9

C9 is an a-globulin. It was isolated by Hadding and Müller-Eberhard[63]. It is an a-globulin with a sedimentation coefficient of 4.5 and a mol. wt. of 79 000. Its serum concentration is said to be less than 10 μg ml^{-1}*.

Of the two components there are a number of reasons for believing C8 to be the one that has the major role in producing lysis. Firstly, C8 fixation alone leads to a slow lysis which has been shown not to be due to traces of C9[64]. Secondly the requirement for C9, in human serum at least, can be abolished by the presence of phenanthrolene or bipyridine, agents which chelate Fe^{2+}[63]. A third reason for so believing is the observation of Stolfi[65] that C8, in certain circumstances, undergoes a change which, while leaving it still capable of binding to $C\overline{567}$ and still capable of subsequently binding C9, renders it haemolytically inactive (see later). Finally, there is a great specificity in the ability of C8 of various species to lyse different erythrocytes. Using human $C\overline{56}$, C7 and C9 in the reactive lysis system it has been shown[66] that, for example, human C8 is the preferred lytic agent for guinea-pig erythrocytes, although it is much less effective on sheep erythrocytes than is guinea-pig C8; and that horse C8 which is quite inactive on sheep erythrocytes gives quite high lytic titres on human and guinea-pig erythrocytes. It is therefore believed that C9 is a co-factor enhancing the lytic activity of C8.

C8 and C9 are bound at the complement fixing site. C8 is believed to bind to $C\overline{567}$; and C9 to C8. However, even after the interaction of C8 and C9, lysis can be prevented by keeping the temperature near 0 °C and by the presence of high concentrations (0.09 M) of EDTA, suggesting that there are further steps in the process.

11.3.5.3.   *The electron microscopic appearance of complement lysis*

The morphological correlates of complement lysis, the characteristic lesions seen on electron microscopy by negative staining techniques, were first described by Borsos, Dourmashkin and Humphrey[67] and have been studied extensively since[68].

The lesions are *ca.* 100 Å in diameter, this varies slightly with the species of complement (88 Å for guinea-pig and 103 Å for human). They are roughly circular with a dark centre surrounded by an electron-lucent ring with a thickness of *ca.* 25 Å, usually showing a discontinuity. When seen in profile in liposomes, the lesions stand proud of the membrane on its 'outer side'[66].

---

* A serum concentration of Ca of 160 μg ml^{-1} has more recently been estimated by Müller-Eberhard and his colleagues

It is uncertain to what extent they should be regarded as true 'holes' in the membrane. The lesions are typical and can be distinguished from the electron microscopic appearance of lysis produced by other agents. Figure 11.2 shows complement lesions in a liposome and by contrast the appearance of lysis by the polyene antibiotic Filimarisin (Upjohn). Lesions can be produced in lipoprotein membranes of all kinds including those of the myxoviruses[68]; in liposomes[61, 69] and in lipid adsorbed on films on bovine serum albumin[68].

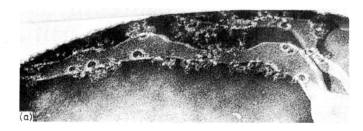

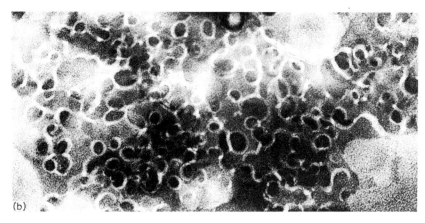

Figure 11.2 (a) Lecithin liposomes that have been lysed by C5–C9 (reactive lysis) showing typical complement lesions. Magnification × 300 000 (Reduced ⅔ on reproduction
(b) Lecithin liposomes that have been lysed by Filimarisin showing lesions that are quite distinct from complement lesions. Magnification × 248 000) Reduced ⅔rds on reproduction)
Electron micrographs were taken by Dr. E. A. Munn

The stage of the complement sequence at which lesions appear has recently become a matter of controversy. Müller-Eberhard and his colleagues[70] originally claimed that reaction as far as C9 was necessary for the lesions to appear. Using the reactive lysis system on liposomes Lachmann et al.[61] similarly showed that the fixation of C567 did not produce lesions but that they appeared, as did the release of trapped marker when C8 and C9 were added to the system. The La Jolla group subsequently revised their opinion and Polley, Müller-Eberhard and Feldman[71] reported that the fixation of C5 was the lesion-producing event, but these observations have not so far been reproduced in other electron-microscopic studies[66, 69]. The reason for the discrepancy is not clear but may lie in the criteria for recognising complement lesions; the morphology of the 'C5 lesions' of Polley et al.[71] being somewhat different from that of the 'typical' complement lesions. Thus, Hesketh et al.[69] have also demonstrated 'ring-like structures' on liposomes treated with antibody and C6-deficient complement (i.e. at the C5 stage) which, however, they consider distinct from the lesions produced with normal complement.

The number of lesions seen on an erythrocyte was equal to the number of functional lesions predicted from single-hit kinetics (e.g. a mean of one lesion per cell when 63% of cells are lysed[67]) only in some circumstances—as when sheep erythrocytes, rabbit IgM antibody and guinea-pig complement were used. On the other hand when human complement was used, a many-fold excess of observed electron-microscopic lesions over predicted functional lesions was seen[73]. At what stage this multiplicity occurs is unknown: whether a multiplicity of $C\overline{567}$ sites are produced per functional hit; whether one $C\overline{567}$ site can activate more than one C8 molecule or whether one C8 molecule can produce clusters of lesions. The first alternative is the most attractive and so far there is certainly no evidence that a lesion can be formed at a site where there is no $C\overline{567}$ fixed, i.e. the C8 stage does not appear to be contagious.

From the work of Humphrey and his group[69, 73] it is clear that the major component of the electron-microscopic lesions is lipid. Thus the lesions cannot be removed by trypsin but are dissolved by chloroform–methanol extraction. However, the presence of a protein component within the lipid cannot be excluded. This would have to be complement protein as typical lesions are formed in pure lipid membranes, and it is likely that the $C\overline{56789}$ complex is the protein basis of the complement lesion.

The lesions are surprisingly stable and, like the grin of the Cheshire cat which could still be seen when the cat had disappeared[74], the lesions can sometimes be seen free of the membrane in which they were formed[66].

If, as seems most likely, the electron-microscopic lesions are a reflection of the functional lesion, this would suggest that the mechanism of lysis involves a micellar rearrangement of the lipid bilayer around some surface-active core. The origin of this core is not known in spite of the considerable effort that has been made in investigating its nature and in obtaining soluble lytic factors from the products of complement activation. Since it became clear that only a phospholipid film and C5∽C9 are required to produce lysis all theories involving membrane proteins or the sodium pump as necessary components of complement lysis have been discarded, and only the lipid substrate and the complement components themselves need to be considered. The role of C8 in determining the specificity of lysis with regard to the cells that are lysed suggests a central role for C8 in the final lytic event, and it can be envisaged either that C8 has some phospholipase activity which generates a detergent from the phospholipid membrane or that a peptide detergent analogous to the bee venom peptide melittin is derived from the C8 itself[176].

The possible phospholipase activity of the complement system has been extensively investigated[66, 75] with essentially negative results. Although using highly sensitive systems, trace amount of phospholipid hydrolysis products have been detected, they appear to be the result and not the cause of lysis. At the present time, therefore, a complement derived detergent seems the more likely explanation. It has, however, so far totally defied isolation.

11.4 HOMEOSTASIS OF COMPLEMENT FIXATION

Homeostatic control of complement fixation is exercised at a number of steps.

11.4.1 C$\bar{1}$ Inhibitor

This material was first described by Lepow *et al.*[76] and was identified by Pensky[77] with the $\alpha2$ neuroaminoglycoprotein originally described by Schultze, Heide and Haupt[78]. It is a stoichiometric inhibitor of a number of serine–histidine esterases found in blood plasma. Besides inhibiting C$\bar{1}$, it also inhibits C1r, plasmin, kininogenase, activated Hageman factor and activated plasma thromboplastin antecedent[79]. Although the reaction of the inhibitor with C$\bar{1}$ is too slow to stop the ongoing complement sequence, it is instrumental in limiting the action of C$\bar{1}$ on C4 and C2 in solution and in preventing the autocatalytic activation of C$\bar{1}$. Deficiency of C$\bar{1}$ inhibitor is associated with hereditary angio-oedema and is discussed below.

11.4.2 The instability of C$\overline{42}$

The instability of C$\overline{42}$ also serves as a homeostatic mechanism limiting the duration of C3 convertase activity at a complement fixation site. A factor accelerating the decay of EAC42 has also been described[80]. Its significance in the complement reaction is unknown.

11.4.3 C3b Inactivator (KAF)

This material was described by Tamura and Nelson[81] as an inhibitor of the haemolytic activity of bound C3b and by Lachmann and Müller-Eberhard[82] as an inactivator of the reactant in bound C3b that reacts with bovine con-glutinin. From the latter property is derived its other name: the *conglutinogen activating factor* or KAF. (Conglutinin is generally abbreviated with a K to avoid confusion with Complement). It has been confirmed that the two activities are properties of the same factor[83].

KAF is a $\beta1$-globulin with a sedimentation coefficient of 6 S and a mol. wt. of *ca.* 100 000. In size and charge KAF is very similar to transferrin, but the two can be separated without great difficulty because of the lower solubility of KAF[84].

The action of KAF on C3b is non-stoichiometric, proceeds extensively in the warm, will inactivate quantities of C3 many times greater than itself and is not consumed in the reaction. The mechanism of action is, therefore, considered to be enzymatic and presumably proteolytic. No fragment of C3b is obviously released during the reaction. However, following KAF action the KAF-treated C3b becomes exquisitely sensitive to trypsin and other similar proteolytic enzymes which then split the molecule.

The functional consequences of KAF action on fixed C3b are: (i) reactivity with conglutinin is acquired; (ii) haemolytic activity is lost; (iii) immune adherence activity is lost; (iv) phagocytosis enhancing activity is lost, (v) The capacity to activate the C3b feed-back pathway (see later) is lost; and (vi) An extremely enzyme-sensitive site is exposed which leads to the hydrolysis of C3b and the 'stripping' of C3b from the cell.

The action of KAF occurs not only on cell bound C3b but also on C3b in the fluid phase. Normal clearance of C3b from the circulation is not seen in the absence of KAF[85].

KAF appears to be of central importance in providing a homeostatic control of C3 activation, particularly of its feed-back role. The genetic absence of KAF gives rise to an immunity deficiency state associated with exhaustion of the factors of the alternative pathway (see below).

11.4.4 The (so-called) 'C6 inactivator'

A further inactivator acting on the complement system was described by Nelson and Biro[86]. They prepared a factor from C6-deficient rabbit serum which was capable of inhibiting the haemolytic activity of EAC1~6. They suggested that this factor was analogous to the C3b inactivator and acted enzymatically upon fixed C6. Since EAC1~6 intermediates are difficult to prepare, relatively little work has been carried out on this inhibitor. However, studies now in progress[87] suggest that a very similar factor acts upon fixed C5 rather than upon fixed C6 and that it is bound to the EAC1~5 intermediate rather than acting enzymatically upon it. Its role in the homeostasis of the C567 step remains to be clarified.

11.4.5 C8i

It is not certain that the C8 analogue, 'C8i' described by Stolfi[65] properly belongs in this section because it is not clear the material occurs naturally *in vivo*. It is, however, a complement inhibitor of great interest even if only for the light it casts on the mode of action of C8. Stolfi described an analogue of C8 that could be prepared by keeping C8 under mildly alkaline conditions or by treating it with small doses of trypsin. This material still has the capacity to bind to EC567; can still deplete C9 from the fluid phase; but it is incapable of producing immune haemolysis. It is, therefore, an efficient inhibitor of the C8 step. Its existence shows that C8 must have three active sites: one binding to C567, one binding C9, and one producing the lytic effect. It remains to be determined whether, and under what conditions, C8i can be formed *in vivo*.

11.5 'NON-CLASSICAL' ACTIVATION OF THE COMPLEMENT SYSTEM

The immune haemolytic reaction described in detail above is the 'classical' complement reaction mechanism, and is initiated by antigen–antibody complexes involving 'complement-fixing' classes of antibody binding C1q and, therefore, giving rise to activation of C1.

There are, however, a variety of other mechanisms that can lead to complement activation. These fall into three major groups.

11.5.1 'Contagion' of complement activation

Complement components activated at a complement fixing site can in certain circumstances spread to the other sites. The two examples of this that are likely to be of *in vivo* significance have already been mentioned. (a) the transfer of bound $C\overline{1}$ from antibody to antibody and (b) the transfer of $C\overline{567}$ (reactive lysis).

11.5.2 'Non-classical' mechanisms for activating C1

(a) Complement-fixing classes of immunoglobulin may be aggregated by agents other than antigen and still behave exactly like antigen-antibody complexes in so far as interaction with C1q is concerned. Such aggregation can be produced by heating or by a variety of chemical procedures (e.g. bisdiazobenzidine or tannic acid treatment). Many forms of particulate matter (e.g. Kaolin and latex) aggregate immunoglobulin on their surfaces. The uric acid crystals formed in gouty joints are believed to do this too[88], a phenomenon that may be of pathogenetic significance. Staphylococcal protein A has the interesting property of reacting with the Fc portion of IgG to give a complement-fixing aggregate[89].

(b) Certain non-immunoglobulin systems can activate C1 by interaction with C1q. Some highly-charged polyanions, DNA[11] and polyinosinic acid[90] have this activity. So do certain bacterial endotoxins[21] and the lipid A derived from them[91]. The complex made between bovine conglutinin (*q.v.*) and its mannose–peptide reactant, the conglutinogen, activates C1, presumably via interaction with C1q[92].

(c) The enzymatic activation of C1s to $C\overline{1}$ normally brought about by C1r can also be effected by plasmin and trypsin[93] and by $C\overline{1}$ itself[76].

All these mechanisms go on to activate the classical pathway as described above and utilise C4 and C2 as well as C1.

11.5.3 Mechanisms for activating C3 that do not require the participation of C1, C4 and C2

From a functional point of view the central reaction of the complement sequence is the fixation of C3. This is the reaction occurring in bulk, involving the component present in the largest amount, and bringing about the most important biological effects. In so far as an analogy can be drawn with blood coagulation, C3 fixation is equivalent to the formation of fibrin and the 'C3 convertase' that splits the native C3 molecule is analogous to thrombin.

Besides $C\overline{42}$, the 'classical' C3 convertase, there are a number of other C3-splitting enzymes that can produce complement activation starting at this point in the cascade. These include serine–histidine esterases such as trypsin, plasmin and thrombin and in the case of the latter two this action may have physiological significance since some C3 is always found on fibrin clotted in fresh serum.

There is, however, a further physiological mechanism for generating a C3-convertase which is believed to be of as great importance *in vivo* as the classical pathway and this will now be discussed in detail.

11.5.4 The 'alternative', 'by-pass', 'properdin' or 'C3 feed back' pathway of complement activation

That a heat-stable component of complement was preferentially destroyed by absorption with yeast cell-wall polysaccharides (zymosan) has been known since 1925 from the studies of Whitehead et al.[46]. This was the third component of complement described and therefore came to be known as C'3. In modern nomenclature this (classical) C'3 comprises the modern C3~9. The mechanism whereby yeast brought about the removal of C'3 was studied in detail by Pillemer and his colleagues in the 1950s (reviewed in Ref. 94). They showed that C3 activation by zymosan required the participation of at least one factor distinct from known complement components and to this factor the name properdin was given. They believed properdin to be a non-antibody and immunologically non-specific material capable of initiating complement activation leading to C3 consumption and pictured this mechanism as of central importance in non-specific immunity. It was later appreciated that the inactivation of C3 by zymosan required, in addition to properdin, two further factors. One of these, factor A, was hydrazine labile and resembled C4, although inactivation studies showed some differences between the properties of factor A and C4[95]. The other, which was heat labile, resembled C2 but again inactivation studies suggested that the two factors were not identical[96]. These findings provided the basis of a suggested alternative pathway of complement fixation not involving the early components, C1, C4 and C2 that are required in immune haemolysis and apparently not requiring antibody. This concept of the properdin system was, however, criticised by Nelson[97, 98] who pointed out that antibodies to yeast cell walls do occur in normal sera and showed that the properdin system was in fact immunologically specific; a point which came to be generally agreed. Nelson further suggested that properdin itself represented not a new specific protein but a mixture of complexes containing natural antibodies and the early-reacting complement components. The topic remained in a confused state until more progress had been made with the fractionation of complement components and more quantitative assay procedures became available. Properdin itself was isolated from human serum by Pensky et al.[99] and has been characterised as a non-immunoglobulin serum β-protein with a sedimentation constant at 5.2 S and a mol. wt. of ca. 230 000. It is antigenically unrelated to other known complement components. Its mechanism of action remains still to be clarified. However, the essential correctness of the view that yeast cell walls as well as bacterial endotoxins, inulin and a number of other polysaccharide substances are capable of leading to the formation of a C3 splitting enzyme without involving C1, C4 and C2 has now been amply confirmed (review in Ref. 100).

11.5.4.1 Modern knowledge of the alternative pathway

Our current information on this pathway is derived principally from the convergence of three distinct lines of study: those concerned with the anti-complementary activity of zymosan, endotoxin and inulin; those concerned with the anticomplementary activity of cobra venom; and those concerned with the consequences of the deficiency or depletion of the C3b inactivator (KAF).

The first line is derived directly from the work of Pillemer and his colleagues. The more precise component assays now available have confirmed that zymosan, endotoxin or suspensions of inulin deplete C3 and later components without detectable depletion of C1, C4 or C2[100]. It has furthermore been shown that by-pass activation requires only Mg″ and not Ca‴[101]. As C1 requires calcium for its activity, this component would seem not to be required in the by-pass reaction. Furthermore, the C3 converting activity of an endotoxin-serum complex could not be inhibited, as could the C3 converting activity of EAC142, by anti-C2 antibody[102]. Furthermore again, this group of 'alternative pathway' activators are capable of converting C3 and depleting later components from the serum of humans genetically deficient in C2[91] and guinea-pigs genetically deficient in C4[103]. The evidence is thus convincing that this group of substances can activate the complement system by a pathway not involving C1, C4 or C2.

Whether the anti-complementary activity of zymosan, endotoxin and similar polysaccharide activators requires immunologically specific (antibody or antibody-like) factors has proved difficult to establish with certainty. There is evidence in favour of their participation. Thus zymosan requires the so-called '0 °C factor' (which is removed from serum by zymosan absorption at 0 °C) in order to inactivate complement[104].

The evidence, in the case of endotoxin was reviewed by Gewurz[100] who believes that the participation of a small amount of natural antibody is likely.

Again it is now clear that aggregates of various classes of immunoglobulin that fail to activate the classical pathway can indeed activate the by-pass. The γ1-immunoglobulins of the guinea-pig[19] and the γ2-immunoglobulins of ruminants[20, 91] are good examples. In man complexes or aggregates of IgA and of IgG4b, which do not activate the classical pathway act as by-pass activators[105]. The balance of the evidence at the present time, therefore, would suggest that some form of natural antibody generally participates in alternate pathway activation.

11.5.4.2 The anticomplementary activity of cobra venom

The anticomplementary activity of cobra venom was described in 1903 by Flexner and Noguchi[106]. However, it was not until 1966 that it was established[107, 108] that the complement inactivating factor was distinct from phospholipase A and that while it acted principally upon C3 in whole serum, its action could not be demonstrated on purified C3. This was shown to require a co-factor, to which the name (cobra-venom factor) C3 proactivator was eventually given. Müller-Eberhard and his colleagues[107] demonstrated that the 7 S cobra-venom protein was converted in serum to a 9 S complex presumably by combination with its co-factor. Fractionation of serum to obtain the co-factor yielded a protein antigenically related to one which had previously been isolated by Haupt and Heide[110] and given the name β2-glycoprotein II and which Boenisch and Alper[111] had also isolated as a component depleted in their patient T.J. of whom more is to be said

below. This protein is now generally abbreviated as GBG (for glycine-rich
β-glycoprotein). During activation of the by-pass, GBG is split into two
fragments GAG (glycine-rich a-glycoprotein) and GGG (glycine-rich γ-
glycoprotein) and this conversion of GBG is often used to monitor alternative
pathway activation. GBG is heat labile and has been shown to have factor
B activity in a properdin system assay[112] where it appears to be the 'C2-like'
component. It is, however, antigenically unrelated to C2 and its serum
concentration (*ca.* 100–200 µg ml^{-1}) is much higher than that of C2 (*ca.*
20 µg ml^{-1}).

There has been considerable controversy—not entirely resolved so far—as
to the relationship between GBG and the Cobra Venom co-factors. It is clear
that the original view of Götze & Müller-Eberhard[113] that GBG binds to
CVF and that this is the only factor required in the generation of the Cobra
Venom Factor C3 convertase is oversimplified. It has been shown that highly
purified GBG does not form a firm complex with CVF[112,114] and it has been
suggested that there may be a separate Cobra Venom Factor binding protein
present as an impurity in GBG[112]. The situation is complicated by the existence
of a further factor that is required for the generation of the CVF-C3 convertase. This factor known as Factor D[114] appears likely to be identical with
the 3S $a2$ euglobulin described as necessary for the alternative pathway and
with (pro)-GBGase (see below).

11.5.4.3 Deficiency of depletion of C3b-inactivator (KAF)

The third line of evidence arose from studies of a unique and intensively
studied patient in Boston, 'T.J.', who has a primary deficiency of C3b
inactivator (KAF)[117,118]. The clinical aspects of this patient are described
further in the section on complement deficiencies. His complement abnormalities are enumerated in Table 11.1, where they are compared with the
effects on normal serum of the immunochemical depletion of KAF *in vitro*.
The effects are parallel and show that the absence of KAF leads to the
spontaneous activation of the alternative pathway as shown by the conversion
of GBG; to the depletion of 'cobra-venom factor C3-proactivator' (i.e. the

Table 11.1 *In vitro* and *in vivo* KAF deficiency

	KAF-depleted serum*	KAF deficiency†
	in vitro	in vivo
KAF activity	0	0
C3	Rapid conversion	Low level conversion producers
C3 detectable on red cells	—	—
GBG	Rapid conversion to GGG and GAG	Low or absent
Cobra venom co-factors	Rapid depletion	Low or not detectable
Levels of C1, C4 and C2	Little depletion	Normal

* Normal human serum precipitated at optimal proportions with purified F(ab')₂ anti-KAF[119]
† Serum from patient T. J.[117,118]

co-factors needed to give rise to the cobra-venom convertase); and to the conversion of C3. These effects of KAF depletion can be attributed to the loss of its inactivation of C3b since if C3 is immunochemically depleted from serum no conversion of GBG or consumption of cobra venom factor C3 proactivator could be produced either by depletion of KAF or by the typical activators of the alternative pathway, zymosan, inulin or immune precipitates using ruminant γ2-antibody. Only cobra-venom factor could give rise to a C3-convertase in the absence of C3. These experiments led to the somewhat paradoxical conclusion that the generation of a C3 convertase by the alternative pathway requires the presence of the principal product of C3 convertase activity, C3b. A similar conclusion has also been reached by Müller-Eberhard and Götze[116] who 'built up' the by-pass convertase from purified components and found that this required a fragment of C3 as well as GBG ('C3 proactivator' in their terminology) and a 3 S a2-euglobulin (C3PA-convertase or pro-GBGase); and has recently been confirmed by Alper *et al.*[120] who found in their, also unique, C3 deficient patient that zymosan was unable to bring about the conversion of GBG.

C3b feed back into the by-pass by being necessary for the activity of the enzyme GBGase which splits GBG. This has been demonstrated by showing that KAF will inhibit the GBGase activity in T.J. serum[118]; and that this GBGase activity can also be removed by the immunochemical depletion of C3 from T.J. serum and restored by the re-addition of more C3[115].

The alternative pathway therefore appears to be a positive feed-back pathway by which C3b generate more C3 convertase. This process is normally controlled by the C3b inactivator (KAF) which destroys the feed-back activity of C3b.

11.5.4.4 The reaction mechanisms of the C3-feed-back cycle

It is difficult at this time to give a picture of the feed-back cycle which is consistent with all the data. The schema given in Figure 11.3 is tentative.

The information on which it draws may be summarised as follows:

(a) There is necessary requirement for C3b for alternate pathway activation by zymosan, inulin, endotoxin or KAF depletion.

(b) Cobra-venom factor, however, can give rise to a C3 convertase in the absence of C3, and is the *only* 'alternative-pathway' activator that can do so. The convertase formed is larger than the usual by-pass convertase and contains GBG antigens. Nevertheless, the addition of CVF to serum does not necessarily give rise to GBG conversion. No GBG conversion is seen if C3 is immunochemically depleted (i.e. all the GBG conversion is feed-back mediated). Even if C3 is present, GBG conversion is not seen if too much CVF is used[115] (i.e. it seems that if all of one of the necessary components is consumed by CVF, it is not available for the feed-back cycle which then fails). It is suggested that the CVF–GBGase complex acts on GBG in a manner analogous with 'ordinary' GBGase but that the products are not released. For this reason the product is large and there is no 'turnover' of GBG.

(c) The cycle involves, besides C3b, a 3 S a2-euglobulin and (probably) a separate cobra-venom factor binding protein. In some way, these three factors (possibly together with yet others) make up 'GBGase' the enzyme which splits GBG t give rise to the by-pass convertase.

(d) In the absence of KAF the cycle activates apparently spontaneously both *in vivo* and *in vitro*.

(e) The point of action of the alternate-pathway activators is not known. They are believed to be concerned (together perhaps with properdin) in generating some initial GBGase, although this could be only an undetectable priming activity. However, it is possible that they generate an evanescent and

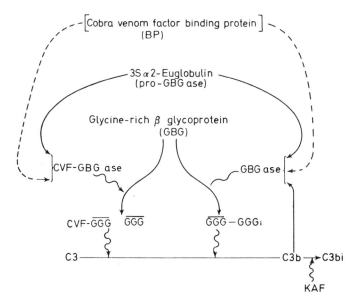

Figure 11.3 The C3-feed-back pathway. The scheme shows the generation of C3-converting enzymes by the C3-feed-back pathway in the right-hand limb and by the cobra-venom factor pathway in the left-hand limb. The curved arrows denote an enzymic effect. The steps are described in the text

entirely different C3-splitting enzyme. For reasons already discussed this is unlikely to be $\overline{C4,2}$.

Nevertheless, it is known that C3b is fixed by the feed-back pathway onto bacterial flagella treated with sheep IgG2 antibody and onto endotoxin and zymosan so that the feed-back convertase is generated on the surface of these feed-back activators.

The feed-back convertase can also be generated in free solution as occurs in KAF-depletion in which case C3b may be fixed to bystander cells or converted entirely in solution.

Note added in proof: Recent reports have shown that properdin undergoes a conversion involving a change in its electrophoretic mobility on activation in the alternative pathway[177] and that properdin together with C3 can 'fire' the C3-feed-back cycle[178].

Although, for the reasons discussed already, $C\overline{42}$ is not a necessary component of the alternative pathway, it can certainly prime the feed-back cycle as shown by the conversion of GBG that occurs in serum undergoing classical pathway activation. However, this is not an efficient way of initiating the feed-back since the amounts of sheep red cells coated with rabbit IgM antibody that are needed to produce GBG conversion are substantially larger than those needed to deplete the early components[91].

11.6 THE BIOSYNTHESIS OF COMPLEMENT COMPONENTS

Current knowledge of the sites of complement component synthesis is summarised in Table 11.2.

Table 11.2   Site of formation of complement components

Components	Site
C1	Intestinal epithelium[71]
C4	Macrophages[49]
C2	Macrophages[49]
C3	Liver[72]
C5	Cells in spleen[173]
C6	Liver[174]
C7	Unknown
C8	Cells in spleen[175]
C9	Liver[109]
Inhibitors	
$C\overline{1}$-inhibitor	Liver[117]
C3b-inactivator (KAF)	Unknown
C3 Feed-back factors	
GBG	Liver[122]

Little is known of what controls the biosynthesis of complement components. It has been recognised for a long time that complement is to some extent an 'acute-phase' reactant and that rises in complement levels, particularly of C3 and of C5 and C6, occur in the acute phase of inflammation. In the case of C3, there is evidence that the presence in the circulation of certain breakdown products of C3 may lead to a slowing of C3 synthesis. Thus in patients with membranoproliferative glomerulonephritis who tend to have C3d circulating and very low levels of C3 there is a normal fractional catabolic rate of administered C3[160, 161]. This suggests strongly that the synthesis rate has been slowed. On the other hand, the KAF-deficient patient[117] who has circulating C3b and very low C3 levels does not appear to have a slow synthetic rate of C3, whereas another patient of Alper *et al.*[162], who has a C3-destroying enzyme in her serum and whose C3 breakdown products go on beyond the C3b stage via KAF treatment to break down to C3c and C3d again, has a slow synthetic rate. If the C3 breakdown products do indeed slow C3 synthesis, it appears to be breakdown products beyond the C3b stage which are responsible.

11.7 THE GENETICS OF THE COMPLEMENT SYSTEM

11.7.1 Genetic polymorphism of complement components

It is only in recent years that genetic markers have been detected on complement components. There is a well-defined group of electrophoretically distinguishable C3 allotypes[117] and C6 allotypes have recently been described. There is a suggestion of similar markers for C4[121]; and for GBG[117]. Unfortunately, no linkage studies are as yet available and it is, therefore, not known to what extent, if any, complement components represent tandem duplications of primordial complement components. In the case of C3, C4 and C5, there are marked similarities in their susceptibility to hydrazine and to potassium thiocyanate and in their reaction patterns during the complement sequence. For these components, it would not be surprising if they were found to derive from a common precursor.

11.7.2 Genetic deficiencies of complement components

A variety of genetic deficiencies in the complement system are now known (see Refs. 117 and 123); these are tabulated in Table 11.3. Isolated complement-component deficiencies have been found in guinea-pigs, rabbits, mice and men. The components involved are different in each species even though in rabbits and mice there are several unrelated strains known with each deficiency, and there are several pedigrees of C2-deficient humans.

In general, these deficiencies of individual complement components are isolated and other complement components occur in normal levels. This is not wholly true of C4-deficient guinea-pigs which have regularly some depression of their C2 levels and a variable depression of C1 levels. The reasons

Table 11.3 Genetic abnormalities of the complement system

Species	Factor deficient	No. of pedigrees known	Clinical state
Man	C1q (not 1° defect)	Many	Hypogammaglobulinaemia
	C1r	2	Renal and skin disease
	C2	Several	Generally healthy
	C3	1	Immunity deficiency
	C5 (Functional deficiency)	Several	Immunity deficiency
	C$\bar{1}$-inhibitor (N.B. heterozygotes)	Many	Hereditary angio-oedema
	C3b-inactivator (KAF)	1	Immunity deficiency
Guinea-pigs	C4	1	Healthy
	A component C3–C9	1	Extinct
Mice	C5	Many	Healthy
Rabbits	C6	Several	Healthy

for this are not known. It has also been found in at least two of the C2-deficient human sera that the levels of GBG are approximately half normal. Again the mechanism for this is unknown.

The C4-deficient guinea-pigs and the C2-deficient humans have an intact alternative pathway as can be shown by the capacity of inulin and zymosan to deplete their sera of the late-acting components (C5∼C9). This presumably accounts for the relatively benign effects of these deficiencies. Although the majority of known C2-deficient subjects have been healthy, there are now at least three C2-deficient patients known who have diseases with immunological overtones; one with glomerulo-nephritis; one with systemic Lupus Erythematosus (SLE)* and one with persistent 'Henoch-Shönlein' purpura. The last patient has been shown to carry in her plasma over a prolonged period structures that closely resemble Mycoplasma and it is possible that she does in fact, have an immunity deficiency albeit of an unusual type[124].

The impeccable good health of the C5-deficient mice and the C6-deficient rabbits is less easy to account for. It seems likely that the C567 stage in the complement reaction is not essential in animals kept under laboratory conditions. There is in these animals, however, some impairment of homograft rejection providing that the transplantation is carried out across a sufficiently wide histocompatibility barrier.

11.7.3 Complement deficiencies in man

C2-deficiency (dealt with above) is the only complement *component* deficiency that occurs with any frequency. The deficiencies in the other components described below are all extremely rare.

11.7.3.1 C1 deficiency

(a) C1q—It has been recorded on several occasions that C1q levels are low in hypogammaglobulinemia particularly of the Swiss type[125, 126]. It, however, now seems likely that this deficiency of C1q is due not to a synthetic defect but to redistribution of C1q between the plasma and the extracellular fluid (perhaps due to a lack of sufficient IgG to complex it) and to increased catabolism[127].

(b) C1r deficiency—One family with C1r deficiency has been described[128] and one further patient is known[129]. This deficiency is accompanied by a serious disease, three siblings in the affected family having died in childhood; two probably from infection and one from a disease resembling SLE. Of the two remaining siblings one has an SLE-like disease and the other has repeated infections and arthralgia. In these C1r-deficient sera the alternate pathway could be shown to be intact; again by showing the consumption of late-acting components by endotoxin. It may therefore be oversimplifying to believe that an intact alternative pathway alone is all that is required complement-wise for the maintenance of good health.

* Systemic Lupus Erythematosus is a disease affecting particularly the skin, joints and kidney where antigen–antibody complexes comprising (mainly nuclear antigens and their respective auto-antibodies produce widespread allergic inflammation around small blood vessels.

11.7.3.2 C3 deficiency

Alper et al.[120] have recently given a preliminary description of a 15-year-old girl with repeated infections who appears to have a total deficiency of C3. It is of some interest that she has normal immunoglobulin levels. Of all complement deficiencies, this is the one which would be expected to produce the most complete picture of complement deprivation and further studies in this patient will no doubt clarify substantially the role of complement in vivo.

11.7.3.3 The functional abnormality of C5

Miller and Nilsson[130] described an opsonic abnormality in children of a family with recurrent infections that could be corrected by the addition of normal C5. The affected subjects had a normal total haemolytic complement and the amount of C5 measured immunochemically was normal as well. These workers attributed the defect to a functional abnormality of C5 but its nature is not established.

11.7.4 Abnormalities of complement inhibitors

11.7.4.1 C1 inhibitor—hereditary angio-oedema

The association of hereditary angio-oedema with the deficiency of $C\overline{1}$ inhibitor was demonstrated by Donaldson and Evans[131] and has been widely confirmed (see Refs. 117 and 132 for review of literature). The disease is transmitted as an autosomal dominant and, in line with this, it has been found that affected subjects have an incomplete deficiency and may show up to 25% of the normal inhibitor level. In the majority of pedigrees there is no antigenically-recognisable protein made by the mutant gene; in about one-fifth of the pedigrees, however, antigenically detectable but inactive protein is made.

The disease is characterised by episodes of angio-oedema (fluid swellings) in the subcutaneous tissues or in the mucosae of the respiratory or alimentary tract. The patches of oedema are generally single and last for 48–72 h. Considerable pain may accompany the attacks, particularly in the abdomen and oedema in the upper respiratory tract is life-endangering. So far as is known attacks are triggered by the local exhaustion of inhibitor, probably as a result of its binding to any of the plasma enzymes with which it can react (see Figure 11.4). When inhibitor is locally exhausted, $C\overline{1}$ activation can occur spontaneously and autocatalytically. As a result, C4 and C2 are broken down and the kinin-like C2 fragment, discussed later, becomes generated. This appears to be the main mediator of the attack. It is less than clear what brings the attacks to an end. Attacks may be treated by the infusion of fresh plasma as source of inhibitor. Successful prophylactic treatment has been

Note added in proof: Single examples of humans deficient in C6 (179) and in C7 (J. Boyer, personal communication) have recently been reported. In neither case did the complement deficiency appear to be producing clinical consequences.

achieved in many cases by the administration of ε-aminocaproic acid which presumably acts by inhibiting the activation of the whole spectrum of plasma enzymes which once activated can consume C$\overline{1}$ inhibitor[132].

11.7.4.2 *C3b inactivator (or KAF) deficiency*

Only one patient with this deficiency has been described (see Ref. 117), but family studies have shown that many of his relatives are heterozygous for the same deficiency[118]. The patient is a young man who has a life-long history of

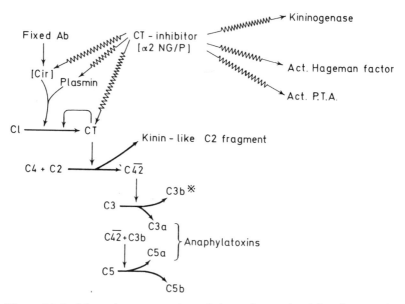

Figure 11.4 Schematic representation of the pathogenesis of hereditary angio-oedemae Jagged arrows denote inhibition of the enzymes concerned. α2-NG/P = α2-neuramino-glycoprotein. PTA = Plasma Thromboplastin Antecedent.
The diagram shows the reaction sequence of the early part of the complement sequence. In the absence of C$\overline{1}$ inhibitor, uncontrolled activation of C$\overline{1}$ can occur with the consequence that C4 and C2 are broken down and the kinin-like C2 fragment formed. Some anaphylatoxin formation is also less likely to result. C$\overline{1}$ inhibitor can be consumed by any of the enzymes it inhibits and activation of any of them may therefore lead to local exhaustion of inhibitor

severe pyogenic infections and also, but probably irrelevantly, suffers from Kleinfelter's syndrome. He has normal immunoglobulins but a severe opsonic defect. He has very low C3 levels and free-circulating C3b in his serum. He breaks down C3 with a fractional catabolic rate of 10% of the plasma pool per hour which is five times the normal rate. He has extremely low levels of GBG and undetectable cobra-venom co-factors. The pathogenesis of these abnormalities have been discussed in the section on the alternate pathway.

11.8 THE BIOLOGICAL EFFECTS OF COMPLEMENT

In spite of the complexity of complement's reaction pattern the biological effects that it produces can be divided into a small number of groups. These are (a) the adherence reactions of fixed complement components to a number of cell types; (b) the production of biologically-active fragments of complement components during the reaction sequence; and (c) the production of the characteristic membrane lesions.

11.8.1 Complement-mediated adherence reactions

These reactions are mediated almost exclusively by fixed C3 in its 'un-KAF-reacted' form.

Bound C3b adheres to the erythrocytes of primates, a reaction which has been known for many years as the 'immune adherence reaction'. An apparently identical adherence occurs to the platelets of a number of non-primate species. Species with immune-adherence-positive platelets include the rabbit, guinea-pig, mouse, rat, cat, dog and horse and immune-adherence-negative species include (besides the primates) pig, ox, sheep and goat[133]. The nature of the adherence reaction is not clearly known. It occurs best at 37 °C and much less at 4 °C and it is inhibited by esters of aromatic amino acids[134]. For this reason it has been thought possible that the adherence was the consequence of some enzymatic reaction of fixed C3b upon the adherent cell. However, it is also possible that a hydrophobic interaction between fixed C3b and the adherent surface is involved. The high degree of specificity in these reactions, however, contrasts strongly with the binding of nascent C3 at complement-fixation sites which is remarkable for its lack of discrimination between potential binding surfaces.

It has been reported[135] that bound C4, if present in sufficient quantity can also mediate immune adherence.

The adherence of bound C3b to phagocytic cells, the so-called 'opsonic adherence' is probably in no way significantly different from immune adherence. Both polymorphs and macrophages adhere to bound C3b. The receptor on neutrophils and on macrophages for C3b is known to be distinct from their receptors for bound IgG[136]. These adherence reactions to phagocytic cells are closely involved in the first stages of phagocytosis and may be among the most important biological actions of complement. The biological significance of the immune-adherence reactions to erythrocytes is less clear but it is likely that this also facilitates the phagocytosis of micro-organisms by holding them against a relatively rigid object, which in cinematographic studies of phagocytosis appears to facilitate ingestion. Immune adherence to platelets is an important step in the complement-mediated release of platelet factor 3 (see later).

A further adherence reaction of bound C3b has been described more recently[137, 138]. This is the adherence of fixed C3b to B lymphocytes. The functional significance of this adherence reaction is not clearly known but has suggested to various workers the possibility that C3 may play a part in the induction of the allergic response. This is discussed in a later section. Whereas the immune-adherence reaction is remarkable for the very small amount of bound C3

(100–1000 molecules cell^{-1}) that is required to bring it about, rosette formation around the B lymphocyte requires substantial amounts of C3b on the complement-coated red cell.

11.8.2   Biologically-active fragments of complement components

11.8.2.1   C2 Kinin

That a kinin-like fragment distinct from bradykinin was produced, probably from C2 during the formation of C3 convertase was reported by Donaldson *et al.*[139, 140] who believed this fragment to be principally responsible for the syndrome of hereditary angio-oedema (q.v.). Although the material has not so far been fully characterised it has been shown to be distinct from bradykinin, C4a, C3a and C5a and to produce permeability effects without involving histamine release[141].

11.8.2.2   C3a

C3a is the small fragment of C3 produced by the action of C3 convertase. It has a mol. wt. of *ca.* 7000 and acts as an anaphylatoxin, i.e. has a capacity to release mediators from mast cells[142]. Identical, or very similar, products can be produced by treatment of C3 with trypsin under very mild conditions or with plasmin[143]. The plasmin fragment was claimed by Ward[144] to have chemotactic activity. The extent to which C3a is a significant chemotactic factor *in vivo* is not certain. C3a is very rapidly broken down in serum by the enzyme described by Bokisch *et al.*[143] as anaphylatoxin inactivator which seems to be identical to kininase or carboxypeptidase B. This enzyme splits off the carboxy terminal arginine and destroys the biological activity of C3a. Presumably because of this enzyme it has not been possible to generate C3a in serum.

11.8.2.3   C5a

C5a is produced during the activation of C5 by C3 convertase and C3b or by trypsin[145]. It has a mol. wt. of *ca.* 15 000 and is believed to be the principal anaphylatoxin. C3a and C5a in their actions on mast cells are non-cross-desensitising whereas each desensitises for itself. This suggests that they either react with mast cells by different receptors and give rise to incomplete mediator release, or, less probably, that different populations of cells have C3a and C5a receptors. C5a has been shown furthermore to be a potent chemotactic factor, and is believed to be the principal chemotactic factor generated in whole serum[146]. However, the recent, and as yet unconfirmed, work of Wissler and his colleagues[147] suggests that chemotactic activity is not a property of the pure anaphylatoxic peptide but requires, in addition, a further peptide component which has been purified and named cocytotaxin. C5a is also broken down by anaphylatoxin inactivator.

11.8.2.4   Leukocyte mobilising factor

A factor with the ability of mobilising polymorphonuclear leucocytes from the bone marrow, that appears to be a product of C3, has been described by Rother[148]. Its relation to other C3 fragments, at the time of writing is not clear.

11.8.2.5   C$\overline{567}$

The trimolecular complex C$\overline{567}$ was the first complement derived factor to be recognised to be chemotactic[149]. It differs from the others in being not a fragment but a macromolecular complex and it has no action as an anaphylatoxin.

It has been suggested that all these chemotactic factors produce their effects by activating a pro-esterase in the polymorph membrane[150].

11.8.3   The membrane lesions of complement

As has already been described, the production of membrane lesions requires only the activity of C5 to C9 and can be brought about not only on all types of cell, but also on artificial membranes. These lesions are responsible for immune haemolysis and for the lysis of nucleated cells by antibody and complement. They are also apparently responsible for platelet factor 3 release from platelets in so far as this is brought about by complement action. Whereas cells that are fully exposed in serum are lysed by the action of complement, in cells that are protected from direct exposure to the extracellular fluid an alternative pattern of reaction has been observed. This is shown as 'complement-mediated lysosomal activation' and was described from studies on the organ culture of chick bones[151]. In this situation it has been shown that growing a chick bone in a culture medium containing antibody against membrane determinants and complement leads to the production of substantial amounts of lysosomal protease with the consequent breakdown of the cartilage matrix. The chondrocytes in the rudiment, however, are not killed as can be shown by restoring the rudiment to normal medium. It will then begin to grow to reform its matrix albeit in an irregular fashion. Until the rudiment becomes severely disorganised, the localisation of complement components in this reaction is restricted to the outermost layer and the lysosomal activation on the inside is presumably due to a mediator release at the surface. Whether this mediator is derived from complement components or from the cells of the periphery remains to be ascertained. The production of lysosomal activation requires the late-acting complement components in so far as it cannot be produced with C6-deficient rabbit serum.

11.8.3.1   Complement-dependent platelet activation

In the rabbit the platelet is immune-adherence positive and therefore adheres to bound C3 at complement-fixation sites. Although this adherence alone brings about the slow release of platelet factor 3 (PF3), much greater release is produced by the further action of $C5 \sim C9$ (i.e. the reactive lysis of the platelets). This mechanism seems to operate in normal blood clotting in the rabbit in as much as C6-deficient rabbits show inadequate pro-thrombin consumption[152] and do not generate PF3 well during clotting in non-wettable containers *in vitro*.

In some conditions such as endotoxin shock, however, this mechanism becomes of major pathogenetic importance. Massive complement activation causes a degree of platelet activation and is sufficient to precipitate disseminated intravascular coagulation. Thus C6-deficient rabbits are substantially resistant, and cobra-venom treated rabbits wholly resistant, to endotoxin shock[153]. In man, although the platelets are immune adherence negative, adherence to a complement-fixation site may occur via the platelet receptor for bound IgG, and a comparable situation can result. 'Massive complement activation' accompanied by disseminated intravascular coagulation is seen in man, for example, in Dengue haemorrhagic fever[154].

11.8.4   The role of complement in the induction of the allergic response

Speculations on the possible involvement of complement in the afferent limb of allergic responses have been put forward from time to time. The observations that in ontogeny complement appears well before antibody, i.e. before it is needed in the efferent limb of the allergic response, suggested that complement might play a role in the production of natural tolerance. Azar *et al.*[155] studied the production of tolerance to aggregate-free IgG in C5 deficient mice and in animals depleted of complement with cobra-venom factor and reported that this was more difficult to achieve. However, although the New Zealand B mouse with its high tendency to develop auto-antibodies is C5 deficient, there is no evidence of failure of self-tolerance in other strains of C5-deficient mice or in C6-deficient rabbits.

The possible role of complement in the induction of antibody formation was suggested by the discovery of the C3 receptor on B lymphocytes[137, 138] and by the observation that a number of the T-independent antigens (endotoxin and pneumoccal polysaccharides) are activators of the alternative pathway of complement fixation. Actual data on the association is confined to the observation of Ellman *et al.*[156] that the C4 deficient guinea-pigs made less antibody in response to low dosage of ovalbumin than did their C4-sufficient controls; and those of Pepys[157] who showed that mice, who had been depleted of complement with cobra-venom factor, showed depressed antibody formation to sheep red cells, and to a smaller extent to ovalbumin, whereas the antibody responses to pneumococcal polysaccharides and polyvinyl pyrrolidone, both T-independent antigens, were normal. He concluded from these findings that complement is required for T-dependent responses and suggested that complement fixation by complexes of antigen and the postulated T-cell 'antibody' allows the complex to be bound on the surface of the B cell via its C3 receptor. Dukor and Hartmann[158] have put forward an alternative

* See Note added in proof, p. 393.

hypothesis, namely that nascent C3 binding to C3 receptor is a non-specific signal required for B-cell proliferation.

There, are however, reasons for believing that complement does not play a *necessary* role in antibody formation. Perhaps the strongest is the existence of the C3-deficient patient with normal levels of immunoglobulins[120] and also of the KAF-deficient patient who has extremely low levels of C3 and has constantly circulating C3b[117] which would be expected to block the C3 receptor on lymphocytes[157]. He, too, has normal levels of immunoglobulin and normal levels of antibodies to the organisms with which he becomes infected. Furthermore, a definitive requirement for complement in *in-vitro* systems for studying antibody formation has not so far been reported. It seems likely therefore that any part complement plays in antibody formation is facultative and potentiating comparable to the role it has in phagocytosis. If one believes that the binding of C3 to the lymphocyte C3 receptor is a signal to the cell, there are at present no good reasons for choosing between models in which it is a 'switching-on' signal and those in which it is a 'switching-off' signal. It is clear that this is an area where more information is needed and will probably be available soon.

11.8.5 Complement as an Auto-antigen—Conglutination

The conglutinating activity of complement has a history only slightly less long than its haemolytic activity. Conglutination is the powerful clumping of complement-coated cells that is produced by a naturally-occurring factor found in the serum of cattle and some other ruminants but not in other types of mammal. This factor was named conglutinin by Bordet and Streng[163]. It has been isolated and found to be an unusual serum protein unrelated antigenically to the immunoglobulins. It shows an extreme degree of molecular asymmetry having a sedimentation coefficient of *ca.* 8 S, a mol. wt. of *ca.* 75 000 and a frictional ratio of *ca.* 4[164]. Conglutinin reacts exclusively with a determinant in KAF-reacted bound C3, and it was this reactivity that gave KAF its name (conglutinogen activating factor)[82]. The determinant is a mannose peptide and is found not only in the fixed C3 of apparently all mammalian species but is found also in the cell walls of yeast and of certain related micro-organisms. The physiological significance of this cross-reactive mannose peptide is unknown. The reaction of the polysaccharide determinant, the conglutinogen, with conglutinin requires calcium ions, another point of difference from most antigen antibody reactions.

Although it is clear that conglutination by bovine conglutinin is not an antigen antibody reaction, antibodies with conglutinin-like activities (immunoconglutinins) can be raised not only by cross-species immunisation with complement coated material but are also found normally in most mammalian species. Coombs[165] first recognised that the 'auto-stimulated' immunoconglutinins were antibodies to hidden determinants in the complement molecule that were exposed upon fixation. In the discussion that follows the term immunoconglutinin is applied only to the autostimulated variety, i.e. to the auto-antibodies that are formed to fix complement.

Such immunoconglutinins occur naturally in man and most mammalian species. Their reactivity is predominantly directed against bound C3. Its reactivity, however, differs from that of conglutinin in that most immunoconglutinins have preferential reaction to native bound C3b over the KAF reacted variety and that even those that react with KAF reactive C3 appear not to react with the conglutinogen in as much as their reaction cannot be inhibited by yeast or conglutinogen fractions prepared from yeast cell walls. Some immunoconglutinins have also been found to react with bound C4 and (in saliva) some are found that react at low titre with bound C567. Serum immunoconglutinins are largely IgM antibodies but, using suitable techniques, immunoconglutinins of other immunoglobulin classes can be detected[167]. The titres of serum immunoconglutinin rise in conditions associated with increased *in vivo* complement fixation, e.g. infectious and auto-allergic disease.

It has been observed more recently[168] that far higher titres of immunoconglutinin than are found in serum are normally present in saliva and apparently also in the jejunal juice. These immunoconglutinins have somewhat different properties from those found in serum. They appear to be large polymers of IgA and their reactivity towards bound complement components differs from that of serum immunoconglutinins in that they are readily inhibited by the presence of complement components in solution. The salivary immunoconglutinins require calcium for their reaction to fixed complement, a very unusual property for an immune reaction. The existence of immunoconglutinins in saliva that react with native C3 casts an interesting light on the nature of immunological tolerance. It seems that in sites that are not exposed to serum proteins it is possible to raise auto-antibodies that react with them. To this extent at least, tolerance would seem to be a local rather than a systemic phenomenon and this must imply that at least the B cells capable of making IgA anti-C3 antibodies are not eliminated fully during tolerance induction.

The significance of bovine conglutinin in cattle is quite obscure. No complement-mediated mechanism appear to be available to cattle by virtue of their conglutinin content that is not also present in other species of mammal. It is perhaps more likely that its significance is related to its activity against yeasts which are present in large numbers in the intestinal tract of ruminants. Immunoconglutinins, on the other hand, have been shown in mice to exert a protective effect against infection with small numbers of virulent organisms[169] and to that extent may serve an adaptive function. The mechanism involved in this protection is most likely to be the aggregating effect on complement-coated particles reducing the active invading dose. It is, however, also possible to show that immunoconglutinins reacting with bound C3 can inhibit the functional ability of the C3; and contrarywise that this same reaction can initiate further sites of complement fixation[170]. Whether the immunoconglutinins found in human allergic disease, therefore, augments or diminishes the allergic process, or neither, remains uncertain. The suggestion that the true function of immunoconglutinins is the clearance of complement fragments from the circulation remains unsubstantiated. The failure of the KAF deficient patient (see earlier) to clear C3b adequately from his circulation although he has high titres of immunoconglutinin directed against it would suggest that immunoconglutinins are not a major mechanism in this respect.

Note added in proof

In support of this point of view Dukor and his colleagues[180] have put forward evidence that cobra venom factor in the presence of C3 sufficent serum is a B-cell mitogen and that it will substitute for T-cell function in the *in vitro* antibody response to sheep erythrocytes.

References

1. W. H. O. Memorandum. "Nomenclature of Complement" (1968). *Bull. Wld. Health Org.*, **39**, 935
2. Macfarlane, R. G. (1969). *Proc. Roy Soc. (London) B.*, **173**, 259
3. Buchner, H. (1889). *Zbl. Bakt. ParasitKde*, **5**, 1–11
4. Bordet, J. (1895). *Ann. Inst. Pasteur*, **9**, 462
5. Bordet, J. (1898). *Ann. Inst. Pasteur*, **12**, 688
6. Mayer, M. M. (1970). *Immunochem.*, **7**, 485
7. Müller-Eberhard, H. J. and Nilsson, U. (1960). *J. Exp. Med.*, **111**, 217
8. Naff, G. B., Pensky, J. and Lepow, I. H. (1964). *J. Exp. Med.*, **119**, 593
9. Lepow, I. H., Naff, G. B., Todd, E. W., Pensky, J. and Hinz, C. F. (1963). *J. Exp. Med.*, **117**, 938
10. Yonemasu, K. and Stroud, R. M. (1971). *J. Immunol.*, **106**, 304
11. Agnello, V., Winchester, R. J. and Kunkel, H. G. (1970). *Immunology*, **19**, 909
12. Sledge, C. R. and Bing, D. H. (1972). *Fed. Proc. (Fed. Amer. Soc. Exp. Biol.)* **31**, 739 (Abstr.)
13. Reid, K. B. M., Lowe, D. M. and Porter, R. R. (1972). *Biochem J.*, **130**, 749
14. Shelton, E., Yonemasu, K. and Stroud, R. M. (1972). *Proc. Nat. Acad. Sci. (USA)*, **69**, 65
15. Müller-Eberhard, H. J. (1969). *Ann. Rev. Biochem.*, **38**, 389
16. Müller-Eberhard, H. J. and Kunkel (1961). *Proc. Soc. Exp. Biol. N.Y.*, **106**, 291
17. Müller-Eberhard, H. J. and Calcott, M. A. (1966). *Immunochemistry*, **3**, 500
18. Augener, W., Grey, H. M., Cooper, N. R. and Müller-Eberhard, H. J. (1971). *Immunochemistry*, **8**, 1011
19. Sandberg, A. L., Osler, A. G., Shin, H. S. and Oliveira, B. (1970). *J. Immunol.*, **104**, 329
20. Feinstein, A. and Hobart, M. J. (1969). *Nature (London)* **223**, 950
21. Müller-Eberhard, H. J., Bokisch, V. A. and Budzko, D. B. (1967). *Immunopathology*, Vol. 6, (P. A. Miescher, editor) (Basel: Schwabe and Co.)
22. Lepow, I. H., Naff, G. B. and Pensky, J. (1965) 74, *CIBA Symposium*, (G. E. W. Wolstenholme and J. Knight, editors) (London: J. and A. Churchill)
23. de Bracco, M. and Stroud, R. M. (1971). *J. Immunol.*, **107**, 310
24. Naff, G. B. and Ratnoff, O. D. (1968). *J. Exp. Med.*, **128**, 571
25. Ratnoff, O. D. and Naff, G. B. (1969). *J. Lab. Clin. Med.*, **74**, 380
26. Bing, D. H. (1971). *Immunochemistry*, **8**, 539
27. Haines, A. L. and Lepow, I. H. (1964). *J. Immunol.*, **92**, 456
28. Kehoe, J. M. and Fougereau, M. (1969). *Nature (London)*, **224**, 1212
29. Borsos, T. and Rapp, H. J. (1965). *Science*, **150**, 505
30. Rapp, H. J. and Borsos, T. (1963). *J. Immunol.*, **91**, 826
31. Borsos, T. and Rapp, H. J. (1965). *J. Immunol.*, **95**, 559
32. Müller-Eberhard, H. J. and Biro, C. E. (1963). *J. Exp. Med.*, **118**, 447
33. Gordon, J., Whitehead, H. R. and Wormall, A. (1926). *Biochem. J.*, **20**, 1028
34. Dalmasso, A. P. and Müller-Eberhard, H. J. (1966). *J. Immunol.*, **97**, 680
35. Patrick, R. A., Taubman, S. B. and Lepow, I. H. (1970). *Immunochemistry*, **7**, 217
36. Budzko, D. B. and Müller-Eberhard, H. J. (1970). *Immunochemistry*, **7**, 227
37. Müller-Eberhard, H. J., Dalmasso, A. P. and Calcott, M. A. (1966). *J. Exp. Med.*, **123**, 33
38. Dalmasso, A. P. and Müller-Eberhard, H. J. (1965). *Fed Proc (Fed. Amer. Soc. Exp. Biol.)* **24**, 466

39. Polley, M. J. and Müller-Eberhard, H. J. (1968). *J. Exp. Med.*, **128**, 533
40. Polley, M. J. and Müller-Eberhard, H. J. (1969). *J. Immunol.*, **102**, 1339
41. Polley, M. J. and Müller-Eberhard, H. J. (1967). *J. Exp. Med.*, **126**, 1013
42. Mayer, M. M., Miller, J. A. and Shin, H. S. (1970). *J. Immunol.*, **105**, 327
43. Donaldson V. H., Ratnoff, O. D., Dias da Silva, W. and Rosen, F. S. (1969). *J. Clin. Invest.*, **48**, 642
44. Gigli, I. and Austen, K. F. (1969). *J. Exp. Med.*, **129**, 679
45. Müller-Eberhard, H. J., Polley, M. J. and Calcott, M. A. (1967). *J. Exp. Med.*, **125**, 359
46. Whitehead, A. R., Gordon, J. and Wormall, A. (1925). *Biochem. J.*, **19**, 618
47. Berry, D. M. and Almeida, J. D. (1968). *J. Gen. Virol.*, **3**, 97
48. Munn, E. A., Feinstein, A. and Lachmann, P. J. (1968). *Brit. Med. Bull.*, **24**, 113
49. Wyatt, H. V., Colten, H. R. and Borsos, T. (1972). *J. Immunol.*, **108**, 1609
50. West, C. D., Davis, N. C., Forestal, J., Herbst, J. and Spitzer, R. (1966). *J. Immunol.*, **96**, 650
51. Pondman, K. W., Hanneman, A. and Wolters, G. (1971). *J. Immunol.*, **107**, 314
52. Nilsson, U. R. and Müller-Eberhard, H. J. (1965). *J. Exp. Med.*, **122**, 277
53. Nilsson, U. R., Tomar, R. H. and Taylor, F. B. Jnr., (1972). *Immunochemistry*, **9**, 709
54. Arroyave, C. M. and Müller-Eberhard, H. J. (1971). *Immunochemistry*, **8**, 995
55. Tedesco, F. and Lachmann, P. J. (1971). *Clin. Exp. Immunol.*, **9**, 359
56. Thompson, R. A. and Lachmann, P. J. (1970). *J. Exp. Med.*, **131**, 629
57. Lachmann, P. J. and Thompson, R. A. (1970). *J. Exp. Med.*, **131**, 643
58. Bitter-Suermann, D., Hadding, U., Melchert, F. and Wellensiek, H. J. (1970). *Immunochemistry*, **7**, 955
59. Hadding, U., Bitter-Suermann and Wellensiek, H. J. (1970). *Immunochemistry*, **7**, 967
60. Goldman, J. N., Ruddy, S. and Austen, K. F. (1972). *J. Immunol.*, **109**, 358
61. Lachmann, P. J., Munn, E. A. and Weissmann, G. (1970). *Immunology*, **19**, 983
62. Manni, J. A. and Müller-Eberhard, H. J. (1969). *J. Exp. Med.*, **130**, 1145
63. Hadding, U. and Müller-Eberhard, H. J. (1969). *Immunology*, **16**, 719
64. Tamura, N., Shimada, A. and Chong, S. (1972). *Immunology*, **22**, 131
65. Stolfi, R. L. (1970). *J. Immunol.*, **104**, 1212
66. Lachmann, P. J., Bowyer, D. E., Dawson, R. M. C., Munn, E. A. and Nicol, P. A. E. (1973). *Immunology*,
67. Borsos, T., Dourmashkin, R. R. and Humphrey, J. H. (1964). *Nature (London)*, **202**, 251
68. Humphrey, J. H. and Dourmashkin, R. R. (1969). *Advan. Immunology*, **11**, 75
69. Hesketh, T. R., Dourmashkin, R. R., Payne Sheila, N., Humphrey, J. H. and Lachmann P. J. (1971). *Nature (London)* **233**, 620
70. Müller-Eberhard, H. J. (1968). *Advan. Immunol.*, **8**, 1
71. Polley, M. J., Müller-Eberhard, H. J. and Feldmann, J. D. (1971). *J. Exp. Med.*, **133**, 53
72. Hesketh, T. R., Payne Sheila, N. and Humphrey, J. H. (1972). *Immunology*, **23**, 705
73. Humphrey, J. H., Dourmashkin, R. R. and Payne, Sheila N. (1967). *Immunopathology* Vol. 5 (P. A. Miescher, editor) (Basel: Schwabe and Co.)
74. Carroll, L. (1869). Alice's Adventures in Wonderland (London: McMillan)
75. Inoue, K. and Kinsky, S. C. (1970). *Biochemistry*, **9**, 4767
76. Lepow, I. H., Ratnoff, O. D. and Levy, L. R. (1958). *J. Exp. Med.*, **107**, 451
77. Pensky, J. and Schwick, H. G. (1969). *Science*, **163**, 698
78. Schultze, H. E., Heide, K. U. and Haupt, H. (1962). *Naturwissenschaften*, **49**, 133
79. Ratnoff, O. D., Pensky, J., Ogston, D. and Naff, G. B. (1969). *J. Exp. Med.*, **129**, 315
80. Opferkuch, W., Loos, M. and Borsos, T. (1971). *J. Immunol.*, **107**, 313 (Abstr.)
81. Tamura, N. and Nelson, R. A. (1967). *J. Immunol.*, **99**, 582
82. Lachmann, P. J. and Müller-Eberhard, H. J. (1968). *J. Immunol.*, **100**, 691
83. Ruddy, S. and Austen, K. F. (1969). *J. Immunol.*, **102**, 533
84. Lachmann, P. J., Aston, W. P. and Nicol, P. A. E. (1973). *Immunochemistry*,
85. Abramson, N., Alper, C. A., Lachmann, P. J., Rosen, F. S. and Jandl, J. H. (1971). *J. Immunol.*, **107**, 19
86. Nelson, R. A., Jr. and Biro, C. E. (1968). *Immunology*, **14**, 527
87. Martin, A. and Lachmann, P. J. Unpublished observations
88. Barnett, E. V., Bienenstock, J. and Block, K. J. (1966). *J. Amer. Med. Assoc.*, **198**, 143
89. Forsgren, A. and Sjoquist, J. (1966). *J. Immunol.*, **97**, 822
90. Yachnin, S., Rosenblum, D. and Chatman, D. (1964). *J. Immunol.*, **93**, 542

91. Nicol, P. A. E. (1973). *Ph.D. Thesis*, University of Cambridge
92. Lachmann, P. J., Elias, D. E. and Moffett, A. (1972). Biological Activities of Complement, 202–214, (D. G. Ingram, editor) (Basel: S. Karger)
93. Ratnoff, O. D. and Naff, G. B. (1967). *J. Exp. Med.*, **125**, 337
94. Lepow, I. H. (1961). *Immunochemical Approaches to Problems* 280–294 (Heideberger and Plescia, editors) (New Brunswick, N.J.: Rutgers University Press)
95. Pensky, J., Wurz, L., Pillemer, L. and Lepow, I. H. (1959). *Z. Immunol.*, **118**, 329
96. Blum, L., Pillemer, L. and Lepow, I. H. (1959). *Z. Immunol.*, **118**, 313
97. Nelson, R. A. (1958). *J. Exp. Med.*, **108**, 515
98. Nelson, R. A. (1961). *Immunochemical Approaches to Problems in Microbiology*, 295 (Heideberger and Plescia, editors) (New Brunswick, N.J.: Rutgers University Press)
99. Pensky, J., Hinz, C. S., Todd, E. W., Wedgewood, R. J., Boyer, J. T. and Lepow, I. H. (1968). *J. Immunol.*, **100**, 142
100. Gewurz, H. (1972). *Biological Activities of Complement*, 56 (D. G. Ingram, editor) (Basel: S. Karger)
101. Sandberg, A. L. and Osler, A. G. (1971). *J. Immunol.*, **107**, 1268
102. Marcus, R. L., Shin, H. S. and Mayer, M. M. (1970). *Fed. Proc. (Fed. Amer. Soc. Exp. Biol.)* **29**, 304
103. Frank, M. M., May, J., Gaither, T. and Ellman, L. (1971). *J. Exp. Med.*, **134**, 176
104. Blum, L. (1964). *J. Immunol.*, **92**, 61
105. Spiegelberg, H. L. and Götze, O. (1972). *Fed. Proc. (Fed. Amer. Soc. Exp. Biol.)* **31**, 655 (Abstr.)
106. Flexner, S. and Noguchi, H. (1903). *J. Exp. Med.*, **6**, 277
107. Müller-Eberhard, H. J., Nilsson, U. R., Dalmasso, A. P., Polley, M. J. and Calcott, M. A. (1966). *Arch. Pathol.*, **82**, 205
108. Nelson, R. A. (1966). *Surv. Opthalmol.*, **11**, 498
109. Rommel, F. A., Goldlust, M. B., Bancroft, F. C., Mayer, M. M. and Tashjian, A. H. Jr. (1970). *J. Immunol.*, **105**, 396
110. Haupt, H. and Heide, K. (1965). *Clin. Chim. Acta*, **12**, 419
111. Boenisch, T. and Alper, C. A. (1970). *Biochem. Biophys. Acta*, **221**, 529
112. Alper, C. A., Goodkofsky, I. and Lepow, I. H. (1972). *J. Exp. Med.*,
113. Götze, O. and Müller-Eberhard, H. J. (1971). *J. Exp. Med.*, **134**, 905
114. Hunsicker, L. G., Ruddy, S. and Austen, K. F. (1972). C3. *Fed. Proc. (Fed. Amer. Soc. Exp. Biol.)* **31**, 788 (Abstr.)
115. Lachmann, P. J. and Nicol, P. A. E. (1973). *Lancet*,
116. Müller-Eberhard, H. J. and Götze, O. (1972). *J. Exp. Med.*, **135**, 1003
117. Alper, C. A. and Rosen, F. S. (1971). *Advan. Immunol.*, **14**, 252
118. Alper, C. A., Rosen, F. S. and Lachmann, P. J. (1972). *Proc. Nat. Acad. Sci. (USA)*, **69**, 2910
119. Nicol, P. A. E. and Lachmann, P. J. (1973). *Immunology*, **24** (in the press)
120. Alper, C. A., Colten, H. R., Rosen, F. S., Rabson, A. R., Macnab, G. and Gear, J. S. A. (1972). *Lancet*, ii 1179
121. Bach, S., Ruddy, S., MacLaren, J. A. and Austen, K. F. (1971). *Immunology*, **21**, 869
122. Alper, C. A. (1972). Personal communication
123. Lachmann, P. J. (1972). Ciba Foundation Symposium: Ontogeny of Acquired Immunity. (R. Porter and J. Knight, editors) (Amsterdam: Associated Science Publishers)
124. Sussman, M., Jones, H. and Lachmann, P. J. (1973). *Clin. Exp. Immunol.*
125. O'Connell, R. M., Enriquez, P., Linman, J. W., Gleich, G. J. and McDuffie, F. C. (1967). *J. Lab. Clin. Med.*, **70**, 715
126. Gewurz, H., Pickering, R. J., Christian, C. L., Snyderman, R., Mergenhagen, S. E. and Good, R. A. (1968). *Clin. Exp. Immunol.*, **3**, 437
127. Kohler, P. F. and Müller-Eberhard, H. J. (1972). *J. Clin. Invest.*, **51**, 868
128. Day, N. K., Geiger, H., Stroud, R., de Bracco, M., Mancado, B., Windhorst, D. and Good, R. A. (1972). *J. Clin. Invest.*, **51**, 1102
129. Pickering, R. J., Naff, G. B., Stroud, R. M., Good, R. A. and Gewurz, H. (1970). *J. Exp. Med.*, **141**, 803
130. Miller, M. E. and Nilsson, U. R. (1970). *New Engl. J. Med.*, **282**, 354
131. Donaldson, V. H. and Evans, R. R. (1963). *Amer. J. Med.*, **35**, 37
132. Hadjiyannaki, K. and Lachmann, P. J. (1971). *Clinical Allergy*, **1**, 221
133. Henson, P. M. (1969). *Immunology*, **16**, 107

134. Basch, R. S. (1965). *J. Immunol.*, **94,** 629
135. Cooper, N. R. (1969). *Science*, **165,** 396
136. Huber, H., Polley, M. J., Linscott, W. D., Fudenberg, H. H. and Müller-Eberhard, H. J. (1968). *Science*, **162,** 1281
137. Lay, W. H. and Nussenzweig, V. (1968). *J. Exp. Med.*, **128,** 991
138. Dukor, P., Bianco, C. and Nussenzweig, V. (1971). *Europ. J. Immunol.*, **1,** 491
139. Donaldson, V. H., Ratnoff, O. D., Dias da Silva, W. and Rosen, F. S. (1969). *J. Clin. Invest.*, **48,** 642
140. Klemperer, M. R., Rosen, F. S. and Donaldson, V. H. (1969). *J. Clin. Invest.*, **48,** 44a
141. Lepow, I. H. (1972). *Biochemistry of the Acute Allergic Reactions'* 205 (K. F. Austen and E. L. Becker, editors) (Oxford: Blackwell Scientific Publications)
142. Silva, W. Dias da., Eisele, J. W. and Lepow, I. H. (1967). *J. Exp. Med.*, **126,** 1027
143. Bokisch, V. A., Müller-Eberhard, H. J. and Cochrane, C. G. (1969). *J. Exp. Med.*, **129,** 1109
144. Ward, P. A. (1967). *J. Exp. Med.*, **126,** 189
145. Jensen, J. A. (1972). *Biological Activities of Complement*, 136. (D. G. Ingram, editor) (Basel: S. Karger)
146. Snyderman, R. and Mergenhagen, S. E. (1972). *Biological Activities of Complement*, 117 (D. G. Ingram, editor) (Basel: S. Karger)
147. Wissler, J. H. (1972). *Europ. J. Immunol.*, **2,** 73, 84, 90
148. Rother, K. (1971). *J. Immunol.*, **107,** 316
149. Ward, P. A., Cochrane, C. C. and Müller-Eberhard, H. J. (1966). *Immunology*, **11,** 141
150. Becker, E. L. (1972). *J. Exp. Med.*, **135,** 376
151. Lachmann, P. J., Coombs, R. R. A., Fell, H. B. and Dingle, J. T. (1969). *Int. Arch. Allergy*, **36,** 469
152. Zimmerman, T. S., Arroyave, C. M. and Müller-Eberhard, H. J. (1971). *J. Exp. Med.*, **134,** 1591
153. Brown, D. L. and Lachmann, P. J. (1973). *Int. Arch. Allergy* (in the press)
154. W. H. O. Report (1973). *Pathogenetic mechanisms in denguehaemorrhagic fever.* Report of an International collaborative study (in the press)
155. Azar, M. M., Ynis, E. J., Pickering, R. J. and Good, R. A. (1968). *Lancet*, I, 1279
156. Ellman, L., Green, I., Judge, F. and Frank, M. (1971). *J. Exp. Med.*, **134,** 162
157. Pepys, M. B. (1972). *Nature New Biol.*, **237,** 157
158. Dukor, P. and Hartmann K-U. (1972). *Europ. J. Immunol.*, (in the press)
159. Colten, H. R. and Wyatt, H. V. (1972). *Biological Activities of Complement*, 244. (D. G. Ingram, editor) (Basel: S. Karger)
160. Alper, C. A. and Rosen, F. S. (1967). *J. Clin. Invest.*, **46,** 2021
161. Peters, D. K., Martin, A., Weinstein, A., Cameron, J. S., Barratt, T. M., Ogg, C. S. and Lachmann, P. J. (1972). *Clin. Exp. Immunol.*, **11,** 311
162. Alper, C. A., Block, K. J. and Rosen, F. S. (1973).
163. Bordet, J. and Streng, O. (1909). *Zbl. Bakt.*, **49,** 260
164. Lachmann, P. J. and Coombs, R. R. A. (1965). Ciba Symposium Complement 242 (Wolstenholme and Knight, editors) (London: J. and A. Churchill)
165. Coombs, R. R. A., Coombs, A. M. and Ingram, D. G. (1961). The serology of conglutination (Oxford: Blackwell)
166. Lachmann, P. J. (1967). *Advan. Immunol.*, **6,** 479
167. Henson, P. M. (1968). *Immunology*, **14,** 697
168. Lachmann, P. J. and Thompson, R. A. (1970). *Immunology*, **18,** 157
169. Ingram, D. G. (1959). *Immunology*, **2,** 345
170. Tedesco, F., Corrocher, R. and Brown, D. L. (1972). *Clin. Exp. Immunol.*, **10,** 685
171. Colten, H. R., Borsos, T. and Rapp, H. J. (1966). *Proc. Nat. Acad. Sci. (USA)*, **56,** 1158
172. Alper, C. A., Johnson, A. M., Birtch, A. G. and Moore, F. D. (1969). *Science*, **163,** 286
173. Phillips, M. E., Rother, U. A., Rother, K. O. and Thorbecke, G. J. (1969). *Immunology* **17,** 315
174. Rother, U. A., Thorbecke, G. J., Stecher-Levin, V. J., Hurlemann, J. and Rother, K. O. (1968). *Immunology*, **14,** 649
175. McConnell, F. I. and Lachmann, P. J. (1973). Unpublished observations.
176. Sessa, G., Freer, J. H., Colacicco, G. and Weissmann, G. (1969). *J. Biol. Chem.*, **244,** 3575
177. McLean, R. H. and Michael, A. F. (1973). *J. Clin. Invest.*, **52,** 634

178. Götze, O. and Müller-Eberhard, H. J. (1973). *J. Immunol.*, (in press)
179. Leddy, J. P., Frank, M. M. Gaither, T., Heusinkveld, R. S., Breckenridge, R. T. and Klemperer, M. R. (1973). *J. Immunol.* (in press)
180. Bitter-Suermann, D., Dukor, P., Gisler, R. H., Schumann, G., Dierich, M., Konig, W. and Hadding, U. (1973). *J. Immunol.* (in press)

Index

Cells *continued*
  precursors, single colony-forming, 44
  receptor sites, antigen recognition and, 330–356
  secreting antibody in mice, 69
  surface, associated functions of linked gene complexes, 323
    immunoglobulin class on, 339–340
    immunoglobulin distribution over, 336–338
  surface markers, histocompatibility (H) antigens and, 258
    identification by, 40
  uninfected, interferon effect on, 26
Chains, in
  a-, 169, 202–205
  γ-, 169, 181, 203–205
  γ1-, 203, 204
  κ-, 201, 202
  λ-, 162, 180, 202, 207, 208
  μ-, 169, 181, 187, 202, 204
Chaotropic agents, 276
Chemotactic agents
  C3a as, 368
  C567 complex as, 389
Chemotactic factor
  C5a as, 370, 388
Chickens
  embryos, cross-tolerance between, 105
  interferon, purification and properties of, 20
  lymphoid cell differentiation in, 248, 249
Chimpanzee histocompatibility antigens, (ChL-A)
  HL-A antigen sharing with, 263
Chloramphenicol, depression of protein synthesis by, 124
Chromosome markers
  and lymphocytes, 48
  for lymphoid cells, 73
Cis integration, mechanisms for, 211, 212
Classical pathway complement components and, 363
Clonal development, 248, 249
Clonal-selection
  and antigen-binding receptors, 338
  for mutant cells, 251
Cobra venom, 378, 379
Combining site, 189, 190, 193
Complement (*See also* C1–C9)
  activation, 376, 377
  binding by Fc region, 182, 183
  biological importance of, 362–393
  and cell-mediated immunity, 69
  components biologically-active fragments of, 388–389
    biosynthesis of, 382, 383
    and the classical pathway, 363
    genetic deficiencies of, 383, 384
    genetic polymorphism of, 383

Complement *continued*
  intermediate complexes of, 363
    sites of formation of, 382
  conglutinating activity of, 391
  deficiencies, 384, 385
  and enzyme-cascade systems, 363
  fixation, assay, HL-A typing by, 302
    C1 fixation and transfer test for, 366
    C1 inhibitor and, 374
    C3b inactivator (KAF) and, 374–375
    C6 inactivator and, 375
    homeostasis of, 373–375
    immunoconglutinins and, 391–392
    initiation of, 364–366
    C5b binding to, 370
  immunochemistry of, 364–373
  inactivator, by zymosan, 378
  inhibitors, abnormalities of, 385, 386
  lesions, composition of, 373
    in a liposome, 371, 372
    and platelet factor, 389
    site of formation of, 373
    stage of appearance of, 372
  lysis, 370–373
  lysosomal activation mediated by, 389
  mediated adherence reactions, fixed C3 and, 387, 388
  membrane lesions of, 389, 390
  platelet activation dependence on, 389, 390
  reaction, reactive lysis and, 370
  receptors for, 55
  role in allergic response induction, 390, 391
    in antibody formation, 390, 391
    in tolerance induction, 117
  sequence, C3 fixation in, 376
  study of membrane damage by, 370
  system, alternate pathway factors in, 363, 364
    genetics of, 383, 386
    non-classical activation of, 375–382
Conformation
  and antigenicity, 145–149
  of immunoglobulin molecules, 171–173
  of lysozyme, 150, 151
  of myoglobin, 150, 152
Congenic strains, production of, 298, 299
Conglutinating activity of complement, 391
Constant regions, 174, 176, 177, 180–185, 201
Contact mutants in active sites, 213
Contact sensitivity and cell-mediated immunity, 85
Copy-choice mechanism and gene expression, 249
Corticosteroids, 122
Covalent intermediates of immunoglobulin classes, 239

Lysozyme *continued*
and immunodominant group, 139
immunological reactivities of, 141, 142
reduced and carboxymethylated, 153

MLR gene and Ir genes, 356
MLR locus, linkage relationships of, 321
MLR response, 321, 322
MN blood group and graft survival, 300
MOPC 104 in mouse constant regions, 180, 181
MOPC 315, 180, 181, 189
MOPC 21 L chain precursor, 242, 243
Macro-complement fixation, measurement of interaction by, 141, 142
Macromolecules, antigenic determinants on, 133
Macrophages
in antibody responses, 66, 75–78
and antigen accessibility, 78
antigen-antibody complexes bound to, 331
as an antigen-concentrating cell, 331
binding of cytophilic antibody to, 69
and B-T cell collaboration, 76
complement C3 receptors of, 331
corticosteroids effect on, 122
and degradation of cellular antigens, 78
immobilisation of, 88
from immune animals, activity of, 77
and the immune response, 44, 330, 331
immunoglobulin G receptors of, 331
induction of antibody synthesis, 77
irradiation effect on, 122
origin from monocytes, 43, 44
participation in T-B cell cooperation, 153
processing of, 77, 78
production of informational RNA, 77
role in antigen recognition, 330, 331
structure and derivation of, 43, 44
tingible-body, in germinal centres, 94, 95
uptake of antigen, 78, 79
Major histocompatibility systems, 320–324, 347, 353
Mammals
B lymphocytes and bone marrow lymphocytes, 42
differentiation of B lymphocytes, 54, 55
lymphoid system, 39
organ equivalent to bursa, 41, 42
origin of lymphocytes in, 50–55
Mast cells, binding of IgE to, 69
Membrane-bound ribosomes, nascent chains on, 233
Membrane damage by complement, study of, 370
Membrane lesions of complement, 389–390
Membrane proteins radioiodination immunoglobulin demonstration by, 337

Membrane turnover, shedding and, 338
Membranoproliferative glomerulonephritis and C3 synthesis rate, 382
Memory
in cell-mediated immunity, 92–94
immunological, 74
Messenger RNA (mRNA), 233–235
translation, and translation initiation factors, 246
in a cell-free system, 242
Methionine tRNA$_F$, initiation of L chain synthesis by, 242
Metmyoglobin, 146–148
Micro-complement fixation, measurement of interaction by, 141, 142
Microbial infection
protection by effector cells, 68
Microcytotoxic assay for HL-A antigens, 260, 261
Microenvironment and maturation of stem cells, 46
Microlymphocytotoxicity assay for HL-A system, 301, 302
Microsomal lipoprotein (MLP) yield by nitrogen decompression, 265
Migration inhibition, 88, 94
Mismatched cross-over mechanism for gene expansion, 221, 222
Mitogens
activation of lymphocytes by, 36
factor, from immune lymphocytes, 75
as interferon inducers, 10
Mixed antiglobulin technique, 333, 339
Mixed lymphocyte reactions, 347, 355–356
Mixed lymphocyte response (MLR), 320–321, 355
Modulation mutants and active sites, 213
Monkeys, interferon, purification, 22
Monoclonal antibodies, isoelectric focusing of, 219
Monoclonal responses, 213–215
Monocytes, 43, 44
Monodispersity of lymphoid HL-A antigens, 275
Mouse
B lymphocyte antigen, 55
differentiation antigens in, 51
genes, 216–218
immunoglobulin-bearing cells in, 339, 340
interferon, purification and properties of, 20, 21
Murine microsomal lipoproteins, 268
Murine sarcoma I cells, 267
Murine spleen cells, 265–267
Murine transplantation antigens, 270
Murine tumour cells, H-antigens from, 265–268
Mutant cells, clonal selection for, 251
Mutation rate measurement by electrophoretic mobility, 223